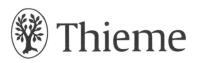

Minimally Invasive Glaucoma Surgery

A Practical Guide

Brian A. Francis, MD, MS
Professor of Ophthalmology
Director of Glaucoma Services
Glaucoma Fellowship Director
Doheny Eye Institute
Rupert and Gertrude Stieger Endowed Chair
Department of Ophthalmology
University of California–Los Angeles
David Geffen School of Medicine
Los Angeles, California

Steven R. Sarkisian, Jr., MD
Clinical Professor
Glaucoma Fellowship Director
Dean McGee Eye Institute
University of Oklahoma
Oklahoma City, Oklahoma

James C. Tan, MD, PhD
Associate Professor of Ophthalmology
Doheny Eye Institute
Department of Ophthalmology
University of California–Los Angeles
David Geffen School of Medicine
Los Angeles, California

With 216 Figures

Thieme
New York • Stuttgart • Delhi • Rio de Janeiro

Executive Editor: William Lamsback
Managing Editor: Elizabeth Palumbo
Editorial Assistant: Haley Paskalides
Director, Editorial Services: Mary Jo Casey
International Production Director: Andreas Schabert
Vice President, Editorial and E-Product Development: Vera Spillner
International Marketing Director: Fiona Henderson
International Sales Director: Louisa Turrell
Director of Sales, North America: Mike Roseman
Senior Vice President and Chief Operating Officer: Sarah Vanderbilt
President: Brian D. Scanlan
Production Editor: Barbara Chernow
Compositor: Carol Pierson, Chernow Editorial Services, Inc.

Library of Congress Cataloging-in-Publication Data

Names: Francis, Brian A., editor. | Sarkisian, Steven R., Jr., editor. |
    Tan, James C., editor.
Title: Minimally invasive glaucoma surgery : a practical guide /
    [edited by] Brian A. Francis, Steven R. Sarkisian, Jr., James C. Tan.
Description: New York : Thieme, [2017] | Includes bibliographical
    references and index.
Identifiers: LCCN 2016029012 (print) | LCCN 2016029906 (ebook) |
    ISBN 9781626231566 (alk. paper) | ISBN 9781626231559
    (eISBN) | ISBN 9781626231559
Subjects: | MESH: Glaucoma—surgery | Minimally Invasive Surgical
    Procedures—methods
Classification: LCC RE871 (print) | LCC RE871 (ebook) | NLM WW
    290 | DDC 617.7/41059--dc23
LC record available at https://lccn.loc.gov/2016029012

Copyright © 2017 by Thieme Medical Publishers, Inc.
Thieme Publishers New York
333 Seventh Avenue, New York, NY 10001 USA
+1 800 782 3488, customerservice@thieme.com

Thieme Publishers Stuttgart
Rüdigerstrasse 14, 70469 Stuttgart, Germany
+49 [0]711 8931 421, customerservice@thieme.de

Thieme Publishers Delhi
A-12, Second Floor, Sector-2, Noida-201301
Uttar Pradesh, India
+91 120 45 566 00, customerservice@thieme.in

Thieme Publishers Rio de Janeiro, Thieme Publicações Ltda.
Edifício Rodolpho de Paoli, 25º andar
Av. Nilo Peçanha, 50 – Sala 2508
Rio de Janeiro 20020-906 Brasil
+55 21 3172 2297

Printed in Germany by CPI, Leck   5 4 3 2

ISBN 978-1-62623-156-6

Also available as an e-book:
eISBN 978-1-62623-155-9

Important note: Medicine is an ever-changing science undergoing continual development. Research and clinical experience are continually expanding our knowledge, in particular our knowledge of proper treatment and drug therapy. Insofar as this book mentions any dosage or application, readers may rest assured that the authors, editors, and publishers have made every effort to ensure that such references are in accordance with **the state of knowledge at the time of production of the book.**

Nevertheless, this does not involve, imply, or express any guarantee or responsibility on the part of the publishers in respect to any dosage instructions and forms of applications stated in the book. **Every user is requested to examine carefully** the manufacturers' leaflets accompanying each drug and to check, if necessary in consultation with a physician or specialist, whether the dosage schedules mentioned therein or the contraindications stated by the manufacturers differ from the statements made in the present book. Such examination is particularly important with drugs that are either rarely used or have been newly released on the market. Every dosage schedule or every form of application used is entirely at the user's own risk and responsibility. The authors and publishers request every user to report to the publishers any discrepancies or inaccuracies noticed. If errors in this work are found after publication, errata will be posted at www.thieme.com on the product description page.

Some of the product names, patents, and registered designs referred to in this book are in fact registered trademarks or proprietary names even though specific reference to this fact is not always made in the text. Therefore, the appearance of a name without designation as proprietary is not to be construed as a representation by the publisher that it is in the public domain.

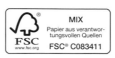

*To our dear wives and children
for their encouragement and endless diversions
as we wrote this book.*

Contents

Section I   Eye Anatomy and Physiology

Section II Clinical Procedures

Video Contents

Preface

This book is designed to help the established or training ophthalmologist navigate the increasing options available for glaucoma surgical treatment. Glaucoma specialists, or those whose practice involves a large percentage of glaucoma patients, need to be familiar with all of these new surgical approaches. But it is the general ophthalmologists who will find this book most helpful, as they are on the front lines of the battle against blindness from glaucoma, and therefore may be performing MIGS procedures in the early stages of glaucoma management. Glaucoma surgical treatment tailored to the patient requires the ability to use the procedures discussed in this book.

Chapter 1 introduces the new treatment options for glaucoma. Then Section I discusses the basic science of our current understanding of the physiological pathways of aqueous formation and drainage, and what happens when they are exploited surgically to reduce intraocular pressure. In many ways, the surgery is driving the science. Technological advances have enabled miniaturization, technical simplification, and other novel ways to shunt aqueous into ocular compartments such as the suprachoroidal space and Schlemm's canal. Moreover, there are new ways to shunt into the more familiar subconjunctival space. These developments have prompted new (and some older) ques

tions about the aqueous humor system: How do collector channels respond to increased aqueous flow following trabecular bypass? How does scarring, that age-old enemy of glaucoma surgery, affect the suprachoroidal space? How does fluid drain from the subconjunctival space? What happens to aqueous secretion and the blood–aqueous barrier years after cyclophotocoagulation? Although many questions lack complete answers, a panel of experts has collected and interpreted the evidence, shared their current thinking, and discussed some important issues unearthed by the surgeries.

Sections II, the clinical chapters, discuss each new procedure, from appropriate selection of patients to surgical technique, management, and prevention of complications, as well as an assessment of the results reported in the medical literature.

Glaucoma surgical treatment is a rapidly evolving field. This book provides a foundation on which the new technologies can be understood and assessed. Then the glaucoma practitioner can decide which technologies to incorporate in his or her practice, based on one's previous experience with similar devices and on a sound basic science understanding of how the body responds to the surgical management of aqueous movement.

Contributors

Iqbal Ike K. Ahmed, MD
Prism Eye Institute
Department of Ophthalmology and Vision Sciences
Trillium Health Partners
University of Toronto
Mississauga, Ontario, Canada

Handan Akil, MD
Research fellow
Ophthalmologist
Doheny Eye Institute
Los Angeles, California

Rachel Alburquerque, MD
Centro Laser
Santo Domingo, Dominican Republic

Evan Allan, MD
Fellow
Dean McGee Eye Institute
Oklahoma City, Oklahoma

Husam Ansari, MD, PhD
Board Certified Ophthalmologist
Ophthalmic Consultants of Boston
Boston, Massachusetts

Esdras Arrieta, MD
Ophthalmic Biophysics Center Bascom Palmer Eye Institute
University of Miami Miller School of Medicine
Miami, FL

Andrew K. Bailey, MD
Clinical Assistant Professor
Department of Ophthalmology
Dean McGee Eye Institute
Oklahoma City, Oklahoma

Juan F. Batlle Pichardo, MD
President
Laser Center in Santo Domingo
Chairman of Blindness Prevention
International Agency for the Prevention of Blindness
  (IAPB)-Vision2020 Latin America
Chief Ophthalmology
Dr. Elias Santana Hospital
Calle Duarte, Dominican Republic

John P. Berdahl, MD
Associate Professor
Vance Thompson Vision
University of South Dakota School of Medicine
Sioux Falls, South Dakota

Michael S. Berlin, MD
Founder and Director
Glaucoma Institute–Beverly Hills
Los Angeles, California

Reay H. Brown, MD
Founder
Atlanta Ophthalmology Associates
Atlanta, Georgia

Igor I. Bussel, MD, MHA
Resident Physician
Department of Ophthalmology
University of Pittsburgh
Eye Center
University of Pittsburgh Medical Center
Pittsburgh, Pennsylvania

Joseph Caprioli, MD
Chief
Glaucoma Division
Professor of Ophthalmology
David May II Chair
University of California–Los Angeles Health
University of California–Los Angeles David Geffin School of
  Medicine
Glaucoma Division
Los Angeles, California

Jessica E. Chan, MD
Metropolitan Ophthalmology Associates
Chevy Chase, Maryland

Anjum Cheema, MD
Department of Ophthalmology
Southeast Permanente Medical Group
Atlanta, Georgia

Vikas Chopra, MD
Doheny Eye Center
University of California–Los Angeles
Arcadia, California

Anne L. Coleman, MD, PhD
Fran and Ray Stark Professor
Department of Ophthalmology
Stein Eye Institute
University of California–Los Angeles
Los Angeles, California

Michael A. Coote, MBBS, FRANZCO
Associate Professor
Center for Eye Research Australia
Royal Victorian Eye and Ear Hospital
Centre for Eye Research Australia (CERA)
Melbourne Australia

Minas Theodore Coroneo, AO, MD, MS, MSc, FRACS
Professor and Chairman
Department of Ophthalmology
University of New South Wales
Prince of Wales Hospital
Sydney, Australia

Francisco Fantes, MD (deceased)
Ophthalmic Biophysics Center
Bascom Palmer Eye Institute
University of Miami Miller School of Medicine
Miami, Florida
Anne Bates Leach Eye Hospital
University of Miami
Miami, Florida

Ronald L. Fellman, MD
Attending Surgeon and Clinician
Glaucoma Associates of Texas
Dallas, Texas

Brian A. Francis, MD, MS
Professor of Ophthalmology
Director of Glaucoma Services
Glaucoma Fellowship Director
Doheny Eye Institute
Rupert and Gertrude Stieger Endowed Chair
Department of Ophthalmology
David Geffen School of Medicine
University of California–Los Angeles
Los Angeles, California

B'Ann T. Gabelt, MS (retired)
Distinguished Scientist
Department of Ophthalmology and Visual Sciences
University of Wisconsin
Madison, Wisconsin

Ivan Goldberg AM, MBBS (Syd), FRANZCO, FRACS
Clinical Associate Professor
Discipline of Ophthalmology
University of Sydney
Head, Glaucoma Unit
Sydney Eye Hospital
Director, Eye Associates
Sydney, Australia

Davinder S. Grover, MD, MPH
Attending Surgeon and Clinician
Glaucoma Associates of Texas
Dallas, Texas

Mohammad Hamid, MD
Glaucoma and Anterior Segment Surgeon
PreciVision Montreal
Saint-Laurent, Quebec, Canada

Paul Harasymowycz, MD, FRCSC
Chief of Glaucoma
University of Montreal
Medical Director
Montreal Glaucoma Institute
Department of Ophthalmology
University of Montreal
Montreal, Quebec, Canada

Melchior Hohensinn, MD
Universidad Miguel Hernández de Elche
Elche, Valencia, Spain

Chi-Hsin Hsu, MD
Director, Glaucoma Service
Department of Ophthalmology
Taipei Medical University
Shuang Ho Hospital
New Taipei City, Taiwan

Alex Huang, MD, PhD
Assistant Professor
Department of Ophthalmology
Doheny Eye Centers
Doheny and Stein Eye Institutes
University of California–Los Angeles
Los Angeles, California

Mark Johnson, PhD
Professor
Departments of Biomedical Engineering, Mechanical
    Engineering, and Ophthalmology
Northwestern University
Evanston, Illinois

Murray Johnstone, MD
Clinical Professor
Department of Ophthalmology
University of Washington
Swedish Hospital Medical Center
Seattle, Washington

Malik Y. Kahook, MD
Slater Family Endowed Chair in Ophthalmology
Vice Chair, Clinical and Translational Research
Chief, Glaucoma Service and Director, Glaucoma Fellowship
Professor of Ophthalmology
University of Colorado Anschutz Medical Campus
Department of Ophthalmology
Aurora, Colorado

Kevin Kaplowitz, MD
Assistant Professor
Department of Ophthalmology
Loma Linda University
Loma Linda, California

Yasushi P. Kato, PhD
Vice President of Research and Development
Innovia LLC
Miami, Florida

Paul L. Kaufman, MD
Ernst H. Bárány Professor of Ocular Pharmacology
Department Chair Emeritus
Department of Ophthalmology and Visual Sciences
School of Medicine and Public Health
University of Wisconsin–Madison
Madison, Wisconsin

Mahmoud A. Khaimi, MD
Clinical Associate Professor
Dean McGee Eye Institute
University of Oklahoma
Oklahoma City, Oklahoma

Paul A. Knepper, MD
Associate Professor
Ophthalmology
Northwestern Medicine
Ann and Robert H. Lurie Children's Hospital of
    Chicago
Chicago, Illinois

Christine L. Larsen, MD
Attending Surgeon
Minnesota Eye Consultants
Minneapolis, Minnesota

Peng Lei, MD
Clinician
Department of Ophthalmology
Kaiser Permanente
Los Angeles, California

Markus Lenzhofer, MD
Fellow
Department of Ophthalmology
Paracelsus Medical University/SALK
Salzburg, Austria

Ridia Lim, MBBS, MPH, FRANZCO
Ophthalmic Surgeon
Glaucoma Service
Sydney Eye Hospital
Sydney, Australia

Shan C. Lin, MD
Professor
University of California, San Francisco
San Francisco California

Nils A. Loewen, MD, PhD
Associate Professor
Department of Ophthalmology
University of Pittsburgh
Pittsburgh, Pennsylvania

Don S. Minckler, MD, MS
Emeritus Professor
Ophthalmology and Glaucoma Service Director
Clinical Professor
Laboratory Medicine (Ophthalmic Pathology)
University of California–Irvine
Orange, California

Peter A. Netland, MD, PhD
Vernah Scott Moyston Professor and Chair
Department of Ophthalmology.
University of Virginia School of Medicine
Charlottesville, Virginia

Robert Noecker, MD, MBA
Ophthalmologist
Ophthalmic Consultants of Connecticut
Fairfield, Connecticut

Paul Palmberg, MD, PhD
Professor of Ophthalmology
Bascom Palmer Eye Institute
University of Miami Miller School of Medicine
Miami, Florida

Jean-Marie Parel, PhD
Ophthalmic Biophysics Center Bascom Palmer Eye
    Institute
University of Miami Miller School of Medicine
Miami, Florida-

Richard K. Parrish II, MD
Edward W. D. Norton, MD, Chair in Ophthalmology
Professor
Associate Dean for Graduate Medical Education
Director, Glaucoma Service
Bascom Palmer Eye Institute
University of Miami Miller School of Medicine
Designated Institutional Official–Jackson Health
    System/Jackson Memorial Hospital
Miami, Florida-

Adalgisa Corona Peralta, MD
Centro Laser
Santo Domingo, Dominican Republic

Leonard Pinchuk, PhD, DsC, NAE
Founder and Chairman Emeritus
InnFocus, Inc.
Ophthalmic Biophysics Center Bascom Palmer Eye
    Institute
University of Miami Miller School of Medicine
Miami, Florida

Herbert A. Reitsamer, MD
Professor and Chairman
Director Research Program Experimental Ophthalmology
Department of Ophthalmology
Paracelsus Medical University/SALK
Salzburg, Austria

Douglas J. Rhee, MD
Chairman
Department of Ophthalmology and Visual Sciences
University Hospital Case Medical Center
Visiting Professor, Ophthalmology
Case Western Reserve University School of Medicine
Director, Eye Institute, University Hospitals
Department of Ophthalmology
Cleveland, Ohio

Grace M. Richter, MD, MPH
Assistant Professor of Ophthalmology, Glaucoma Division
University of Southern California Roski Eye Institute
Keck School of Medicine
University of Southern California
Los Angeles, California

Isabelle Riss, MD
Pôle Ophtalmologique de la Clinique Mutualiste
Cedex, France

Sruthi Sampathkumar, MD
Research Associate
Department of Ophthalmology
Case Western Reserve University
Cleveland, Ohio

John R. Samples, MD
Glaucoma Consultant
Eye Clinic
Portland, Oregon

Thomas W. Samuelson, MD
Founding Partner and Attending Surgeon
Minnesota Eye Consultants
Adjunct Associate Professor of Ophthalmology
University of Minnesota
Minneapolis, Minnesota

Steven R. Sarkisian, Jr., MD
Clinical Professor
Glaucoma Fellowship Director
Dean McGee Eye Institute
University of Oklahoma
Oklahoma City, Oklahoma

Kurt Scavelli
Research Fellow
Department of Ophthalmology
University Hospitals Case Medical Center
Cleveland, Ohio

Joel S. Schuman, MD, FACS
Chairman
Eye Center
University of Pittsburgh Medical Center
Pittsburgh, Pennsylvania

Donald Schwartz, MD
Assistant Clinical Professor
Department of Ophthalmology
University of Southern California Keck School of Medicine
Long Beach, California

Manjool Shah, MD
Clinical Instructor
Department of Ophthalmology and Visual Sciences
Glaucoma, Cataract, and Anterior Segment Disease
Kellogg Eye Center
University of Michigan
Ann Arbor, Michigan

Arsham Sheybani, MD
Assistant Professor
Department of Ophthalmology
Washington University of Medicine
St. Louis, Missouri

Kuldev Singh, MD
Professor
Department of Ophthalmology
Stanford University Medical Center
Stanford Byers Eye Institute
Stanford, California

Arthur J. Sit, SM, MD
Consultant
Department of Ophthalmology
Associate Professor
College of Medicine
Mayo Clinic
Rochester, Minnesota

Joel M. Solano, MD
Associate Professor
Vance Thompson Vision
University of South Dakota School of Medicine
Sioux Falls, South Dakota

James C. Tan, MD, PhD
Doheny Eye Center University of California–Los Angeles
Arcadia, California

Carol B. Toris, PhD
Professor
Department of Ophthalmology
Case Western Reserve University
Cleveland, Ohio

Ramya N. Swamy, MD, MPH
Assistant Professor
Ophthalmology
University of California–Los Angeles Health
Los Angeles, California

Vanessa Vera, MD
Department of Ophthalmology and Vision Sciences
University of Toronto
Toronto, Ontario, Canada

Steven D. Vold, MD
Founder
Vold Vision
Fayetteville, Arkansas

Bruce A. Weber, MBA
InnFocus, Inc.
Miami, FL

Robert N. Weinreb, MD
Chairman and Distinguished Professor of Ophthalmology
Director of the Shiley Eye Center
Director of the Hamilton Glaucoma Center
Morris Gleich, MD, Chair of Glaucoma
University of California–San Diego
La Jolla, California

Tony Wells, MBBS FRANZCO
Wells Orthodonics, LLC
Evansville (East), Indiana

Amy D. Zhang, MD
Assistant Professor
Glaucoma Service, University Hospitals Eye Institute
Case Western Reserve University School of Medicine
Cleveland, Ohio

1 New Options in the Treatment of Glaucoma

Brian A. Francis, Steven R. Sarkisian, Jr., and James C. Tan

Case Presentations

Case 1

A 71-year-old woman with a history of primary open-angle glaucoma with severe optic nerve and visual field damage presented with uncontrolled intraocular pressure (IOP) on maximum tolerated medications. The cup-to-disk (C/D) ratio was 0.9 to 0.95 with superior and inferior thinning of the rim and corresponding dense superior and inferior arcuate scotomas. Despite this, visual acuity was 20/30, but 20/400 in the fellow eye, making her functionally monocular. The IOP was 19 to 21 on three topical medications, including a prostaglandin analogue, β-blocker, and carbonic anhydrase inhibitor. The patient had an allergy to α-agonists. The visual field was showing slow but steady progression over a 3-year period, with a mean deviation slope of −1.6. After the patient provided appropriate informed consent, the decision was made to proceed with a trabeculectomy with mitomycin.

The surgery was uneventful, and after 3 months of follow-up the IOP was 12 to 14 on no glaucoma medications. The conjunctival bleb was diffuse, but cystic and avascular at the limbus. Three years following surgery, the patient experienced a decline in vision, with pain and redness. She was seen emergently and diagnosed with blebitis and possible endophthalmitis due to the presence of vitreous cells. The vision was 20/400, and a small hypopyon was present with a mild amount of purulent discharge. The patient underwent emergent pars plana vitrectomy with intravitreal fortified antibiotics (gentamicin and Ancef). A culture was taken and eventually grew *Streptococcus* species that was sensitive to the treating antibiotics. Despite this, the vision dropped to light perception, and 2 weeks later the patient underwent repeat vitrectomy, this time via endoscopic guidance because the cornea was opacified. The endoscopic view demonstrated dense fibrinous purulent material throughout the vitreous cavity. This was removed, except for a dense plaque that was adherent to the macula. Despite eventual control of the infection, the vision remained at light perception only.

Case 2

A 78-year-old Caucasian woman with primary open-angle glaucoma and moderate to severe optic nerve damage and visual field loss presented with uncontrolled IOP on maximum tolerated medications. The visual acuity was 20/70 with a 3+ nuclear sclerotic cataract (**Fig. 1.1**). The IOP was 24 mm Hg on a prostaglandin analogue and fixed combination of β-blocker and carbonic anhydrase inhibitor. The patient underwent surgery with a Baerveldt glaucoma implant 350 (Abbott Medical Optics, Santa Ana, CA) and combined phacoemulsification cataract extraction.

Six weeks after surgery, the ligature occluding the tube opened and the patient developed hypotony and a flat anterior chamber. Ultrasonography demonstrated a mixed choroidal effusion and hemorrhage, without central touch but with a decrease in vision to 20/400 and an IOP of 25. The patient was placed on topical steroids and atropine 1%. Despite medical treatment and eventual resolution of the choroidal fluid, the anterior chamber remained very shallow. The patient was lost to follow-up for 2 months, and returned with corneal decompensation and bullous keratopathy, with an IOP of 5. A tube exchange was performed with removal of the Baerveldt implant and placement of an Ahmed glaucoma valve (New World Medical, Rancho Cucamonga, CA) to increase the IOP to more physiological levels. The patient refused further surgery until 2 years later, when a penetrating keratoplasty was performed. At last follow-up, the IOP was 15 on a fixed combination of β-blocker and carbonic anhydrase inhibitor, but the cornea transplant had rejected and vision was now light perception (**Fig. 1.2**).

Introduction to the Novel Glaucoma Procedures

Traditional glaucoma filtration surgery relies on the shunting of aqueous humor to the subconjunctival space, either through a perilimbal scleral opening (as in trabeculectomy) or through a tube shunt to an external reservoir in the equatorial area. Techniques have advanced in these procedures so that they are quite successful in lowering the IOP with an improving safety profile. However, as these unfortunate case presentations exhibit, significant postoperative risks exist, such as late-onset bleb infection or endophthalmitis, hypotony maculopathy, choroidal effusion or hemorrhage, flat anterior chamber, corneal damage, diplopia, and cataract formation.[1]

These risks may be acceptable to a patient with advanced glaucoma and rapidly progressing visual field loss to prevent blindness, but they are not appropriate for a patient with mild to moderate disease or one who wishes to reduce the medication burden. Recently, a new category of glaucoma surgery has developed—minimally invasive glaucoma surgery (MIGS),[2] also called microincisional and microinvasive glaucoma surgery.

The basic tenets of MIGS procedures are an ab interno surgical approach that uses a small incision and spares the conjunctiva and sclera (**Table 1.1**). The surgery should be minimally traumatic with minimal tissue disruption. The safety profile is excellent, especially as compared with more traditional glaucoma filtration surgery. Recovery should be rapid, with good preservation of vision. The IOP is lowered to "physiological levels" or usually in the mid-teens (**Table 1.2**).

When conceptualizing existing and new glaucoma surgical techniques, it is helpful to categorize them by the method of action. In this book, we shall elucidate four different pathways by which we can manipulate aqueous movement to lower the IOP in a minimally invasive fashion: trabecular, or Schlemm's canal;

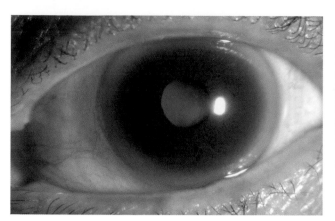

Fig. 1.1 Preoperative slit-lamp photograph prior to combined aqueous tube shunt implantation and cataract extraction (visual acuity = 20/70; IOP = 24).

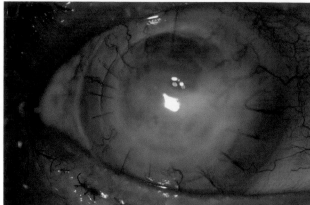

Fig. 1.2 Postoperative slit-lamp photograph showing failed penetrating keratoplasty, flat anterior chamber with iridocorneal touch, and Ahmed valve (visual acuity is light perception only, IOP = 15).

the suprachoroidal space; aqueous humor production; and the subconjunctival space. **Fig. 1.3** illustrates different ways that the canal or the suprachoroidal space can be altered to increase outflow.

Trabecular Outflow Surgery

Schlemm's canal procedures include several Food and Drug Administration (FDA)-approved treatments that involve either a trabeculotomy by internal approach or some type of trabecular micro-bypass that uses a stenting device that remains in the canal. Both types of canal surgery are designed to reduce the outflow resistance caused by the diseased trabecular meshwork. One of the ways to perform an ab interno trabeculotomy involves the use of the Trabectome (NeoMedix, Tustin, CA). The Trabectome accomplishes this by removing a 90- to 180-degree portion of the trabecular meshwork via a plasma thermocautery handpiece. Other methods of performing an ab interno trabeculotomy include a gonioscopy-assisted transluminal trabeculotomy (GATT), or a trabeculotomy using the TRAB360 device (Sight Sciences, Inc., Menlo Park, CA). Finally, there is another technique that does not perform a trabeculotomy but rather uses a laser to make holes in the trabecular meshwork. This is called Excimer Laser Trabeculotomy (Coherent, Santa Clara, CA).

The only FDA-approved device used to bypass the trabecular meshwork at this time is the iStent (Glaukos, Laguna Hills, CA).

The iStent accomplishes this by the placement of a small titanium stent through the trabecular meshwork that allows aqueous to flow from the anterior chamber into Schlemm's canal. Another device for performing a trabecular bypass is the Hydrus implant (Ivantis, Irvine, CA).

Typically, trabecular outflow surgery is used to treat mild to moderate glaucoma in patients with a target IOP in the mid-teens.

These procedures are easily combined with cataract surgery and are commonly used in this setting of combined surgery. They can also be used as a stand-alone procedure (off-label with iStent). Schlemm's canal surgery has changed the way we approach glaucoma treatment, shifting the surgical treatment paradigm to earlier in the disease process.

Future advances in this area will focus on stent design, with multiple stent placements and larger stents to open more of the canal. Individual mapping of the trabecular outflow system will match outflow collector channels with targeted placement of stents. Pharmacological treatment will be used to modulate fibrosis and to maintain the patency of the distal outflow pathway.

Suprachoroidal Outflow Surgeries

The suprachoroidal space is a potential pathway for enhancing aqueous outflow. The pressure gradient between the anterior chamber and the suprachoroidal space enables the potential flow of fluid in this direction. Although there are no FDA-

Table 1.1 Basic Principles of Minimally Invasive Glaucoma Surgery

- Surgical approach: ab interno, small incision, conjunctiva sparing

- Minimal trauma and tissue disruption

- Very high safety profile

- Rapid visual recovery

- Easily combined with phacoemulsification cataract surgery

- Moderate to high IOP-lowering capabilities

Table 1.2 Methods of Lowering Intraoperative Pressure with Minimally Invasive Glaucoma Surgery

- Trabecular outflow or Schlemm's canal Surgery (Trabectome, NeoMedix; iStent, Glaukos; Trab360, Sight Sciences, Inc.; GATT; excimer laser trabeculostomy (ELT); Hydrus*, Ivantis)

- Suprachoroidal space (Cypass*, Transcend; Supra*, Glaukos; Gold Shunt*, Solx)

- Aqueous humor production (endoscopic cyclophotocoagulation; Beaver Visitec International)

- Subconjunctival space (XEN*, Aquesys; MicroShunt*, Innfocus)

*Not approved by the Food and Drug Administration.

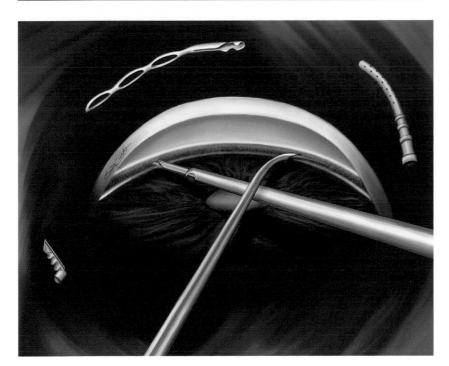

Fig. 1.3 A selection of minimally invasive glaucoma surgery (MIGS) devices. Clockwise from left outside the eye: the first generation iStent, the Hydrus, the CyPass. Inside the eye: The Trabectome is pointed to the left; the TRAB 360 is pointed to the right.

approved devices in this area, two are currently in trials in the United States: Supra (Glaukos) and CyPass (Transcend Medical, Menlo Park, CA). This surgery involves the placement of a small stent in the potential plane between the scleral spur and the ciliary body band that establishes a communication between the anterior chamber and the suprachoroidal space. Like Schlemm's canal procedures, it is performed via an ab interno approach that spares the conjunctiva and combines well with cataract extraction. The patient population is also very similar, aimed at mild to moderate glaucoma patients with a target IOP in the mid-teens. Future research is likely to involve stent design and modulation of healing to prevent fibrosis and closure of the distal end of the stent.

Aqueous Humor Production Surgery

Lowering of aqueous humor production is performed by laser treatment of the ciliary processes, or cyclophotocoagulation. The transscleral approach is performed by the external application of energy via a handheld probe placed near the corneal limbus. Because of the tissue destruction involved, this approach is not considered a MIGS procedure.

In contrast, endoscopic cyclophotocoagulation (ECP) (Beaver Visitec International, Waltham, MA) involves the application of laser energy directly to the ciliary epithelium via an internal, endoscopic approach. Because of the lower energy requirements and decrease in tissue damage, many surgeons consider this procedure to be part of the MIGS category.

When used in combination with cataract extraction, ECP involves the treatment of 270 degrees or more of the ciliary processes via a temporal corneal incision. The energy delivery is usually lower and thus results in moderate IOP lowering with high safety and rapid recovery. ECP can also be used more aggressively to treat glaucoma refractory to filtration surgery. In these cases, 330 to 360 degrees of the ciliary processes are usually treated with a higher amount of energy delivered. ECP can also be performed via a pars plana approach and with treatment of the pars plana tissue (ECP Plus) for greater efficacy. The safety

profile is still high, but with a longer recovery period and more postoperative inflammation.

Subconjunctival Filtration Surgery

The subconjunctival space is the pathway used by traditional glaucoma filtration surgery, and it is debatable whether it falls into the MIGS spectrum. Depending on one's definition of MIGS, the formation of a filtration bleb may exclude this category. There are currently no FDA-approved devices in this group, but several are under investigation. The XEN implant (AqueSys Inc., Aliso Viejo, CA) is a collagen shunt that passes from the anterior chamber to the subconjunctival space. It is implanted using an ab interno approach with or without the help of antifibrotic agents (mitomycin C). The InnFocus Micro Shunt (InnFocus, Miami, FL) is a small stent made of poly(styrene-block-isobutylene-block-styrene) (SIBS) also connecting the anterior chamber to the subconjunctival space, but it is implanted via an external approach with conjunctival dissection and application of antifibrotics.

The goal of these procedures is to duplicate the IOP-lowering capabilities of trabeculectomy while decreasing the risks of hypotony and bleb-related infections. Therefore, they may be appropriate for patients with more advanced glaucoma disease, requiring a lower target IOP.

In summary, the advent of MIGS has the potential to substantially change the way we treat glaucoma patients. With these alternatives in our treatment armamentarium, we are beginning to treat glaucoma as a surgical disease in its earlier stages. Thus, surgery is now being considered in much the same way as medical or laser therapy, rather than as a last resort. Glaucoma treatment can be more tailored to meet a patient's disease characteristics and therapeutic needs. Using the four categories of glaucoma surgical treatment (Schlemm's canal, suprachoroidal space, aqueous humor production, and subconjunctival space), we can treat patients with the most appropriate surgical intervention, based on their anatomy, disease status, and treatment history. In addition, we can potentially combine surgeries that utilize different pathways for greater IOP reduction. For example, a Schlemm's canal procedure can be combined with a suprachoroidal shunt or an aqueous humor-decreasing procedure.

Conclusion

This book begins with a basic science section delving into our current understanding of physiological pathways of aqueous formation and drainage and what happens when they are exploited surgically to reduce intraocular pressure. In many ways, the surgery is driving the science. Technological advances have enabled miniaturization, technical simplification and novel ways to shunt aqueous into ocular compartments, such as the suprachoroidal space and Schlemm's canal. Moreover, there are new ways to shunt into the more familiar subconjunctival space. These developments have prompted new (and some older) questions about the aqueous humor system. How do collector channels respond to increased aqueous flow following trabecular bypass? How does scarring—that age-old enemy of glaucoma surgery—affect the suprachoroidal space? How does fluid really drain from the subconjunctival space? What happens to aqueous secretion and the blood aqueous barrier years after cyclophotocoagulation? While many lack complete answers, our panel of experts has collected and interpreted the evidence, shared their current thinking, and espoused on some important questions unearthed by the surgeries.

The clinical section is designed to familiarize the reader with each new procedure in its entirety, from appropriate selection of patients to surgical technique, management and prevention of complications, and knowledge of the results contained in the medical literature.

We understand that this is a rapidly evolving field; however, this book is intended to be a foundational trunk from which branches will grow and evolve as these technologies mature and come into broader use. Our goal is to help the reader to understand the available tools to individualize care for each glaucoma patient and be able to adapt with each new device's commercial release based on previous experience with predicate devices and a sound basic science understanding of how the body responds to the surgical management of aqueous movement.

References

1. Gedde SJ, Schiffman JC, Feuer WJ, Herndon LW, Brandt JD, Budenz DL; Tube versus Trabeculectomy Study Group. Treatment outcomes in the Tube Versus Trabeculectomy (TVT) study after five years of follow-up. Am J Ophthalmol 2012;153:789–803.e2

2. Saheb H, Ahmed II. Micro-invasive glaucoma surgery: current perspectives and future directions. Curr Opin Ophthalmol 2012;23:96–104

Section I   Eye Anatomy and Physiology

2 Structure and Mechanisms of Trabecular Outflow

Kurt Scavelli, Amy D. Zhang, Carol Toris, and Douglas J. Rhee

The trabecular outflow pathway is the eye's main site of aqueous humor (AH) drainage. It is responsible for 60 to 95% of AH outflow depending on the age of the patient and the health of the eye. The remaining drainage occurs through the uveoscleral pathway. The trabecular outflow pathway is located at the iridocorneal angle, and it is composed of the trabecular meshwork (TM), endothelial lining of Schlemm's canal, collector channels, and aqueous veins **(Fig. 2.1).** The trabecular outflow pathway is a key site of intraocular pressure (IOP) regulation and a critical pathway in the pathogenesis of primary open-angle glaucoma (POAG).

Trabecular Meshwork

As AH exits the anterior chamber through the trabecular outflow pathway, it first traverses the three layers of the TM. The TM is located in a semicircular groove on the inner aspect of the sclera known as the scleral sulcus. The TM attaches anteriorly to the peripheral cornea at Schwalbe's line and inserts posteriorly into the scleral spur.[1] Attachment of the TM together with the ciliary muscle to the scleral spur is important in regulating the trabecular outflow pathway, as this arrangement allows ciliary muscle contraction to widen the TM. Structurally, the TM is a sponge-like network of connective tissue composed of trabecular beams, which contain a core of collagen and elastin fibers. Lining the trabecular beams are TM endothelial cells. The cells on the outer layers of the TM are phagocytic in nature and are believed to help remove cellular debris from the AH.[1]

The TM serves two main functions in the eye. First, it filters the AH, removing any cellular or pigment debris that can disrupt drainage of AH through the trabecular outflow pathway. Second, it acts as a path of resistance for the regulation of outflow facility and ultimately IOP. Histologically, the TM can be separated into three regions that differ in structure: the uveal meshwork, the corneoscleral meshwork, and the juxtacanalicular tissue (JCT).

Uveal Meshwork

The uveal meshwork is the innermost region of the trabecular meshwork. It originates at the anterior aspect of the ciliary body and inserts at the peripheral cornea. The uveal meshwork is composed of one to three layers of trabecular beams and has relatively large intertrabecular spaces, which provide minimal resistance to AH outflow.[2]

Corneoscleral Meshwork

The corneoscleral meshwork forms the middle region of the TM and extends from the scleral spur to Schwalbe's line. This region is composed of eight to 15 layers of trabecular beams, which are thicker than the uveal meshwork, resulting in smaller intertrabecular spaces that confer a greater resistance to AH outflow.[2]

Juxtacanalicular Tissue

The JCT is the thinnest (2–20 μm) and outermost portion of the TM and is located directly adjacent to the endothelial lining of Schlemm's canal. It has a unique architecture compared with that of the other regions of the TM, in that it is not composed of trabecular beams. The JCT is a dynamic and complex region made up of loose connective tissue supported by an incomplete basement membrane with TM cells surrounded by a fibrillar extracellular matrix (ECM).[1,3] Compared with the other regions of the TM, it has relatively low porosity, and it functions as the main point of resistance for the TM outflow pathway. Within the ECM of the JCT, there are nonstructural elements called matricellular proteins, such as secreted protein acidic and rich in cysteine (SPARC) and thrombospondin-1 (TSP-1). Matricellular proteins are secreted by cells of the ECM and aid in cellular communication with the ECM.[4-6] A prominent structural change in the TM of patients with POAG is an increase in the fibrillar content in the ECM of the JCT.[7] Due to the increased deposition of ECM in patients with POAG and the importance that ECM turnover plays in managing outflow facility, matricellular proteins have become an important focus for determining the pathogenesis of POAG.

Schlemm's Canal

After passing through the TM, AH drains into Schlemm's canal. Schlemm's canal is a collecting channel deep to the TM in the scleral sulcus. The inner wall of Schlemm's canal is formed by a layer of endothelial cells. As AH flows by transcellular transport into the inner wall endothelium, giant vacuoles develop and bulge into the lumen of the canal[8,9] **(Fig. 2.2).** The giant vacuoles in Schlemm's canal are hypothesized to be involved in regulating the resistance of AH outflow. The outer wall of Schlemm's canal has a single layer of endothelium and contains outlet channels that drain directly into the episcleral veins.

Physiology of Trabecular Meshwork Outflow

The flow of AH through the TM outflow pathway is a pressure-dependent process. At steady-state IOP, the combination of flow of AH across the trabecular and uveoscleral outflow pathway is at the same rate as its production from the ciliary body.[9] In pathological processes, such as aging and POAG, the steady-state IOP can shift. The increase in IOP in these two examples is due to an increase in resistance across the TM outflow pathway.[10,11] Three major mechanisms govern outflow resistance across the

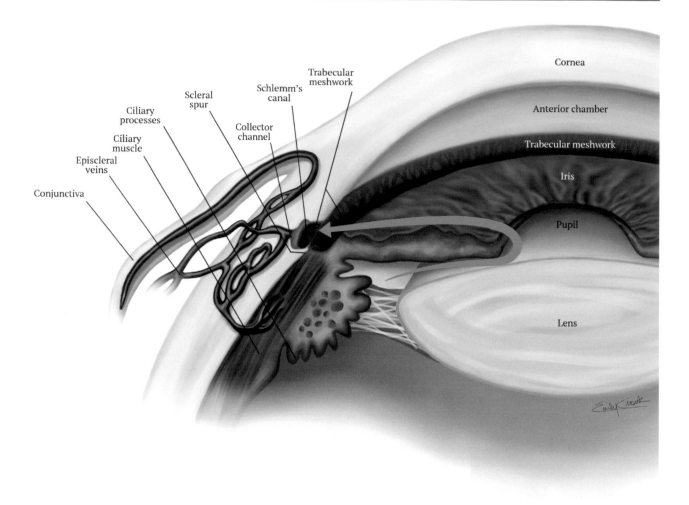

Fig. 2.1 Aqueous humor (AH) is produced from the ciliary body in the posterior chamber and passes into the anterior chamber through the pupil. The majority of AH exits the anterior chamber through the trabecular outflow pathway, which is located at the iridocorneal angle. In the trabecular outflow pathway, AH flows through the trabecular meshwork, which drains into Schlemm's canal. The outer wall of Schlemm's canal contains outlet collector channels that drain into the episcleral veins.

TM outflow pathway. The *transcellular* route is the flow of AH as it leaves the JCT and enters vacuoles in the inner-wall endothelial cells of Schlemm's canal. The *paracellular* route is the flow of AH passing between the inner-wall endothelial cells of Schlemm's canal. The third mechanism of resistance is the ECM turnover that occurs in the JCT region[12] (**Fig. 2.3**). Because of the electrical charge of many of the structural components, the JCT ECM provides resistance to water and ions.

Extracellular Matrix Turnover

Flow of AH through the TM is a dynamic process that requires regulation of outflow resistance to maintain a stable IOP. Homeostatic regulation of outflow resistance is believed to be triggered by cellular monitoring of changes in stretch or distortion of the TM. Cellular signals then alter ECM turnover in the TM to shift its balance toward higher or lower resistance.[9,13] Matricellular proteins, such as SPARC, may be key intermediates in the regulation of ECM turnover as they are highly expressed following cellular stress and are involved in ECM regulation in other tissues. Alteration in the regulation of ECM turnover is believed to be key in the pathogenesis of POAG. Patients with POAG characteristically display increased deposition of ECM in the JCT region

of the TM.[7] Multiple studies have shown that patients with POAG have elevated levels of transforming growth factor-β_2 (TGF-β_2), which increases ECM synthesis in the TM.[14,15]

Contractile Influence on Trabecular Outflow

The trabecular outflow pathway receives contractile forces from the ciliary body and scleral spur. Tendons of the ciliary muscle extend anteriorly and attach to the scleral spur; they are continuous with the ECM of the TM. As a result, contraction of the ciliary muscle posteriorly displaces the scleral spur and widens the trabecular meshwork, which enlarges the intertrabecular pores and decreases outflow resistance (**Fig. 2.4**). The cells of the scleral spur also have a contractile phenotype and receive parasympathetic innervation.[16,17] Given the attachment of the TM to the scleral spur, a change in scleral spur cell tone would likely affect outflow resistance. Furthermore, there is evidence to suggest a contractile phenotype for TM cells as well, and studies have shown that TM cells can modify outflow resistance by changing cellular tone and altering the contractile nature of the JCT–Schlemm's canal region.[18,19]

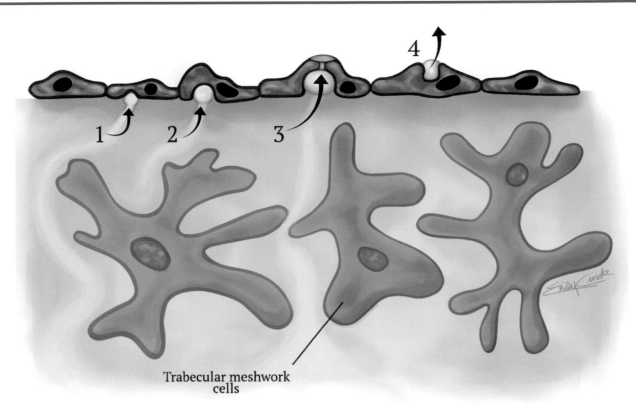

Trabecular meshwork
cells

Fig. 2.2 One way that AH enters into Schlemm's canal is by transcellular transport into the inner wall endothelium of Schlemm's canal. As AH enters the endothelial cell *(1,2)* it generates a vacuole that bulges into the lumen of the canal. Fusion of the vacuole to the basal membrane of the endothelial cells generates a transcellular route for AH to enter into Schlemm's canal *(3)*. As the AH flows into Schlemm's canal, the vacuole regresses *(4)*.

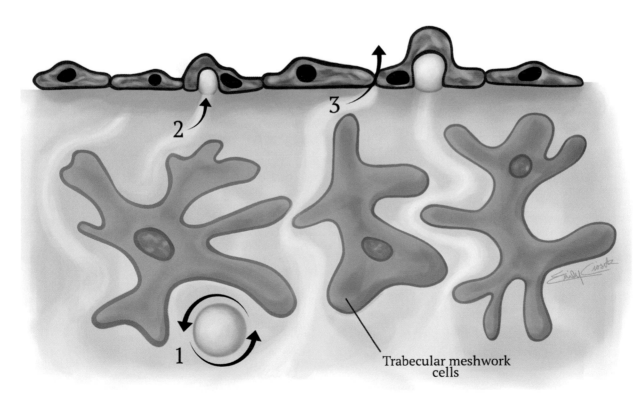

Trabecular meshwork
cells

Fig. 2.3 Three mechanisms of resistance to AH outflow in the trabecular meshwork outflow pathway: *1*, extracellular matrix turnover occurs in the juxtacanalicular tissue region. *2*, the transcellular route is the flow of AH as it leaves the JCT and enters vacuoles in the inner wall endothelial cells of Schlemm's canal. The vacuoles provide resistance to outflow. *3*, the paracellular route is the flow of AH passing between the inner wall endothelial cells of Schlemm's canal.

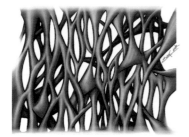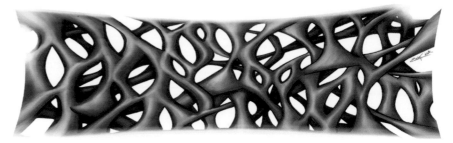

Fig. 2.4 Contraction of the ciliary muscle causes the scleral spur to displace posteriorly. Because the trabecular meshwork originates from the scleral spur, this displacement results in widening of the pores of the trabecular meshwork to facilitate increased outflow of AH.

Segmental Flow

Although the TM is present circumferentially around the anterior chamber, AH does not exit the anterior chamber uniformly throughout the 360 degrees of the iridocorneal angle. Instead, there are select areas of the TM that receive a large percentage of AH outflow and other areas that receive little or none—a concept that is referred to as segmental flow.[20,21] On gonioscopy, one can see evidence of segmental flow by observing segmental pigmentation of the iridocorneal angle. Experimentally, segmental flow has been demonstrated through the perfusion of cationic ferritin or fluorescent beads in enucleated eyes or animal models.[21,22] It is hypothesized that AH preferentially flows through the TM in areas with greater porosity and close proximity to collector channel ostia. However, no particular geographic pattern to segmental flow through the TM has been identified, which hints at a dynamic nature to the process. It is important to fully elucidate segmental flow through the TM for determination of optimal device placement when using implants designed to bypass the trabecular meshwork and shunt AH between Schlemm's canal and the anterior chamber.

Effect of Aging on the Trabecular Meshwork

Aging is a strong and important risk factor for the development of POAG. The prevalence of POAG increases greatly beginning at the age of 60 in Caucasian patients and age 40 in African-American and Hispanic patients.[10] Therefore, it is not surprising that there are characteristic changes that occur in the TM as people age. On histological examination, there is a decrease in the cellularity and an increase in cellular senescence of the TM.[23,24] Furthermore, there is an increase in the thickness of the trabecular beams and an increase in the deposition of extracellular proteoglycans.[7] It is hypothesized that aging of TM cells along with decreased cellularity leads to their decreased function, resulting in decreased phagocytosis of debris and dysregulation of the ECM of the TM. These changes in the architecture of the TM result in a decrease in the size of the intertrabecular spaces, causing greater outflow resistance and subsequent elevated IOP.

Trabecular Meshwork in Primary Open-Angle Glaucoma

The TM is the anatomic location of the pathogenesis of POAG. Morphologically, the outer TM in eyes with POAG is similar to that of age-matched controls,[7] but the JCT shows dysregulation of the ECM, specifically an increased number of sheath-derived plaques of the elastic fibers. Interestingly, the amount of plaque in the JCT correlates with the severity of optic nerve damage in patients

with POAG, but it does not correlate with elevation of IOP.[25] Other characteristics of the trabecular outflow pathway in patients with POAG are an increase in the intrinsic stiffness of the TM and a decrease in the porosity of the endothelial lining of Schlemm's canal.[26,27] Each of these pathological changes contributes to the increase in resistance to outflow facility in patients with POAG.

A key mediator of the ECM dysregulation in POAG is TGF-β_2. TGF-β_2 is found in significantly higher than normal concentrations in the AH of patients with POAG, and it is a known mediator of abnormal ECM deposition/fibrosis.[14,15,28,29] In perfused human cadaveric anterior chambers, TGF-β_2 increases IOP. SPARC has been demonstrated as a downstream regulator of TGF-β_2-mediated ocular hypertension.[30] Given SPARC's known role in the regulation of ECM, it is believed to be an important protein in both TM normal physiology and the pathogenesis of POAG. Other proteins, such as connective tissue growth factor, cochlin, gremlin, and frizzled proteins also have some regulatory role.[31–35]

Modifying the Trabecular Meshwork Outflow Pathway

Modifying TM outflow to decrease the outflow resistance and interrupt the disease pathophysiology are the foci of modern therapeutic investigation. The site of most resistance is presumed to be the inner-wall endothelial layer of Schlemm's canal and the juxtacanalicular region. Historically, there have been studies that decreased the TM resistance by disrupting the microfilaments that are part of the ECM of the TM. The various agents that were examined included cytochalasins, ethylenediaminetetraacetic acid (EDTA) and H-7, an agent that disrupts the actin cytoskeleton.[36] Sulfhydryl reagents, iodoacetamide, N-ethylmaleimide, and ethacrynic acid that alter the cellular membrane of the endothelial lining of Schlemm's canal also decrease outflow resistance.[37–39] Novel drugs that alter the resistance of the TM are in clinical trials. These drugs focus on different components of the ECM.

Rho-associated coiled coil-forming protein kinase (ROCK) inhibitors target the actin cytoskeleton. They are believed to decrease outflow resistance by affecting the contractile properties of TM and by actomyosin regulation. Currently, there are four compounds that are in phase II or III testing that show IOP lowering in the range of 3.7 to 6.2 mm Hg, with the major side effect being ocular hyperemia.[40]

Latrunculins are macrolides that inhibit actin polymerization of the cells of the trabecular meshwork. Their proposed mechanism of action is thought to involve the expansion of space between the trabecular collagen beams and the inner wall of Schlemm's canal as well as increasing the space between the inner wall cells. Lactrunculin B compound (Inspire Pharmaceuticals, Raleigh, NC; drug INS-115622) in phase I trials, reported IOP lowering of 4 mm Hg, with the drug being well tolerated.[41]

Adenosine receptor agonists are thought to increase TM outflow by shrinking the cellular volume as well as altering the structure of the extracellular matrix. Trabodenoson (Inotek Pharmaceuticals, Lexington, MA; drug INO-8875) is a selective adenosine-1 agonist in phase I/II trials that is well tolerated and provides a statistically significant reduction in IOP.[42] It is thought to increase the upregulation of proteases that digest proteins that can obstruct the flow of aqueous humor through the TM.

Ways to reduce IOP without chronic topical dosing are being offered by minimally invasive glaucoma surgery (MIGS). Some procedures are designed to overcome the increase in outflow resistance present in glaucomatous TM by bypassing the TM and providing direct access to Schlemm's canal (e.g., iStent, Glaukos, Laguna Hills, CA; and Hydrus, Ivantis, Irvine, CA). Another approach involves removal of a section of the TM and with it the resistance to outflow in that region (Trabectome, NeoMedix, Tustin, CA). Dilation of the Schlemm's canal is thought to decrease resistance and IOP (canaloplasty).

References

1. Tamm ER. The trabecular meshwork outflow pathways: structural and functional aspects. Exp Eye Res 2009;88:648–655

2. Shaarawy T, Sherwood MB, Crowston JG. Glaucoma: Medical Diagnosis and Therapy. New York: Saunders/Elsevier; 2009:40–46

3. Acott TS, Kelley MJ. Extracellular matrix in the trabecular meshwork. Exp Eye Res 2008;86:543–561

4. Bornstein P. Thrombospondins as matricellular modulators of cell function. J Clin Invest 2001;107:929–934

5. Flügel-Koch C, Ohlmann A, Fuchshofer R, Welge-Lüssen U, Tamm ER. Thrombospondin-1 in the trabecular meshwork: localization in normal and glaucomatous eyes, and induction by TGF-beta1 and dexamethasone in vitro. Exp Eye Res 2004;79:649–663

6. Rhee DJ, Fariss RN, Brekken R, Sage EH, Russell P. The matricellular protein SPARC is expressed in human trabecular meshwork. Exp Eye Res 2003;77:601–607

7. Tektas OY, Lütjen-Drecoll E. Structural changes of the trabecular meshwork in different kinds of glaucoma. Exp Eye Res 2009;88:769–775

8. Garron LK, Feeney ML, Hogan MJ, McEwen WK. Electron microscopic studies of the human eye. I. Preliminary investigations of the trabeculas. Am J Ophthalmol 1958;46(1 Pt 2):27–35

9. Levin LA, Adler FH. Adler's Physiology of the Eye. Edinburgh: Saunders/Elsevier; 2011:274–307

10. Caprioli J. Glaucoma: a disease of early cellular senescence. Invest Ophthalmol Vis Sci 2013;54:ORSF60-7

11. Gabelt BT, Kaufman PL. Changes in aqueous humor dynamics with age and glaucoma. Prog Retin Eye Res 2005;24:612–637

12. Chatterjee A, Villarreal G Jr, Rhee DJ. Matricellular proteins in the trabecular meshwork: review and update. J Ocul Pharmacol Ther 2014;30:447–463

13. Bradley JM, Vranka J, Colvis CM, et al. Effect of matrix metalloproteinases activity on outflow in perfused human organ culture. Invest Ophthalmol Vis Sci 1998;39:2649–2658

14. Picht G, Welge-Luessen U, Grehn F, Lütjen-Drecoll E. Transforming growth factor beta 2 levels in the aqueous humor in different types of glaucoma and the relation to filtering bleb development. Graefes Arch Clin Exp Ophthalmol 2001;239:199–207

15. Tripathi RC, Li J, Chan WF, Tripathi BJ. Aqueous humor in glaucomatous eyes contains an increased level of TGF-beta 2. Exp Eye Res 1994;59:723–727

16. Tamm E, Flügel C, Stefani FH, Rohen JW. Contractile cells in the human scleral spur. Exp Eye Res 1992;54:531–543

17. Tamm ER, Koch TA, Mayer B, Stefani FH, Lütjen-Drecoll E. Innervation of myofibroblast-like scleral spur cells in human monkey eyes. Invest Ophthalmol Vis Sci 1995;36:1633–1644

18. Tian B, Geiger B, Epstein DL, Kaufman PL. Cytoskeletal involvement in the regulation of aqueous humor outflow. Invest Ophthalmol Vis Sci 2000;41:619–623

19. Wiederholt M, Thieme H, Stumpff F. The regulation of trabecular meshwork and ciliary muscle contractility. Prog Retin Eye Res 2000;19:271–295

20. Swaminathan SS, Oh DJ, Kang MH, et al. Secreted protein acidic and rich in cysteine (SPARC)-null mice exhibit more uniform outflow. Invest Ophthalmol Vis Sci 2013;54:2035–2047

21. Hann CR, Bahler CK, Johnson DH. Cationic ferritin and segmental flow through the trabecular meshwork. Invest Ophthalmol Vis Sci 2005;46:1–7

22. Swaminathan SS, Oh DJ, Kang MH, Rhee DJ. Aqueous outflow: segmental and distal flow. J Cataract Refract Surg 2014;40:1263–1272

23. Alvarado J, Murphy C, Polansky J, Juster R. Age-related changes in trabecular meshwork cellularity. Invest Ophthalmol Vis Sci 1981;21:714–727

24. Grossniklaus HE, Nickerson JM, Edelhauser HF, Bergman LA, Berglin L. Anatomic alterations in aging and age-related diseases of the eye. Invest Ophthalmol Vis Sci 2013;54:ORSF23-7

25. Gottanka J, Johnson DH, Martus P, Lütjen-Drecoll E. Severity of optic nerve damage in eyes with POAG is correlated with changes in the trabecular meshwork. J Glaucoma 1997;6:123–132

26. Johnson M, Chan D, Read AT, Christensen C, Sit A, Ethier CR. The pore density in the inner wall endothelium of Schlemm's canal of glaucomatous eyes. Invest Ophthalmol Vis Sci 2002;43:2950–2955

27. Last JA, Pan T, Ding Y, et al. Elastic modulus determination of normal and glaucomatous human trabecular meshwork. Invest Ophthalmol Vis Sci 2011;52:2147–2152

28. Inatani M, Tanihara H, Katsuta H, Honjo M, Kido N, Honda Y. Transforming growth factor-beta 2 levels in aqueous humor of glaucomatous eyes. Graefes Arch Clin Exp Ophthalmol 2001;239:109–113

29. Ochiai Y, Ochiai H. Higher concentration of transforming factor-beta in aqueous humor of glaucomatous eyes and diabetic eyes. Jpn J Ophthalmol 2002;46:249–253

30. Kang MH, Oh DJ, Kang JH, Rhee DJ. Regulation of SPARC by transforming growth factor β2 in human trabecular meshwork. Invest Ophthalmol Vis Sci 2013;54:2523–2532

31. Abreu JG, Ketpura NI, Reversade B, De Robertis EM. Connective-tissue growth factor (CTGF) modulates cell signalling by BMP and TGF-beta. Nat Cell Biol 2002;4:599–604

32. Browne JG, Ho SL, Kane R, et al. Connective tissue growth factor is increased in pseudoexfoliation glaucoma. Invest Ophthalmol Vis Sci 2011;52:3660–3666

33. Bhattacharya SK, Gabelt BT, Ruiz J, Picciani R, Kaufman PL. Cochlin expression in anterior segment organ culture models after TGFbeta2 treatment. Invest Ophthalmol Vis Sci 2009;50:551–559

34. Wordinger RJ, Fleenor DL, Hellberg PE, et al. Effects of TGF-beta2, BMP-4, and gremlin in the trabecular meshwork: implications for glaucoma. Invest Ophthalmol Vis Sci 2007;48:1191–1200

35. Wang WH, McNatt LG, Pang IH, et al. Increased expression of the WNT antagonist sFRP-1 in glaucoma elevates intraocular pressure. J Clin Invest 2008;118:1056–1064

36. Kaufman PL. Enhancing trabecular outflow by disrupting the actin cytoskeleton, increasing uveoscleral outflow with prostaglandins, and understanding the pathophysiology of presbyopia interrogating Mother Nature: asking why, asking how, recognizing the signs, following the trail. Exp Eye Res 2008;86:3–17

37. Epstein DL, Hashimoto JM, Anderson PJ, Grant WM. Effect of iodoacetamide perfusion on outflow facility and metabolism of the trabecular meshwork. Invest Ophthalmol Vis Sci 1981;20:625–631

38. Epstein DL, Patterson MM, Rivers SC, Anderson PJ. N-ethylmaleimide increases the facility of aqueous outflow of excised monkey and calf eyes. Invest Ophthalmol Vis Sci 1982;22:752–756

39. Lindenmayer JM, Kahn MG, Hertzmark E, Epstein DL. Morphology and function of the aqueous outflow system in monkey eyes perfused with sulfhydryl reagents. Invest Ophthalmol Vis Sci 1983;24:710–717

40. Wang SK, Chang RT. An emerging treatment option for glaucoma: Rho kinase inhibitors. Clin Ophthalmol 2014;8:883–890

41. Ritch R, Zink RC, et al. Latrunculin B (ins115644) reduces intraocular pressure (IOP) in ocular hypertension (OHT) and primary open angle glaucoma (POAG). Invest Ophthalmol Vis Sci 2010;51:6432

42. Kim N, Supuran C, et al. INO-8875, an adenosine A1 agonist, lowers intraocular pressure through the conventional outflow pathway. Invest Ophthalmol Vis Sci 2010;51:3238

3 How Does Trabecular Bypass Affect the Relationship Between Schlemm's Canal Pressure and Episcleral Venous Pressure?

Arthur J. Sit

Aqueous humor exiting the anterior chamber through the trabecular (conventional) outflow system must pass through two primary regions of resistance: (1) the trabecular meshwork (TM) and inner wall of Schlemm's canal; and (2) the distal outflow system consisting of collector channels, aqueous veins, and ultimately the episcleral veins. For the distal outflow system, the pressure difference between Schlemm's canal and the episcleral veins is the driving force for fluid flow. By reducing TM resistance, trabecular bypass surgery may alter this pressure difference, with long-term consequences on surgical efficacy.

A relevant point to consider is how much of the total fluid resistance is proximal to and how much is distal to Schlemm's canal. In nonhuman primates, direct measurement of Schlemm's canal pressure and episcleral venous pressure (EVP) suggests that only 10% of resistance is distal.[1] In human cadaver eyes, Grant[2,3] demonstrated that 75% of outflow resistance was proximal to Schlemm's canal. However, as reported by Rosenquist et al,[4] the perfusion pressures used by Grant in his original experiments were too high to be physiological, given that EVP in cadaver eyes is zero. A perfusion pressure of 25 mm Hg would result in a pressure drop from the anterior chamber to the episcleral veins that is much higher than normal. Assuming an intraocular pressure (IOP) of 15 mm Hg and an EVP of around 7 to 8 mm Hg, the pressure drop should be only 7 to 8 mm Hg instead of 25 mm Hg. When the more physiological perfusion pressure of 7 mm Hg was used, only 50% of total resistance was eliminated by a complete 360-degree trabeculotomy. Therefore, the pressure in Schlemm's canal could be expected to be approximately equal to the mean of IOP and EVP in normal eyes.

Trabecular bypass surgery can theoretically provide a low resistance path from the anterior chamber to Schlemm's canal. If successful, the pressure in Schlemm's canal would be expected to be nearly equal to the anterior chamber pressure, at least in the region of the surgery. If the distal resistance and EVP remain constant, the pressure difference between Schlemm's canal and the episcleral veins would be expected to rise in most cases. For example, if EVP is 7 mm Hg, IOP is 21 mm Hg, and 50% of the total outflow resistance is proximal to Schlemm's canal, then the difference in Schlemm's canal pressure and EVP would be expected to be half of the IOP–EVP difference, or 7 mm Hg. Removal of half of the TM resistance would be expected to result in a 33% decrease in the IOP–EVP difference, resulting in an IOP of 16.3 mm Hg. The difference in Schlemm's canal pressure and EVP would therefore increase to 9.3 mm Hg. The effect of increasing the pressure difference between Schlemm's canal and the

episcleral veins is unknown. However, it is possible that distal outflow system resistance and EVP are dynamic, just like the resistance in the TM, and they affect the long-term efficacy of MIGS procedures.

There is significant evidence that homeostatic mechanisms in the TM work to regulate IOP.[5] It is possible that other homeostatic mechanisms in the distal outflow pathway perform a similar function, and serve to prevent hypotony. Increased flow through a small segment of the outflow system could potentially result in shear-induced vessel constriction.[6] Because resistance varies with diameter to the fourth power, even a small change in vessel diameter could have a significant effect on resistance. In this case, the pressure difference between Schlemm's canal and the episcleral veins would increase further. It is also possible that increased flow results in a regional alteration in EVP. The episcleral vascular plexus contains multiple arteriovenous anastomoses,[7] and alteration of these connections could modify EVP on a regional basis to maintain IOP. In this case, the pressure difference between Schlemm's canal and the episcleral veins would be maintained, but the back pressure would be increased. Further research is required to elucidate the true nature of the relationship between Schlemm's canal pressure and EVP after MIGS, and this may play an important role in determining the efficacy of these devices and procedures.

References

1. Mäepea O, Bill A. Pressures in the juxtacanalicular tissue and Schlemm's canal in monkeys. Exp Eye Res 1992;54:879–883

2. Grant WM. Further studies on facility of flow through the trabecular meshwork. AMA Arch Opthalmol 1958;60(4 Part 1):523–533

3. Grant WM. Facility of flow through the trabecular meshwork. AMA Arch Opthalmol 1955;54:245–248

4. Rosenquist R, Epstein D, Melamed S, Johnson M, Grant WM. Outflow resistance of enucleated human eyes at two different perfusion pressures and different extents of trabeculotomy. Curr Eye Res 1989;8:1233–1240

5. Acott TS, Kelley MJ, Keller KE, et al. Intraocular pressure homeostasis: maintaining balance in a high-pressure environment. J Ocul Pharmacol Ther 2014;30:94–101

6. Segal SS. Regulation of blood flow in the microcirculation. Microcirculation 2005;12:33–45

7. Kiel JW. The ocular circulation. In: Granger DN, Granger JP, eds. Synthesis Lectures on Integrated Systems Physiology: From Molecule to Function to Disease. San Rafael, CA: Morgan & Claypool Life Sciences; 2010

4 What Role Do Collector Channels Play in Determining Outcomes of Trabecular Bypass Surgery?

Mark Johnson and Joel S. Schuman

Modern research into the pathogenesis of elevated intraocular pressure (IOP), which is characteristic of glaucoma, has focused on the deeper aspect of the trabecular meshwork and the endothelial lining of the inner wall of Schlemm's canal. Less attention has been paid to the collector channels and aqueous veins, as these vessels are not thought to be responsible for the altered hydrodynamics of the glaucomatous aqueous outflow pathway.[1,2] However, the flow resistance of these vessels may have an important role in determining the outcome of certain types of trabecular bypass surgery.

The bulk of aqueous outflow resistance is generated in the trabecular meshwork and inner wall of Schlemm's canal. It has been anticipated that procedures that bypass the trabecular meshwork (e.g., ab interno trabeculectomy and trabecular bypass procedures) would lower the IOP to levels not much higher than that of episcleral venous pressure; however, such procedures do not lower the IOP to the extent that was expected. This is likely due to the flow resistance of the collector channels and aqueous veins.

As aqueous humor flows out of Schlemm's canal, it enters into the collecting channels that connect the canal with the aqueous and episcleral veins, thus establishing venous return. The collector channels and aqueous veins have diameters that are many micrometers across, and the use of Poiseuille's law leads to the conclusion that these vessels should have negligible flow resistance.[3] However, experimental support for this conclusion is mixed. Mäepea and Bill[4,5] measured pressures in Schlemm's canal of primate eyes and found that the pressures were little different from the episcleral venous pressures, in agreement with Poiseuille's law. However, several other investigators have perfused enucleated primate and human eyes before and after a 360-degree trabeculotomy that would be expected to eliminate all flow resistance proximal to the collector channels and aqueous veins.[6-11] All of these studies have shown that at least 25% of outflow resistance remains after this procedure, in contrast to what would have been predicted theoretically. This has been demonstrated with sinusotomy as well.[12] It is possible that contractile cells surrounding these vessels[13] may locally constrict vessel size and increase their flow resistance.

The effect of this collector channel resistance is magnified when a partial trabeculotomy is done or a stent is inserted into Schlemm's canal. In such procedures, most aqueous flow bypasses the trabecular meshwork and enters into Schlemm's canal, or is exposed directly to the collector channel ostia themselves. The flow passing through those segments of Schlemm's canal nearest these openings is much higher than occurs normally. Furthermore, because there is substantial flow resistance in the collector channels, all of the flow cannot travel through just one or two collector channels, and thus flow may have to travel a sig-nificant extent through Schlemm's canal before exiting through the collector channels. These effects can generate a significant pressure drop in Schlemm's canal, in contrast to the normal physiological situation[14] in which the flow resistance of Schlemm's canal is negligible. This resistance is in addition to that generated by the collector channels, and thus it is not surprising that use of the trabectome or stents in Schlemm's canal leads to higher than expected postsurgical IOP.

Thus, when looking to lower aqueous outflow resistance by removing or bypassing the trabecular meshwork, it might be advisable to consider measures that also reduce the distal flow resistance in the collector channels and aqueous veins.

References

1. Johnson M, Erickson K. Mechanisms and routes of aqueous humor drainage. In: Albert DM, Jakobiec FA, ed. Principles and Practice of Ophthalmology. Philadelphia: Saunders; 2000:2577–2595

2. Johnson M. What controls aqueous humour outflow resistance? Exp Eye Res 2006;82:545–557

3. Rosenquist R, Epstein D, Melamed S, Johnson M, Grant WM. Outflow resistance of enucleated human eyes at two different perfusion pressures and different extents of trabeculotomy. Curr Eye Res 1989;8:1233–1240

4. Mäepea O, Bill A. The pressures in the episcleral veins, Schlemm's canal and the trabecular meshwork in monkeys: effects of changes in intraocular pressure. Exp Eye Res 1989;49:645–663

5. Mäepea O, Bill A. Pressures in the juxtacanalicular tissue and Schlemm's canal in monkeys. Exp Eye Res 1992;54:879–883

6. Grant WM. Further studies on facility of flow through the trabecular meshwork. AMA Arch Opthalmol 1958;60(4 Part 1):523–533

7. Grant WM. Experimental aqueous perfusion in enucleated human eyes. Arch Ophthalmol 1963;69:783–801

8. Ellingsen BA, Grant WM. Trabeculotomy and sinusotomy in enucleated human eyes. Invest Ophthalmol 1972;11:21–28

9. Van Buskirk EM, Grant WM. Lens depression and aqueous outflow in enucleated primate eyes. Am J Ophthalmol 1973;76:632–640

10. Peterson WS, Jocson VL. Hyaluronidase effects on aqueous outflow resistance. Quantitative and localizing studies in the rhesus monkey eye. Am J Ophthalmol 1974;77:573–577

11. Van Buskirk EM. Trabeculotomy in the immature, enucleated human eye. Invest Ophthalmol Vis Sci 1977;16:63–66

12. Schuman JS, Chang W, Wang N, de Kater AW, Allingham RR. Excimer laser effects on outflow facility and outflow pathway morphology. Invest Ophthalmol Vis Sci 1999;40:1676–1680

13. deKater A, Shahsafaei A, Epstein D. Localization of smooth muscle and nonmuscle actin isoforms in the human aqueous outflow pathway. Invest Ophthalmol Vis Sci 1992;33:424–429

14. Johnson MC, Kamm RD. The role of Schlemm's canal in aqueous outflow from the human eye. Invest Ophthalmol Vis Sci 1983;24:320–325

5 Segmental Aqueous Outflow and Trabecular Bypass

Alex Huang

Aqueous humor is produced at the ciliary processes, moves into the anterior chamber, passes through the trabecular meshwork (TM) into Schlemm's canal (SC), and then into collector channels, intrascleral venous plexuses, and finally the aqueous and episcleral veins, where it joins the systemic venous circulation.[1–3] This two-dimensional perspective of conventional outflow pathway organization gives the impression that aqueous outflow occurs uniformly around the circumference of SC and then radially away from the limbus, but this is not necessarily the case. The introduction of minimally invasive glaucoma surgery (MIGS) to bypass discrete regions of the TM has made it important and clinically relevant to better characterize the nature of segmental aqueous outflow, during which the outflow rate through different regions of the conventional pathway and around the circumference of the eye may vary.

Segmental outflow has been described in different species and by different methods. Introduction of labeled microbead tracers into the anterior chamber has shown segmental outflow through the TM in species such as rodents, cows, and humans.[4–12] It suggests the presence of high-flow and low-flow regions in the TM attributable to the influence of extracellular matrix components such as proteoglycans and their regulators.[10,11] Even outflow across Schlemm's endothelium may be segmental and influenced by Rho-kinase inhibition.[12] A unifying funneling theory has been proposed to explain the dynamics of segmental outflow through TM and SC regions.[13] However, recall that the molecular weight of water is different from that of microbeads, with the latter likely utilizing different cellular mechanisms to facilitate phagocytic transcellular or paracellular movement. Although it is not clear how closely the path of microbead outflow mimics that of water or aqueous humor, it does indicate that segmental passage through the TM is possible.

To study post-TM pathways, canalography and channelography have been performed in real time following injection of tracers through a cannula inserted into SC during human glaucoma surgery.[14–16] Although the delivery of tracers under pressure and the access route used by these techniques may not be physiological, they nevertheless reveal an outflow path from SC onward that agrees with our morphological understanding of the conventional outflow route distal to TM.

Ideally, to capture physiologically relevant segmental outflow, outflow imaging should be performed live, in real time, and at relatively physiological perfusion pressures. Visualization of the aqueous outflow tract around the eye's limbal circumference should be possible, and findings should reflect outflow behavior in the whole conventional outflow tract from anterior chamber to episcleral veins.

We are developing aqueous angiography as a novel real-time outflow imaging method.[17] The method is based on general principles of retinal intravenous angiography, wherein fluorescein (or other tracer agents) is introduced into the peripheral veins to study retinal and choroidal blood flow. In aqueous angiography, 2.5% fluorescein (as described by the American Academy of Ophthalmology for capsular staining during cataract surgery[18]) is introduced intracamerally at physiological pressures. Aqueous angiography in an enucleated pig (**Fig. 5.1**) and in cow and human eyes demonstrates regions of positive and negative signal, reflecting segmental aqueous outflow in these models. The fluorescein route traversed encompasses the whole conventional outflow tract, including the TM. We are using this technique to determine relative outflow rates around the circumference of the eye ex vivo and in vivo, and the technique may have potential for human translation.

The MIGS trabecular bypass stents are typically placed nasally during surgery, but it is not clear if this approach best exploits segmental outflow in each eye, as the distribution and organization of distal outflow structures and the nature of flow in different parts of the system may vary from eye to eye, possibly explaining the variable success reported of the trabecular bypass procedures. It may be that customizing bypass location to suit segmental outflow features of each eye will enhance the success of these surgeries.

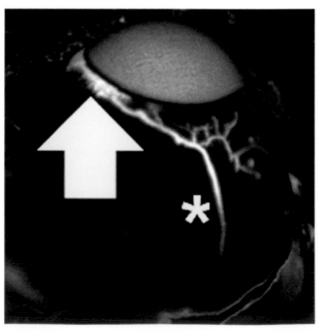

Fig. 5.1 Aqueous angiography in a pig eye, in which segmental outflow *(arrow)* is seen in the limbal region where collector channels reside leading distally to an episcleral vein *(asterisk)*. Fluorescence imaging was performed with the Heidelberg Spectralis.

Financial Disclosure

Alex Huang receives financial support in the form of research materials from Glaukos Corporation and Heidelberg Engineering.

References

1. Johnson M. What controls aqueous humour outflow resistance? Exp Eye Res 2006;82:545–557

2. Swaminathan SS, Oh DJ, Kang MH, Rhee DJ. Aqueous outflow: segmental and distal flow. J Cataract Refract Surg 2014;40:1263–1272

3. Ashton N. Anatomical study of Schlemm's canal and aqueous veins by means of neoprene casts. Part I. Aqueous veins. Br J Ophthalmol 1951;35:291–303

4. Chang JY, Folz SJ, Laryea SN, Overby DR. Multi-scale analysis of segmental outflow patterns in human trabecular meshwork with changing intraocular pressure. J Ocul Pharmacol Ther 2014;30:213–223

5. Battista SA, Lu Z, Hofmann S, Freddo T, Overby DR, Gong H. Reduction of the available area for aqueous humor outflow and increase in meshwork herniations into collector channels following acute IOP elevation in bovine eyes. Invest Ophthalmol Vis Sci 2008;49:5346–5352

6. Swaminathan SS, Oh DJ, Kang MH, et al. Secreted protein acidic and rich in cysteine (SPARC)-null mice exhibit more uniform outflow. Invest Ophthalmol Vis Sci 2013;54:2035–2047

7. Ethier CR, Chan DW. Cationic ferritin changes outflow facility in human eyes whereas anionic ferritin does not. Invest Ophthalmol Vis Sci 2001;42:1795–1802

8. Lu Z, Overby DR, Scott PA, Freddo TF, Gong H. The mechanism of increasing outflow facility by rho-kinase inhibition with Y-27632 in bovine eyes. Exp Eye Res 2008;86:271–281

9. Gong H, Francis A. Schlemm's canal and collector channels as therapeutic targets. In: Samples JR, Ahmed I, eds. Surgical Innovations in Glaucoma. New York: Springer; 2014

10. Vranka JA, Bradley JM, Yang YF, Keller KE, Acott TS. Mapping molecular differences and extracellular matrix gene expression in segmental outflow pathways of the human ocular trabecular meshwork. PLoS ONE 2015;10:e0122483

11. Keller KE, Bradley JM, Vranka JA, Acott TS. Segmental versican expression in the trabecular meshwork and involvement in outflow facility. Invest Ophthalmol Vis Sci 2011;52:5049–5057

12. Sabanay I, Gabelt BT, Tian B, Kaufman PL, Geiger B. H-7 effects on the structure and fluid conductance of monkey trabecular meshwork. Arch Ophthalmol 2000;118:955–962

13. Overby DR, Stamer WD, Johnson M. The changing paradigm of outflow resistance generation: towards synergistic models of the JCT and inner wall endothelium. Exp Eye Res 2009;88:656–670

14. Aktas Z, Tian B, McDonald J, et al. Application of canaloplasty in glaucoma gene therapy: where are we? J Ocul Pharmacol Ther 2014;30:277–282

15. Grieshaber MC, Pienaar A, Olivier J, Stegmann R. Clinical evaluation of the aqueous outflow system in primary open-angle glaucoma for canaloplasty. Invest Ophthalmol Vis Sci 2010;51:1498–1504

16. Grieshaber MC. Ab externo Schlemm's canal surgery: viscocanalostomy and canaloplasty. Dev Ophthalmol 2012;50:109–124

17. Saraswathy S, Tan JCH, Francis BA, Hinton DR, Weinreb RN, Huang AS. Aqueous angiography: a real-time, physiologic, and comprehensive aqueous humor outflow imaging technique. Manuscript in submission

18. Jacobs DS, Cox TA, Wagoner MD, Ariyasu RG, Karp CL; American Academy of Ophthalmology; Ophthalmic Technology Assessment Committee Anterior Segment Panel. Capsule staining as an adjunct to cataract surgery: a report from the American Academy of Ophthalmology. Ophthalmology 2006;113:707–713

6 Pulsatile Aqueous Outflow Observations to Guide Glaucoma Surgery

Murray Johnstone

Acqueous outflow is pulsatile, and clinicians can see the pulsations. This simple and well-accepted insight[1,2] provides clinicians with a wealth of information to use in surgical management.[3–5] This information includes direct surveillance of mechanisms controlling aqueous outflow,[6] outflow abnormalities in glaucoma,[3,7] surgical technique decisions,[8] and the effects of outflow surgery.[9] Powerful clinical tools to take advantage of these insights are within immediate reach of every surgeon, and include a slit lamp, careful observation, and patience.[4,5] Pulsatile aqueous outflow provides important clues to the functional properties of the outflow system, and its health along the entire outflow pathway from the trabecular meshwork (TM) to the episcleral veins (**Fig. 6.1**).

Pulsatile Flow Origin and Implications

Pulsatile aqueous outflow synchronous with the ocular pulse[10,11] originates in Schlemm's canal (SC; **Fig. 6.1a**).[5] Such pulsatility has clearly defined requirements[12,13]: (1) a reservoir or chamber represented by SC; (2) deforming tissue represented by the TM to change reservoir dimensions; and (3) oscillatory compressive forces represented by the ocular pulse (**Fig. 6.1a**), blinking, and eye movement, each creating a pulse that deforms the trabecular tissue.

The clinical signs of pulsatile outflow indicate that the TM has sufficient elasticity and compliance to deform[14–16] and to change the SC reservoir dimensions[17]; the collector channels are able to open[18]; the intrascleral channels are patent; and both the anterior chamber (AC) and SC pressures are in a delicately poised equilibrium with the episcleral venous pressure (EVP).

In glaucoma patients, pulsatile outflow is harder to see, and in advanced glaucoma it may be absent, likely due to loss of trabecular tissue elasticity.[7] This loss is associated with pathologically reduced outflow. In this scenario, the intraocular pressure (IOP) becomes more variable as the TM responds less and less effectively to the hemodynamic forces driving pulsatile outflow.

Normally, pulsatile outflow is segmental, seen in some regions of the ocular circumference but not in others. The location of segmental pulsatile flow remains unchanged for an individual, probably for a lifetime.[3] In eyes with glaucoma, retention of pulsatile features in these regions suggests function at these aqueous vein locations is only partially compromised and it is possible that these pulsatile segments lend themselves to being exploited by minimally invasive trabecular bypass surgery. In contrast, absence of pulsatile flow in these locations suggests minimally invasive glaucoma surgery (MIGS) may be less likely to succeed.

How Do We Find Aqueous Veins?

The distribution of aqueous veins is highly asymmetric, with 87% seen in the inferior quadrants, of which 58% lie in the inferior nasal quadrant at or below the midline (**Fig. 6.2**).[4,19] Typically only one to three aqueous veins are present in an eye, a finding that should not be surprising because the average aqueous vein has a flow volume of ~ 1 µL/min. The volume of flow per aqueous vein may explain why just two aqueous veins are needed to cope with trabecular outflow.[5,20] Aqueous veins at times carry primarily aqueous humor (*1–3* in **Fig. 6.1b**) making them almost transparent; at other times aqueous veins carry primarily blood (*4,5* in **Fig. 6.1b**), making them look red (**Fig. 6.3**); either condition can make the aqueous veins difficult to recognize.[4]

A great aid in determining the presence and distribution of aqueous veins is to apply very gentle pressure through the lower lid to transiently and slightly raise the IOP. Often, a bolus of aqueous will then be seen entering a vessel previously containing solely blood (*4,5* in **Fig. 6.1b** and **Fig. 6.3**). In a quick dynamic response, blood rapidly refills the aqueous vein within seconds. The rapid transition from blood-filled to an aqueous-filled lumen and back again to a blood-filled lumen signals that the vessel is an aqueous vein.

In a vessel containing primarily aqueous humor (*1–3* in **Fig. 6.1b**), the previously mentioned exertion of gentle pressure forces a little aqueous humor through the TM, into the venous collector system, and out of the eye, reducing the IOP transiently. When IOP falls below the homeostatic set point,[7] aqueous humor no longer flows into the aqueous vein; instead blood fills the previously clear aqueous vein. Within a few seconds, however, the IOP rises again to the homeostatic set point, restoring a pressure gradient and driving aqueous outflow into the aqueous veins. Aqueous humor then enters and displaces blood in the aqueous vein.

Once the aqueous veins are identified (**Fig. 6.3**), the many manifestations of pulsatile aqueous outflow are readily observed, including intermittent boluses of blood from tributary veins, pulsatile laminar flow, and trilaminar flow (**Figs. 6.1** and **6.3**).

Surgical Value

Clues from observing outflow clinically may have predictive value that can be used in the operating room to position minimally invasive bypass surgical devices at segments in which the distal outflow system exhibits relatively physiological behavior.[8] It is postulated that enhancing outflow in these segments makes trabecular bypass procedures more effective.

Observing fluid enter the aqueous veins by pressuring the eye right after inserting a trabecular bypass device ensures that a

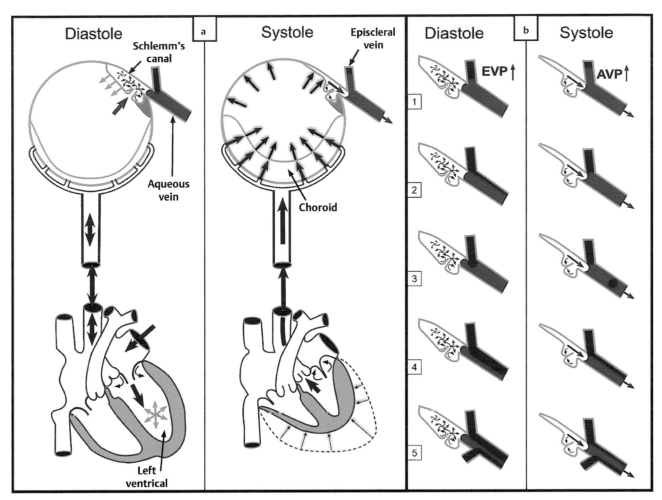

Fig. 6.1 **(a)** *Right panel*: source of pulsatile aqueous flow. Choroidal vasculature expansion during systole causes a transient intraocular pressure (IOP) increase that distends the trabecular meshwork (TM; *green diaphragm*) forcing it outward into Schlemm's canal (SC) to create a pulsatile wave of aqueous that enters the aqueous humor–filled *(navy blue)* aqueous vein. **(a)** *Left panel:* the IOP drops in diastole, as indicated by *double-headed arrows*. The TM recoils, reducing pressure in SC, allowing aqueous humor in the anterior chamber (AC) to enter SC. **(b)** (*Left* and *right*) Scenarios showing different appearances *(1–5)* of a pulsatile wave of aqueous humor *(navy blue)* during diastole *(left)* and systole *(right)*. **(b)** *Left panel*: during diastole episcleral venous pressure (EVP) is slightly higher than aqueous vein pressure (AVP), resulting in a relatively increased EVP (EVP↑). EVP↑ causes blood *(red)* from a tributary episcleral vein to move toward its branch point with the aqueous vein *(1)* or into the aqueous mixing vein *(2–5)*. **(b)** *Right panel*: during systole, AVP is relatively high (AVP↑). AVP↑ causes transient aqueous movement *(navy blue)* toward a tributary episcleral vein *(1)*; transient elimination of a lamina of blood *(2; red)*; sweeping of a bolus of blood into the aqueous stream *(3)*; an oscillating increase in the diameter of the aqueous component of a persistent aqueous lamina *(4)*; or an oscillating trilaminar aqueous flow wave where an aqueous vein joins two episcleral veins *(5)*.

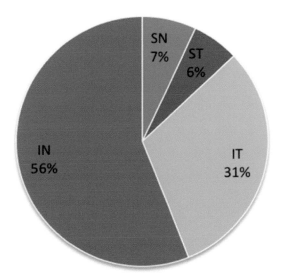

Fig. 6.2 Frequency distribution of aqueous veins in each eye quadrant: superior nasal (SN), superior temporal (ST), inferior temporal (IT), and inferior nasal (IN). (Modified from De Vries S. De Zichtbare Afvoer Van Het Kamerwater. Amsterdam: Dukkerij Kinsbergen; 1947: 90.)

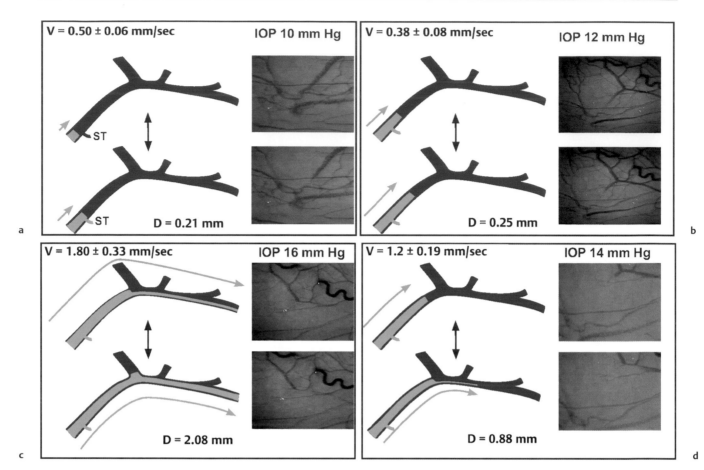

Fig. 6.3 Sequential images illustrating pulsatile aqueous humor outflow in the aqueous veins in response to IOP changes after a H_2O drinking test in a 59-year-old man. As IOP increases, [add comma] the length of a column of aqueous humor in an aqueous vein increases as the aqueous humor advances, along with mixing occurring in the vein previously containing blood. In addition, the oscillations with each pulse wave increase, resulting in a larger volume of aqueous humor (an increased stroke volume [V]) entering the vein during each systole. This same type of increase in stroke volume occurs after the introduction of outflow medications, resulting in an increase in total outflow that precedes pressure reduction. **(a)** Baseline IOP is 10 mm Hg. Aqueous humor column elongation (*D*) demonstrates that the distance traveled of the aqueous wave front along the aqueous vein in systole is small. A standing transverse wave oscillates, resulting in discharge of aqueous into a small venous tributary (ST) in systole only. **(b)** At a higher IOP of 12 mm Hg, an increased pulse wave results in greater aqueous column elongation in systole. The aqueous column moves further away (distally) from the aqueous vein's scleral exit point. The venous tributary (ST) is now filled in both diastole and systole. **(c)** At an IOP of 14 mm Hg, aqueous pulse wave velocity and column elongation increase yet further during systole. **(d)** The trend continues as the IOP increases further to 16 mm Hg.

direct connection with the venous system has been established[9]; observing late postoperative aqueous outflow into an aqueous vein in the same area provides assurance that the procedure has had an intended and enduring effect.

References

1. Ascher KW. Aqueous veins. Am J Ophth 1942;25:31–38

2. Goldmann H. Abfluss des Kammerwassers beim Menschen. Ophthalmologica 1946;111:146–152

3. Ascher KW. The Aqueous Veins: Biomicroscopic Study of the Aqueous Humor Elimination. Springfield, IL: Charles C. Thomas; 1961:251

4. Johnstone M, Jamil A, Martin E. Aqueous veins and open angle glaucoma. In: Schacknow PN, Samples JR, eds. The Glaucoma Book. New York: Springer; 2010:65–78

5. Johnstone M, Martin E, Jamil A. Pulsatile flow into the aqueous veins: manifestations in normal and glaucomatous eyes. Exp Eye Res 2011;92: 318–327

6. Johnstone MA. The aqueous outflow system as a mechanical pump: evidence from examination of tissue and aqueous movement in human and non-human primates. J Glaucoma 2004;13:421–438

7. Johnstone MA. A new model describes an aqueous outflow pump and explores causes of pump failure in glaucoma. In: Grehn H, Stamper R, eds. Essentials in Ophthalmology: Glaucoma II. Heidelberg: Springer; 2006

8. Saheb H, Ahmed II. Micro-invasive glaucoma surgery: current perspectives and future directions. Curr Opin Ophthalmol 2012;23:96–104

9. Fellman RL, Grover DS. Episcleral venous fluid wave: intraoperative evidence for patency of the conventional outflow system. J Glaucoma 2014;23:347–350

10. Coleman DJ, Trokel S. Direct-recorded intraocular pressure variations in a human subject. Arch Ophthalmol 1969;82:637–640

11. Phillips CI, Tsukahara S, Hosaka O, Adams W. Ocular pulsation correlates with ocular tension: the choroid as piston for an aqueous pump? Ophthalmic Res 1992;24:338–343

12. LaBarbera M, Vogel S. The design of fluid transport systems in organisms. Am Sci 1982;70:54–60

13. Zamir M, Ritman E. The Physics of Pulsatile Flow. Biological Physics Series. New York: AIP Press, Springer-Verlag; 2000:174

14. Johnstone MA, Grant WG. Pressure-dependent changes in structures of the aqueous outflow system of human and monkey eyes. Am J Ophthalmol 1973;75:365–383

15. Li P, Reif R, Zhi Z, et al. Phase-sensitive optical coherence tomography characterization of pulse-induced trabecular meshwork displacement in ex vivo nonhuman primate eyes. J Biomed Opt 2012;17:076026

16. Li P, Shen TT, Johnstone M, Wang RK. Pulsatile motion of the trabecular meshwork in healthy human subjects quantified by phase-sensitive optical coherence tomography. Biomed Opt Express 2013;4:2051–2065

17. Johnstone MA. Intraocular pressure regulation: findings of pulse-dependent trabecular meshwork motion lead to unifying concepts of intraocular pressure homeostasis. J Ocul Pharmacol Ther 2014;30:88–93

18. Hariri S, Johnstone M, Jiang Y, et al. Platform to investigate aqueous outflow system structure and pressure-dependent motion using high-resolution spectral domain optical coherence tomography. J Biomed Opt 2014;19:106013

19. De Vries S. De Zichtbare Afvoer Van Het Kamerwater. Amsterdam: Dukkerij Kinsbergen; 1947

20. Stepanik J. Measuring velocity of flow in aqueous veins. Am J Ophthalmol 1954;37:918–922

7 The Effect of Ultrasound on Aqueous Dynamics

Donald Schwartz

Ultrasound has several beneficial attributes that are potentially useful in medical treatment. Most ophthalmologists are familiar with phacoemulsification, whereby ultrasound is used to create cavitation and destroy lens nucleus material. Besides its vibrational effect, ultrasound has other noteworthy effects. Ultrasound has an associated thermal effect, which as cataract surgeons are aware, must be mitigated with constant irrigation. Another possible effect found with low-frequency ultrasound is the ability to trigger intracellular activities through a stretch effect within the trabecular meshwork (TM).[1]

The use of ultrasound as a treatment for glaucoma began with the work of Jackson Coleman's group at Cornell.[2,3] His device became commercialized in the 1980s as one of the first uses of ultrasound in medicine, known as the Sonocare Therapeutic Ultrasound System (Sonocare, Ridgewood, NJ). This method of treatment used high-intensity focused ultrasound (HIFU). The ultrasound was focused on the ciliary body to decrease the production of aqueous by thermal destruction of ciliary body processes. Later, it was thought that there might be an additional effect on outflow due to thinning of the scleral wall. Comorbidities of intractable uveitis, scleral wall thinning, and even phthisis resulted in the abandonment of this device.

More recently, EyeTechCare of Lyon, France, developed a more refined device to decrease aqueous production using HIFU.[4] This device (EyeOP1) offers a more precise technique to ablate the ciliary body to treat intransigent glaucoma. It has a circular attachment ring with six piezoelectric precisely aimed transducers to titrate the amount of tissue treated, thereby decreasing the potential for significant adverse effects.

The use of a nonfocused ultrasound for its vibrational effects in clearing trabecular meshwork debris was proposed and tested by Bjorn Svedbergh in Sweden in the 1990s with some limited and temporary effect on intraocular pressure (IOP).[5] A mechanical oscillatory device, Deep Wave Trabeculoplasty (DWP), is being developed to use a sonic (non-ultrasound) frequency applied externally to stretch the trabecular meshwork.[6] It is in early studies.

Beginning in 2006, I began developing a low-power, low-frequency, focused ultrasound device to lower the IOP[7,8] **(Fig. 7.1)**. This Therapeutic Ultrasound for Glaucoma (TUG; EyeSonix, Long Beach, CA) device is designed to yield a combined vibrational and mild, controlled hyperthermic effect within the trabecular meshwork. The induced hyperthermia would be mild and less than 45°C; above this temperature, tissue thermal damage and pain occur,[9] but just below it, only a mild inflammatory response occurs. It was thought that the cytokine cascade arising by this mild thermally induced inflammation lowers the IOP,[10–12] as might also occur after phacoemulsification surgery.[13–17]

This application has been developed to enhance the outflow of aqueous humor and lower the IOP in mild to moderate open-angle glaucoma **(Fig. 7.2)**. Early clinical studies in human patients showed at least 20% IOP lowering in over 80% of those treated.[7] This included patients with insufficiently controlled IOP by medicines, in whom the therapeutic effect lasted at least 6 months. Examinations of over 80 treated patients have revealed scant side effects, with the most common being a post-treatment inflammatory reaction on day 1 similar to that seen after selective laser trabeculoplasty (SLT). Here, mild ocular irritation typically accompanies moderate conjunctival injection and rare mild anterior chamber flare without cells on slit-lamp examination.[18]

Although originally thought to enhance outflow solely by its thermal effect on trabecular meshwork microanatomy,[8] as was believed with argon laser trabeculoplasty (ALT),[19,20] recent studies indicate ultrasonically induced IOP lowering occurs by mechanisms similar to SLT (and probably its predecessor, ALT), namely by the triggering of a cytokine cascade.[21] This cytokine cascade may lower IOP by increasing matrix metalloproteinases, inducing macrophage activity, and altering intercellular connections in the juxtacanalicular meshwork.[22–25] It may be that common cytokine pathways mediate the IOP lowering of TUG ultrasound and SLT therapies for glaucoma.

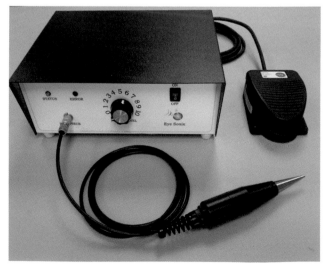

Fig. 7.1 Working Therapeutic Ultrasound for Glaucoma (TUG) prototype.

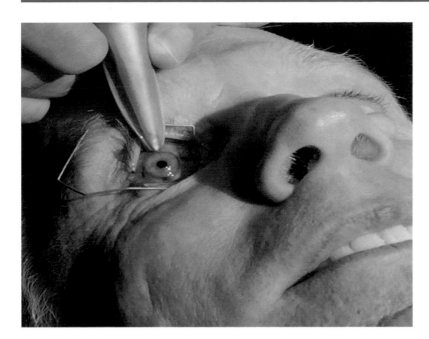

Fig. 7.2 Treatment with the TUG device at the limbus.

Disclosure

Donald Schwartz is the founder and owner of EyeSonix

References

1. Wang N, Chintala SK, Fini ME, Schuman JS. Ultrasound activates the TM ELAM-1/IL-1/NF-kappaB response: a potential mechanism for intraocular pressure reduction after phacoemulsification. Invest Ophthalmol Vis Sci 2003;44:1977–1981

2. Silverman RH, Vogelsang B, Rondeau MJ, Coleman DJ. Therapeutic ultrasound for the treatment of glaucoma. Am J Ophthalmol 1991;111:327–337 Erratum in: Am J Ophthalmol 1991;112:105

3. Valtot F, Kopel J, Haut J. Treatment of glaucoma with high intensity focused ultrasound. Int Ophthalmol 1989;13:167–170

4. Aptel F, Charrel T, Lafon C, et al. Miniaturized high-intensity focused ultrasound device in patients with glaucoma: a clinical pilot study. Invest Ophthalmol Vis Sci 2011;52:8747–8753

5. Svedbergh B, personal communication

6. Ocutherix. www.ocutherix.com. Accessed January 23, 2015

7. Schwartz D, Samples J, Korosteleva O. Therapeutic ultrasound for glaucoma: clinical use of a low frequency, low power ultrasound for lowering intraocular pressure. J Ther Ultrasound 2014;2:15

8. Samples JR, Ahmed IIK, eds. Surgical Innovations in Glaucoma. New York: Springer; 2014:227

9. Roti Roti JL. Cellular responses to hyperthermia (40-46 degrees C): cell killing and molecular events. Int J Hyperthermia 2008;24:3–15

10. Haveman J, Geerdink AG, Rodermond HM. Cytokine production after whole body and localized hyperthermia. Int J Hyperthermia 1996;12:791–800

11. Katschinski DM, Wiedemann GJ, Longo W, d'Oleire FR, Spriggs D, Robins HI. Whole body hyperthermia cytokine induction: a review, and unifying hypothesis for myeloprotection in the setting of cytotoxic therapy. Cytokine Growth Factor Rev 1999;10:93–97

12. Robins HI, Kutz M, Wiedemann GJ, et al. Cytokine induction by 41.8 degrees C whole body hyperthermia. Cancer Lett 1995;97:195–201

13. Poley BJ, Lindstrom RL, Samuelson TW. Long-term effects of phacoemulsification with intraocular lens implantation in normotensive and ocular hypertensive eyes. J Cataract Refract Surg 2008;34:735–742

14. Bowling B, Calladine D. Routine reduction of glaucoma medication following phacoemulsification. J Cataract Refract Surg 2009;35:406–407, author reply 407

15. Shingleton BJ, Laul A, Nagao K, et al. Effect of phacoemulsification on intraocular pressure in eyes with pseudoexfoliation: single-surgeon series. J Cataract Refract Surg 2008;34:1834–1841

16. Pohjalainen T, Vesti E, Uusitalo RJ, Laatikainen L. Phacoemulsification and intraocular lens implantation in eyes with open-angle glaucoma. Acta Ophthalmol Scand 2001;79:313–316

17. Mierzejewski A, Eliks I, Kałuzny B, Zygulska M, Harasimowicz B, Kałuzny JJ. Cataract phacoemulsification and intraocular pressure in glaucoma patients. Klin Oczna 2008;110:11–17

18. Schwartz D. Therapeutic Ultrasound for Glaucoma. Presented at the Glaucoma Research Foundation, Glaucoma 360, San Francisco, February 2015

19. Worthen DM, Wickham MG. Argon laser trabeculotomy. Trans Am Acad Ophthalmol Otolaryngol 1974;78:OP371–OP375

20. Wise JB, Witter SL. Argon laser therapy for open-angle glaucoma. A pilot study. Arch Ophthalmol 1979;97:319–322

21. Kelley M. Personal communication on TNF triggering by TUG device in porcine eyes

22. Bradley JM, Anderssohn AM, Colvis CM, et al. Mediation of laser trabeculoplasty-induced matrix metalloproteinase expression by IL-1beta and TNFalpha. Invest Ophthalmol Vis Sci 2000;41:422–430

23. Alvarado JA, Alvarado RG, Yeh RF, Franse-Carman L, Marcellino GR, Brownstein MJ. A new insight into the cellular regulation of aqueous outflow: how trabecular meshwork endothelial cells drive a mechanism that regulates the permeability of Schlemm's canal endothelial cells. Br J Ophthalmol 2005;89:1500–1505

24. Zhang X, Schroeder A, Callahan EM, et al. Constitutive signalling pathway activity in trabecular meshwork cells from glaucomatous eyes. Exp Eye Res 2006;82:968–973

25. Wang N, Chintala SK, Fini ME, Schuman JS. Activation of a tissue-specific stress response in the aqueous outflow pathway of the eye defines the glaucoma disease phenotype. Nat Med 2001;7:304–309

8 Sonic Effect on Aqueous Outflow

Malik Y. Kahook

The treatment of glaucoma typically follows the same sequence of topical drops, followed by laser trabeculoplasty (LT) and incisional surgery. There are advantages and disadvantages to each of these approaches. Topical therapy is very safe but patients demonstrate poor adherence. More invasive approaches, such as trabeculectomy and glaucoma drainage device implantation, are more effective at lowering the intraocular pressure (IOP) but entail a higher rate of complications. LT, often used as a bridge treatment between medication and invasive therapy, has been shown to be moderately effective and safe. However, the IOP lowering that results post-LT wanes over time, and repeat treatments are not as effective as the primary therapy. In an effort to enhance adherence and IOP lowering outcomes, there have been multiple attempts to innovate new treatment modalities that can bridge the gap between using topical drops and the more invasive therapies while also allowing for repeatable treatments over the lifetime of the patient.

Deep wave trabeculoplasty (DWT) is an investigational therapy intended to reduce IOP in patients with open-angle glaucoma and ocular hypertension. The DWT device **(Fig. 8.1)** applies focal mechanical oscillation (low amplitude, sonic frequency) to the surface of the eye proximate to the limbal region and ante-

rior to the trabecular meshwork (TM). In healthy eyes, IOP homeostasis is in part regulated by a pressure-induced stretch of conventional outflow cells, resulting in release of adenosine triphosphate (ATP) and downstream effects on TM cell contractility, extracellular matrix turnover, and the barrier function of Schlemm's canal. External scleral deflection with the DWT device is thought to stretch conventional outflow tissues, triggering ATP release and signaling cascades that increase outflow facility and lower IOP. Preclinical studies **(Table 8.1** and **Fig. 8.2)** and a first-in-human study have demonstrated that DWT has a very favorable safety and efficacy profile.

In a first-in-humans clinical trial, 30 patients with primary open-angle glaucoma (baseline washed-out IOP of 22 to 36) were enrolled and followed for 3 months. In each subject, one eye was randomized to DWT treatment (single unilateral treatment) and the fellow eye served as control. Medication was washed out for 1 month prior to treatment. At follow-up visits, rescue medical therapy for elevated IOP could be administered in either eye at the discretion of the investigator. Prior to treatment and at all follow-up visits, IOP was measured, and routine slit-lamp exams were performed. The treated eyes had a statistically significant reduction of IOP at each of the follow-up visits compared with

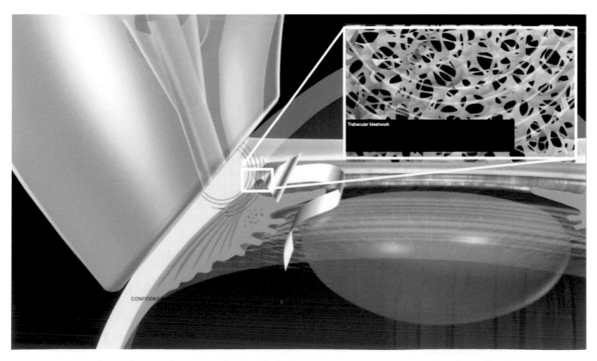

Fig. 8.1   The deep wave trabeculoplasty oscillating tip is placed at the limbus proximate to the underlying trabecular meshwork.

Table 8.1 Results of a 1-Month Study of Intraocular Pressure (IOP) Reduction in Brown Norway Rats in One Eye, with the Contralateral Eye Serving as Control[1]

	Study	Control
Rat A	(27, 26, 24, 22)	(28, 28, 27, 29)
Rat B	(28, 26, 25, 21)	(29, 30, 29, 29)
Rat C	(27, 24, 23, 23)	(27, 27, 28, 27)
Rat D	(28, 27, 25, 22)	(29, 29, 27, 28)
Rat E	(29, 26, 26, 20)	(30, 28, 28, 27)
Rat F	(27, 26, 25, 22)	(26, 27, 27, 28)
Rat G	(30, 29, 27, 23)	(29, 29, 28, 29)
Rat H	(31, 30, 28, 21)	(26, 26, 27, 28)
Rat J	(27, 26, 27, 20)	(26, 25, 25, 26)

Overall treatment eyes:
Baseline (BL): 28.22 ± 1.48   after 2 months: 26.67 ± 1.80   after 15 months: 25.56 ± 1.59   after 1 week: 21.56 ± 1.13
Overall control eyes:
BL: 27.78 ± 1.47   after 2 months: 27.67 ± 1.49   after 15 months: 27.33 ± 1.05   after 1 week: 27.89 ± 0.99

Treated eyes:	$p = 0.06$ BL vs 2 months	$p = 0.002$ BL vs 15 months	$p < 0.001$ BL vs 1 week
Control eyes:	$p = 0.88$ BL vs 2 months	$p = 0.47$ BL vs 15 months	$p = 0.85$ BL vs 1 week

1. Intraocular pressure is measured in mmHg.

baseline, with a mean IOP reduction of 26% at the 3-month visit **(Fig. 8.3)**. Dependence on medication also decreased significantly from a mean baseline of two medications to mean of 0.6 medications at last follow-up. The control eyes required restarting of medications at a higher rate and earlier timeline due to the lack of IOP control. These results illustrate the IOP-lowering and medication-reducing capabilities of this treatment modality. However, longer follow-up and a head-to-head trial compared with an active control (such as laser trabeculoplasty) are needed to reach definitive conclusions.

Compared with LT, minimally invasive glaucoma surgery (MIGS), and traditional glaucoma surgery, DWT is less invasive, results in no permanent tissue damage, and preserves the possibility of using other treatment options. Compared with drugs, DWT eliminates compliance issues, reduces the number of medications required, and defers more invasive surgery. Because of its promising safety and efficacy profile, and because of its noninvasive nature, DWT has promise as a viable second-line treatment option after drugs and before more invasive glaucoma procedures. If long-term safety, efficacy, and repeatability can be

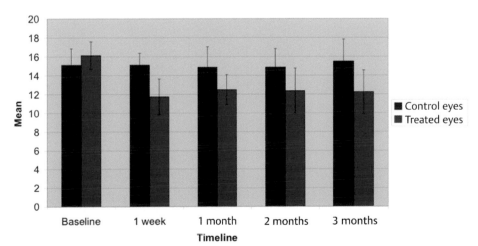

Fig. 8.2 A 3-month study in New Zealand white rabbits with treated eyes demonstrating a decrease in intraocular pressure (IOP) from 16.13 ± 1.46 mm Hg to 12.25 ± 2.31 mm Hg, representing a 3.88 mm Hg (24%) decrease in IOP. IOP in the untreated contralateral control eyes was not statistically different from baseline.

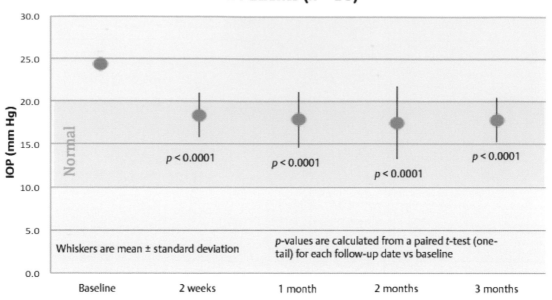

Fig. 8.3 Treated human eyes experienced a sustained decrease in IOP over 3 months.

demonstrated, DWT has promise as a first-line treatment alternative to topical medications. Further studies are underway and should shed light on how this novel treatment modality can benefit glaucoma patients in years to come.

Disclosure

Malik Y. Kahook is the inventor of, and holds two patents on, sonic therapy.

9   Structure and Mechanisms of Uveoscleral Outflow

Alex Huang and Robert N. Weinreb

Astute observations led to the notion that there were separate drainage routes for aqueous humor from the eye. First, it was noted that the episcleral venous hematocrit was lower than that of the peripheral venous hematocrit, leading to the idea that episcleral blood was either diluted by a fluid exiting the eye or that blood cells were being removed into the eye.[1] The dilutional theory eventually led to the discovery of the conventional trabecular outflow pathway—the first drainage route.[2] Anders Bill[3] then observed in 1965 that when radioactive albumin (^{125}I-labeled) was injected into the anterior chamber of macaque monkeys, 20% of the total radioactivity could not be recovered from the conventional pathway **(Fig. 9.1)**. Thus, a second drainage route had to exist, and the search for this mystery fraction led to the discovery of the uveoscleral outflow pathway. Today, this second drainage route, or uveoscleral outflow pathway, represents a major medical and possibly surgical therapeutic target for intraocular pressure (IOP) reduction to treat glaucoma.[4]

Species Differences, Direct Measurements, and Serendipity

Uveoscleral outflow is difficult to measure. The direct method to measure it uses tracers, such as radioactive proteins,[3,5,6] India ink,[7] and fluorescent dextrans.[8,9] A tracer is introduced into the eye, and the final tracer concentration is measured in the peripheral blood. Uveoscleral outflow is then calculated after correction for the peripheral distribution and the amount delivered into the anterior chamber.[6,10] The direct method is more easily accomplished in animals than in humans, although it has been performed in a small number of human eyes with intraocular tumors[11] prior to enucleation.

The direct method has been used to calculate uveoscleral outflow in a variety of animals **(Table 9.1)**. As a percentage of total outflow, some species demonstrate very little uveoscleral outflow (cat and rabbit), some demonstrate intermediate outflow (dog and human), and some demonstrate greater outflow (monkey). As such, it may have been fortuitous that Anders Bill chose to work first with monkeys.

Age Differences, Indirect Measurements, and Serendipity

To facilitate the measurement and study of uveoscleral outflow, indirect methods that are more feasible for human application have been developed. All indirect methods utilize the Goldmann equation with or without applying aqueous suppressants to calculate parameters of the aqueous dynamic.[12]

The simplest mathematical model of the basic Goldmann equation ($IOP = F_{in}(R) + EVP$)[13] predicts IOP as a function of aqueous humor production (F_{in}; μL/min), resistance of trabecular outflow (R; mm Hg * min/μL), and episcleral venous pressure (EVP; mm Hg), but it does not account for uveoscleral outflow. To account for uveoscleral outflow, a modified Goldmann equation can be formulated where the variable F of the basic equation is expanded to include uveoscleral outflow (F_u). Thus, the Goldmann equation is re-expressed as $IOP = (F_{in} - F_u)(R) + EVP$.[14]

Trabecular outflow is said to be pressure-dependent as it occurs down a pressure gradient (increased outflow with increased IOP), but uveoscleral outflow is considered to be pressure-independent, being little influenced by IOP in a typical physiological range. The pressure independence of uveoscleral outflow does not imply that this pathway is without resistance. Rather, the anatomy of the uveoscleral outflow pathway is such that resistance along this drainage route within the intraocular space is not influenced much by physiologically relevant IOPs so that uveoscleral outflow becomes better modeled by the F variable above.

With the modified Goldmann equation, one can calculate F_u after IOP is measured by applanation tonometry, F_{in} is calculated by fluorophotometry,[15] R is determined by Schiotz tonometry,[16] and EVP is estimated by manometry.[17] Of course, the limitation of this indirect method lies in the assumptions used to determine each of the parameters of the modified Goldmann equation, as all are estimated indirectly. Although the equation estimates uveoscleral outflow, particularly in humans, a critical observer is careful to acknowledge these limitations and potential sources of error when using indirect means to calculate uveoscleral outflow.

Uveoscleral outflow, as measured by direct and indirect methods, varies with age. Uveoscleral outflow determined in eyes with tumors in older people (54 and 65 years old)[11] was found to be quite low, but subsequent studies have found that uveoscleral outflow may be nearly 40% higher in younger than older people.[18] This agrees with Anders Bill's fortuitous original descriptions of uveoscleral outflow in young macaque monkeys[6] that were later confirmed in monkeys stratified by age.[19] The influence of age on uveoscleral outflow is relevant, as glaucoma is itself age related. Uveoscleral outflow may also be lower in glaucoma dogs[19] and ocular hypertensive humans.[20]

Anatomy of Uveoscleral Outflow

The term *uveoscleral*, which has grown out of the variety of methods used to define it, including Anders Bill's original descriptions, correctly reflects the nature of the pathway. Uveoscleral outflow occurs by bulk flow of aqueous humor through the ciliary muscle into the supraciliary space and then into the choroid and suprachoroidal clefts, subsequently leaving the eye via the perivascular spaces of the emissarial scleral channels or directly through permeable scleral collagen bundles **(Fig. 9.2)**.

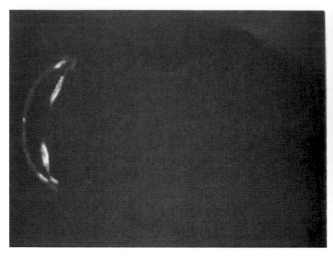
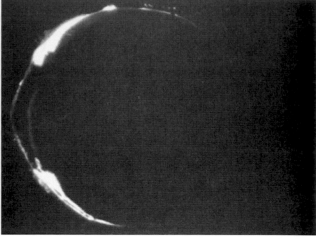

a

b

Fig. 9.1 Uveoscleral outflow in monkey autoradiograms demonstrate accumulation of radiolabeled tracer in the uveoscleral outflow pathway of cynomolgus monkey. **(a)** Pilocarpine treatment. **(b)** Atropine treatment.

(From Bill A. Effects of atropine and pilocarpine on aqueous humour dynamics in cynomolgus monkeys *(Macaca irus)*. Exp Eye Res 1967;6:120–125. Reprinted with permission from Elsevier.)

Various morphological considerations are important to mention. The monkey eye with greater uveoscleral outflow has a ciliary muscle that is well developed, supporting multiple functions with three different portions that are apparent as fibers running in different directions.[21,22] Contraction of the longitudinal muscle under parasympathetic control pulls the scleral spur and stretches the trabecular meshwork to increase trabecular outflow capacity. The circular muscle, also under parasympathetic control, contracts the diameter of the circular ciliary muscle ring to loosen tension on the zonules and allow accommodation according to the Helmholtz theory of accommodation.[23] While in a relaxed state, the intermuscular connective tissue of the monkey ciliary muscle is sparse with large spaces felt to permit bulk flow down the tract.[24] These spaces diminish with muscular contraction, and this may underlie the decrease in uveoscleral outflow seen with pilocarpine **(Fig. 9.1)**; see Contractile Regulators of Uveoscleral Outflow, below.[24] By comparison, although histological and electron microscopic studies of the rabbit ciliary muscle show large empty spaces similar to those in primates, frozen sections avoiding the use of organic solvents demonstrate large amounts of hyaluronan filling these spaces, possibly reflecting a barrier to uveoscleral outflow and explaining the monkey and rabbit difference **(Fig. 9.3)**.[25]

With increasing age, accommodative ability is diminished in primates, and the large intermuscular spaces in the ciliary muscle change. Large clumps of pigmented cells fill these spaces in monkeys **(Fig. 9.4)**.[26] In humans, increased connective tissue

deposition occurs, and the large intermuscular spaces seen in young ciliary muscle are lost **(Fig. 9.5)**.[21] In the distal portions of choroid and sclera, the electron density of the elastic fibers is increased, the choroidal elastin is diminished, and the collagen is more cross-linked and thicker, giving the impression of plate formation in the sclera.

Table 9.1 Species Differences in Uveoscleral Outflow

Species	Uveoscleral Outflow as Percentage of Total Outflow (%)	PMID Citation Number
Monkey	35–60	5001096[12]
Cat	3	2678147[13]
Rabbit	3–8	5982257[14] and 1559555[15]
Dog (beagle)	15	2578758[16]
Human	4–14	5130270[11]

Source: Modified from Alm A, Nilsson SF. Uveoscleral outflow–a review. Exp Eye Res 2009;88:760–768.

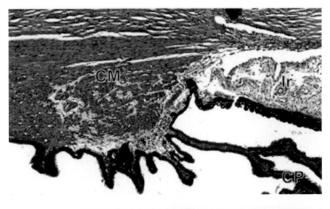

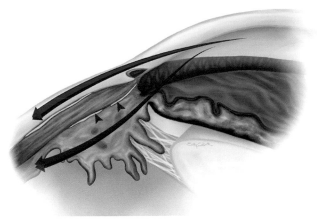

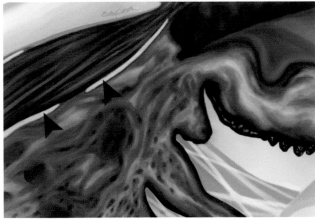

Fig. 9.2 Anatomy of anterior uveoscleral outflow. **(a)** Normal anatomy near the angle and ciliary body in a 34-year-old man (Masson stain.) CM, ciliary muscle; CP, ciliary process; Ir, iris. (From Alm A, Nilsson SF. Uveoscleral outflow—a review. Exp Eye Res 2009;88:760–768. Reprinted with permission from Elsevier). **(b)** Clefts within the ciliary muscles *(arrowheads)* support uveoscleral outflow. Illustration of normal anatomy. *Blue arrow* depicts conventional outflow, and *red arrow* depicts uveoscleral outflow. **(c)** Enlarged illustration of ciliary body with clefts *(arrowheads)*.

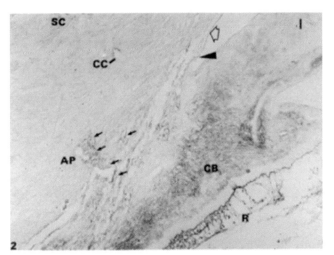

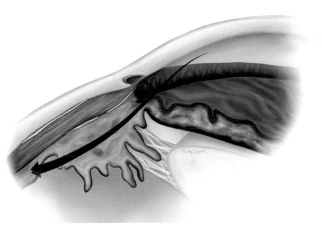

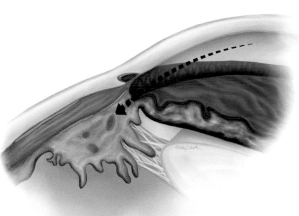

Fig. 9.3 Uveoscleral outflow in rabbit. **(a)** The rabbit ciliary body is filled with hyaluronan *(pink)*. AP, aqueous plexus; CB, ciliary body; CC, collector channel; I, iris; R, remnant of vitreous; Sc, sclera. (From Lutjen-Drecoll E, Schenholm M, Tamm E, Tengblad A. Visualization of hyaluronic acid in the anterior segment of rabbit and monkey eyes. Exp Eye Res 1990;51:55–63. Reprinted with permission from Elsevier.) **(b)** Illustration of normal uveoscleral outflow anatomy and clefts. *Red arrow* depicts uveoscleral outflow. **(c)** Illustration of rabbit anatomy with clefts full of hyaluronan *(pink)*. *Red arrow* depicts uveoscleral outflow.

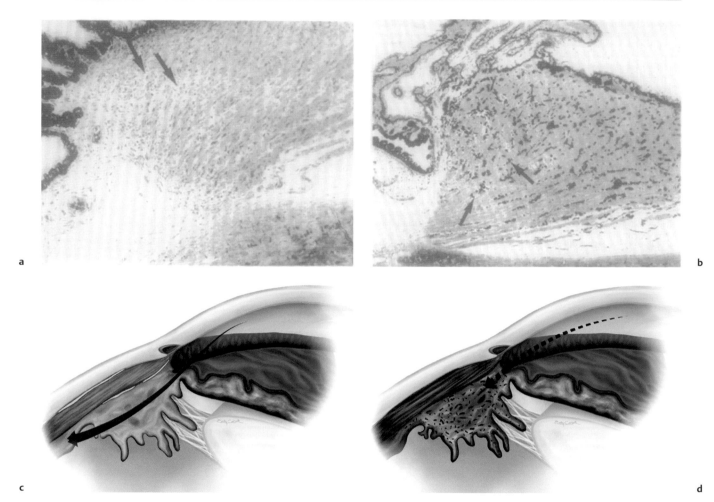

Fig. 9.4 Uveoscleral outflow in monkey with age. **(a)** The young monkey ciliary body demonstrates clefts *(arrows)*. **(b)** The clefts are missing and replaced with pigment in the older monkey ciliary body *(arrows)*. **(a,b** from Lutjen-Drecoll E, Tamm E, Kaufman PL. Age changes in rhesus monkey ciliary muscle: light and electron microscopy. Exp Eye Res 1988;47:885–899 Reprinted with permission from Elsevier.) **(c)** Illustration of young monkey uveoscleral outflow and anatomy. *Red arrow* depicts uveoscleral outflow. **(d)** Old monkey demonstrating pigment deposition *(black spots)*. *Red arrow* depicts uveoscleral outflow.

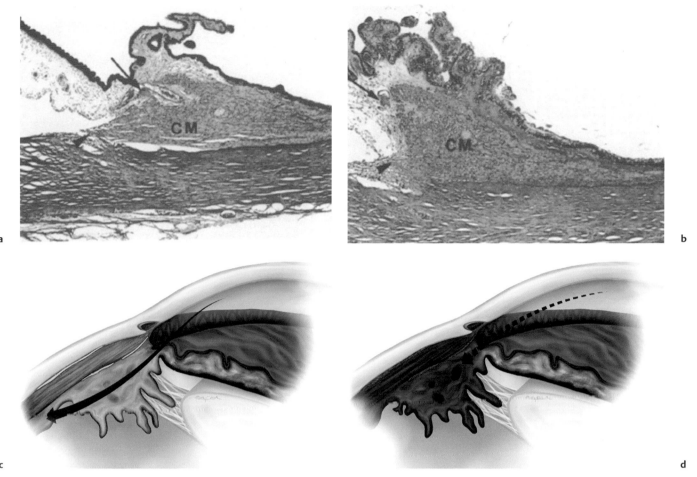

a   b

c   d

Fig. 9.5 Uveoscleral outflow in human with age. **(a)** The young human ciliary body demonstrates clefts *(arrow)*. CM, ciliary muscle. **(b)** The clefts are missing and replaced with extracellular matrix in the older human ciliary body. **(a,b** from Tamm S, Tamm E, Rohen JW. Age-related changes of the human ciliary muscle. A quantitative morphometric study. The arrowhead points to the scleral spur. Mech Aging Dev 1992;62:209–221. Reprinted with permission from Elsevier.) **(c)** Illustration of young human uveoscleral outflow *(red arrow)* and anatomy. **(d)** Illustration of old human demonstrating extracellular matrix deposition (increased blue coloration). *Red arrow* depicts uveoscleral outflow.

Interestingly, in glaucoma, ciliary muscle sheaths and tendons are thickened and have plaque-like deposits so that muscle fibers appear fused **(Fig. 9.6)**.[27] These pathological changes may explain the uveoscleral outflow abnormalities seen in glaucoma dogs[28] and human ocular hypertensive[20] eyes, mentioned above.

Taken together, species and age data suggest that large intermuscular spaces in the ciliary muscle represent the starting point of·the uveoscleral outflow pathway for aqueous humor exiting the anterior chamber. They may play roles in limiting the rate of outflow and also development of pathology leading to higher IOP.

Contractile Regulators of Uveoscleral Outflow

Key factors in regulating uveoscleral outflow are ciliary muscle contraction and extracellular matrix (ECM) dynamics.

Pilocarpine (a muscarinic agonist) and atropine (a muscarinic antagonist) respectively contract and relax components of the ciliary muscle (longitudinal, circular, and radial), reflecting parasympathetic control of the muscle complex and the unique muscarinic paradox influencing total aqueous humor outflow. In primates, muscarinic activation (pilocarpine) contracts the longitudinal ciliary muscle, opening the trabecular meshwork

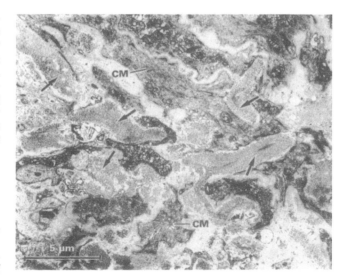

Fig. 9.6 Electronic microscopic image of glaucomatous changes in ciliary body and muscle. *Arrows* indicate plaque-like deposits. (From Lutjen-Drecoll E, Shimizu T, Rohrbach M, Rohen JW. Quantitative analysis of "plaque material" between ciliary muscle tips in normal- and glaucomatous eyes. Exp Eye Res 1986;42:457–465. Reprinted with permission form Elsevier.)

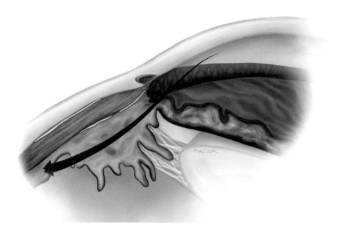
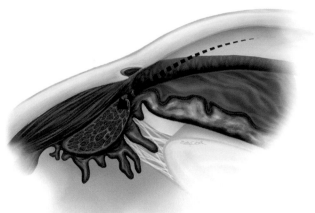

a

b

Fig. 9.7 Contractile regulators of uveoscleral outflow. **(a)** Illustration of normal anatomy and uveoscleral outflow. *Red arrow* depicts uveoscleral outflow. **(b)** Illustration of diminished uveoscleral outflow and anatomy after pilocarpine treatment. *Arrow* depicts uveoscleral outflow. Note the increased muscular contraction and absent ciliary body clefts.

and increasing outflow facility by the trabecular route.[29] However, circular ciliary muscle contraction decreases intermuscular spaces, leading to decreased uveoscleral outflow **(Fig. 9.7)**.[11,30] Direct measurements in human eyes show uveoscleral outflow comprising 4 to 14% of total outflow, with this changing to 0 to 3% after pilocarpine and 4 to 27% after atropine.[11]

Prostaglandins and Matrix Regulators of Uveoscleral Outflow

Prostaglandins that are a mainstay in IOP-lowering glaucoma treatment increase uveoscleral outflow by altering ECM homeostasis. Critical to understanding this was the use of ciliary muscle cultures[31] that had presented the main players for prostaglandin-mediated uveoscleral outflow: (1) prostaglandin receptors, (2) ECM, and (3) prostaglandin-regulated matrix metalloproteinases (MMPs) to modify the ECM. Prostaglandin-binding sites and prostaglandin receptors (eg, FP, EP) have been found in the ciliary muscle itself.[32,33] This is important, as receptor subtypes influence prostaglandin binding and likely ocular hypotensive responses to various agents.

The ECM of the ciliary muscle is composed of collagen (subtypes I, III, IV, and VI), fibronectin, elastin, and laminins.[34] In ciliary muscle cultures, each of these matrix proteins is expressed and organized above and below the cells themselves, allowing for a testable system.[35,36] In addition, MMPs are found in the uveoscleral outflow pathway. MMPs are a family of neutral proteases that degrade various ECM proteins in a peptide sequence-specific manner.[37] Their activity is balanced by α_2-microglobulin or tissue inhibitor of metalloproteinases (TIMPs).[37] Importantly, many MMPs, such as MMP-1, -2, -3, and -9, are known to carry an activator protein 1 (AP-1) transcriptional regulatory element in their promoters.[38] Prostaglandins are known to stimulate c-Fos, a DNA-binding protein that directly stimulates AP-1–containing genes, thus linking prostaglandins to MMPs.[39]

Putting this all together, all key components for prostaglandin-mediated regulation of uveoscleral outflow are located in the ciliary body and muscle. Prostaglandin $F_{2\alpha}$ ($PGF_{2\alpha}$) treatment of ciliary muscle cultures (at 20–200 nM concentrations that match well with estimated prostaglandin concentrations in the aqueous humor after topical application[38]) induces expression of c-Fos to stimulate AP-1.[39] AP-1 can then increase MMPs in vitro (causing elevated MMP-1 as detected by enzyme-linked immunoassays and MMP-1, -2, -3, and -9 by zymography[40]) and in vivo

(elevated MMP 1–3 are seen in ciliary muscle and iris root after topical $PGF_{2\alpha}$[41]). This is associated with decreased type I and III collagen in vitro[36] and in vivo.[42] Reduced type IV and VI collagen with otherwise unchanged morphology may also be seen after topical prostaglandin therapy[43] in vivo **(Fig. 9.8)**.[44] Thus, there is evidence that prostaglandins bind to prostaglandin receptors in the uveoscleral outflow pathway to increase expression of MMPs, alter ECM, and create widened spaces for uveoscleral outflow.

Prostaglandin analogues now serve as first-line medical therapies to lower IOP in a compliance-friendly once-daily dosing regimen. Prostaglandin analogues are stratified by receptor specificity (travoprost FP >> EP specific; latanoprost FP > EP; bimatoprost FP = EP) and presence or absence of preservative (tafluprost).[43,45] The greater latanoprost affinity for FP than EP receptors implicates FP receptors as the agent's dominant mechanism for lowering IOP.[43,45] Toris et al[12] calculated that latanoprost induced a 100% increase in uveoscleral outflow in 22 normal and ocular hypertensive patients. The once-daily dosing, slower onset of action, and delayed recovery of IOP elevation after cessation agrees with a mechanism of action that requires time for gene expression changes and ECM remodeling. Despite pilocarpine and prostaglandins having conflicting actions on uveoscleral outflow, combining the agents still has partially additive effects on IOP lowering.[46]

Why a Uveoscleral Pathway and Possibly a Uveolymphatic Role?

If the conventional trabecular outflow pathway sufficiently establishes a rigid eye to maintain stable optics, and simultaneously prevents blood influx into the eye to prevent a cloudy media, one can ask why is it even necessary to have a second door for aqueous drainage by uveoscleral outflow. Recent identification of lymphatics[47] **(Fig. 9.9)** in the ciliary body and choroid contradicts previous notions that the eye and orbit lack lymphatics. It indicates a possible connection between the uveoscleral outflow pathway and lymphatic system, which traditionally is considered to play roles in maintaining tissue fluid balance and immune surveillance. Identification of lymphatics used to be based on morphological features, but new markers such as lymphatic vessel endothelial hyaluronic acid receptor (LYVE-1) and podoplanin now enable more rapid and accurate detection of lymphatic vessels in tissue.[47] Immunohistochemical detection

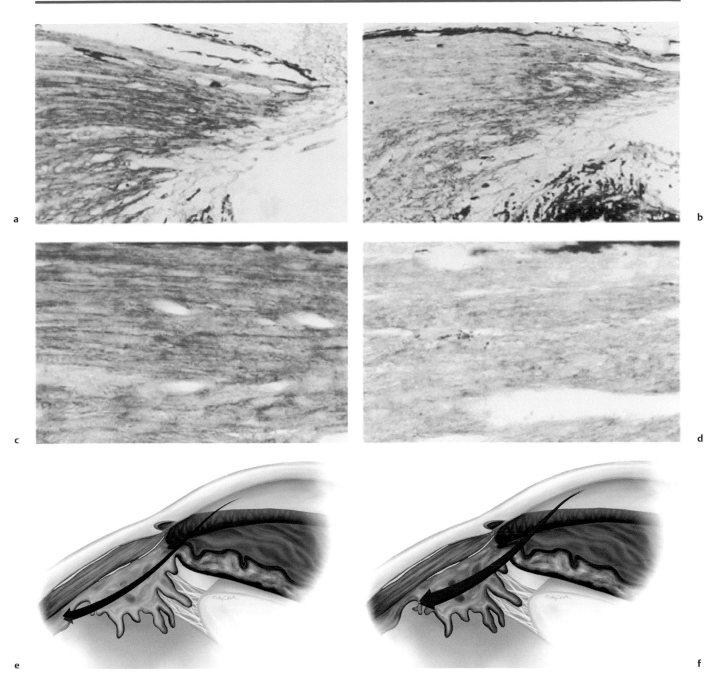

Fig. 9.8 Extracellular matrix (collagen 4) decreases in monkey ciliary body after topical prostaglandin treatment. **(a,c)** Control and **(b,d)** latanoprost treatment. **(c,d)** High magnification. (From Ocklind A. Effect of latanoprost on the extracellular matrix of the ciliary muscle. A study on cultured cells and tissue sections. Exp Eye Res 1998;67:179–191. Reprinted with permission from Elsevier.) **(e)** Illustration of normal anatomy and uveoscleral outflow *(red arrow)*. **(f)** Illustration of uveoscleral outflow *(red arrow)* after prostaglandin treatment. *Blue coloration* represents extracellular matrix.

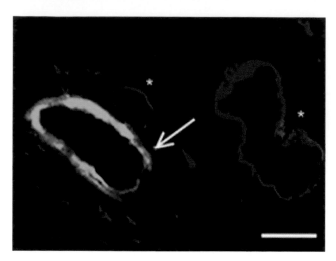

Fig. 9.9 The uveolymphatic pathway. D2–40–labeled lymphatic channel *(green; indicated by arrow)* is distinct from collagen IV labeling for a blood vessel *(red; indicated by asterisk).* (From Yucel YH, Johnston MG, Ly T, et al. Identification of lymphatics in the ciliary body of the human eye: a novel "uveolymphatic" outflow pathway. Exp Eye Res 2009;89:810–819. Reprinted with permission from Elsevier.)

of intraocular LYVE-1 and podoplanin along the uveoscleral outflow tract combined with head/neck lymph node recovery of intracamerally injected ^{125}I-labeled albumin hint at a possible "uveolymphatic pathway."[47] This is further supported by latanoprost-mediated enhancement of this phenomenon using intracamerally delivered fluorescent Q-dots.[48]

In addition to asking why a uveoscleral pathway should exist, one can also ask why a "uveolymphatic pathway" is necessary. Large proteins and even larger red blood cells can pass through the trabecular meshwork.[49] Subsequent episcleral venous passage carries these constituents to lymphatic organs such as the spleen. An example of the complex and unique relationship between trabecular outflow and the immune system is altered antigen processing and immune responses, as seen with anterior chamber-associated immune deviation (ACAID).[50] Therefore, delivering proteins from the uveoscleral outflow pathway to the lymphatics and lymph nodes may reflect an alternative functional relationship between the eye and immune system.

Future Directions for Exploiting the Uveoscleral Outflow Pathway (Medical and Surgical)

The immediate future of uveoscleral outflow therapeutic manipulation revolves around new prostaglandin analogues and surgeries to enhance uveoscleral outflow.

Future medical enhancements of uveoscleral outflow may involve drug delivery innovations as well as multiple-mechanism single agents. Examples of new drug delivery approaches include drug-impregnated punctual plugs[51] or nanoparticulate platforms.[52] One example of a single-dual mechanism drug is latanoprostene bunod, which chemically combines a prostaglandin analogue with a nitric oxide (NO) donor felt to improve trabecular outflow. In a phase 2b trial, it was demonstrated to be more effective than latanoprost alone in lowering IOP.[53] As such, this and similar agents could beneficially and synergistically modify combinations of uveoscleral outflow, aqueous production, and trabecular outflow.

Traditionally, the surgical enhancement of uveoscleral outflow occurred by intentionally or unintentionally creating cyclodialy-

sis clefts.[54] Clefts produced by a cyclodialysis spatula or trauma can increase outflow of aqueous humor to the suprachoroidal space, bypassing the uveoscleral outflow rate-limiting step of the ciliary muscle.[55] Although creating a cleft with a cyclodialysis spatula is unpredictable, inserting a shunt such as SOLX's (Waltham, MA) gold shunt, Transcend Medical's (Menlo Park, CA) CyPass, or Glaukos's (Laguna Hills, CA) iStent Supra that are currently under investigation[56] may be more predictable. However, it is not known currently whether introduction of a foreign body into the suprachoroidal space will lead to fibrosis and increase resistance to outflow.

References

1. Thomassen TL, Perkins ES, Dobree JH. Aqueous veins in glaucomatous eyes. Br J Ophthalmol 1950;34:221–227
2. Goel M, Picciani RG, Lee RK, Bhattacharya SK. Aqueous humor dynamics: a review. Open Ophthalmol J 2010;4:52–59
3. Bill A. The aqueous humor drainage mechanism in the cynomolgus monkey (Macaca irus) with evidence for unconventional routes. Invest Ophthalmol 1965;4:911–919
4. Alm A, Nilsson SF. Uveoscleral outflow—a review. Exp Eye Res 2009;88: 760–768
5. Bill A, Hellsing K. Production and drainage of aqueous humor in the cynomolgus monkey (Macaca irus). Invest Ophthalmol 1965;4:920–926
6. Bill A. Conventional and uveo-scleral drainage of aqueous humour in the cynomolgus monkey (Macaca irus) at normal and high intraocular pressures. Exp Eye Res 1966;5:45–54
7. Fine BS. Observations on the drainage angle in man and rhesus monkey: a concept of the pathogenesis of chronic simple glaucoma. a light and electron microscopic study. Invest Ophthalmol 1964;3:609–646
8. Gelatt KN, Gum GG, Williams LW, Barries KP. Uveoscleral flow of aqueous humor in the normal dog. Am J Vet Res 1979;40:845–848
9. Lindsey JD, Weinreb RN. Identification of the mouse uveoscleral outflow pathway using fluorescent dextran. Invest Ophthalmol Vis Sci 2002;43: 2201–2205
10. Gabelt BT, Kaufman PL. Prostaglandin F2 alpha increases uveoscleral outflow in the cynomolgus monkey. Exp Eye Res 1989;49:389–402
11. Bill A, Phillips CI. Uveoscleral drainage of aqueous humour in human eyes. Exp Eye Res 1971;12:275–281
12. Toris CB, Camras CB, Yablonski ME. Effects of PhXA41, a new prostaglandin F2 alpha analog, on aqueous humor dynamics in human eyes. Ophthalmology 1993;100:1297–1304
13. Brubaker RF. Goldmann's equation and clinical measures of aqueous dynamics. Exp Eye Res 2004;78:633–637
14. Larsson L-I, Alm A. Clinical aspects of uveoscleral outflow. In: Alm A, Kaufman PL, Kitazawa Y, Lutjen-Drecoll E, Stjernschantz J, Weinreb RN, eds. Uveoscleral Outflow: Biology and Clinical Aspects. London: Mosby-Wolfe; 1998:73–86
15. Jones RF, Maurice DM. New methods of measuring the rate of aqueous flow in man with fluorescein. Exp Eye Res 1966;5:208–220
16. Moses RA, Becker B. Clinical tonography; the scleral rigidity correction. Am J Ophthalmol 1958;45:196–208
17. Sit AJ, Ekdawi NS, Malihi M, McLaren JW. A novel method for computerized measurement of episcleral venous pressure in humans. Exp Eye Res 2011;92:537–544
18. Toris CB, Yablonski ME, Wang YL, Camras CB. Aqueous humor dynamics in the aging human eye. Am J Ophthalmol 1999;127:407–412
19. Gabelt BT, Gottanka J, Lütjen-Drecoll E, Kaufman PL. Aqueous humor dynamics and trabecular meshwork and anterior ciliary muscle morphologic changes with age in rhesus monkeys. Invest Ophthalmol Vis Sci 2003;44:2118–2125
20. Toris CB, Koepsell SA, Yablonski ME, Camras CB. Aqueous humor dynamics in ocular hypertensive patients. J Glaucoma 2002;11:253–258
21. Tamm S, Tamm E, Rohen JW. Age-related changes of the human ciliary muscle. A quantitative morphometric study. Mech Ageing Dev 1992;62: 209–221
22. Lutjen-Drecoll E. Normal morphology of the uveoscleral outflow pathways. In: Alm A, Kaufman PL, Kitazawa Y, Lutjen-Drecoll E, Stjernschantz J,

Weinreb RN, eds. Uveoscleral Outflow: Biology and Clinical Aspects. London: Mosby-Wolfe; 1998:7–24

23. Hartridge H. Helmholtz's Theory of Accommodation. Br J Ophthalmol 1925;9:521–523

24. Barany E, Rohen J. Localized contraction and relaxation within the ciliary muscle of the vervet monkey (Cercopithecus ethiops). In: Rohen J, ed. The Structure of the Eye, Second Symposium. Stuttgart: FK Schattauer Verlag; 1965:287–311

25. Lütjen-Drecoll E, Schenholm M, Tamm E, Tengblad A. Visualization of hyaluronic acid in the anterior segment of rabbit and monkey eyes. Exp Eye Res 1990;51:55–63

26. Lütjen-Drecoll E, Tamm E, Kaufman PL. Age changes in rhesus monkey ciliary muscle: light and electron microscopy. Exp Eye Res 1988;47:885–899

27. Lütjen-Drecoll E, Shimizu T, Rohrbach M, Rohen JW. Quantitative analysis of "plaque material" between ciliary muscle tips in normal and glaucomatous eyes. Exp Eye Res 1986;42:457–465

28. Barrie KP, Gum GG, Samuelson DA, Gelatt KN. Quantitation of uveoscleral outflow in normotensive and glaucomatous Beagles by 3H-labeled dextran. Am J Vet Res 1985;46:84–88

29. Bartels SP, Neufeld AH. Mechanisms of topical drugs used in the control of open angle glaucoma. Int Ophthalmol Clin 1980;20:105–116

30. Bill A. Effects of atropine and pilocarpine on aqueous humour dynamics in cynomolgus monkeys (Macaca irus). Exp Eye Res 1967;6:120–125

31. Korbmacher C, Helbig H, Coroneo M, et al. Membrane voltage recordings in a cell line derived from human ciliary muscle. Invest Ophthalmol Vis Sci 1990;31:2420–2430

32. Ocklind A, Lake S, Wentzel P, Nistér M, Stjernschantz J. Localization of the prostaglandin F2 alpha receptor messenger RNA and protein in the cynomolgus monkey eye. Invest Ophthalmol Vis Sci 1996;37:716–726

33. Csukas S, Bhattacherjee P, Rhodes L, Paterson CA. Prostaglandin E2 and F2 alpha binding sites in the bovine iris ciliary body. Invest Ophthalmol Vis Sci 1993;34:2237–2245

34. Weinreb RN, Lindsey JD, Luo XX, Wang TH. Extracellular matrix of the human ciliary muscle. J Glaucoma 1994;3:70–78

35. Lindsey JD, Kashiwagi K, Kashiwagi F, Weinreb RN. Prostaglandin action on ciliary smooth muscle extracellular matrix metabolism: implications for uveoscleral outflow. Surv Ophthalmol 1997;41(Suppl 2):S53–S59

36. Lindsey JD, Kashiwagi K, Kashiwagi F, Weinreb RN. Prostaglandins alter extracellular matrix adjacent to human ciliary muscle cells in vitro. Invest Ophthalmol Vis Sci 1997;38:2214–2223

37. Murphy G, Docherty AJ. The matrix metalloproteinases and their inhibitors. Am J Respir Cell Mol Biol 1992;7:120–125

38. Lindsey JD, Weinreb RN. Effects of prostaglandins on uveoscleral outflow. In: Alm A, Kaufman PL, Kitazawa Y, Lutjen-Drecoll E, Stjernschantz J, Weinreb RN, eds. Uveoscleral Outflow: Biology and Clinical Aspects. London: Mosby-Wolfe; 1998:41–56

39. Lindsey JD, To HD, Weinreb RN. Induction of c-fos by prostaglandin F2 alpha in human ciliary smooth muscle cells. Invest Ophthalmol Vis Sci 1994;35:242–250

40. Weinreb RN, Kashiwagi K, Kashiwagi F, Tsukahara S, Lindsey JD. Prostaglandins increase matrix metalloproteinase release from human ciliary smooth muscle cells. Invest Ophthalmol Vis Sci 1997;38:2772–2780

41. Gaton DD, Sagara T, Lindsey JD, Gabelt BT, Kaufman PL, Weinreb RN. Increased matrix metalloproteinases 1, 2, and 3 in the monkey uveoscleral outflow pathway after topical prostaglandin F(2 alpha)-isopropyl ester treatment. Arch Ophthalmol 2001;119:1165–1170

42. Sagara T, Gaton DD, Lindsey JD, Gabelt BT, Kaufman PL, Weinreb RN. Topical prostaglandin F2alpha treatment reduces collagen types I, III, and IV in the monkey uveoscleral outflow pathway. Arch Ophthalmol 1999;117:794–801

43. Stjernschantz J, Selen G, Ocklind A, Resul B. Effects of latanoprost and related prostaglandin analogues. In: Alm A, Kaufman PL, Kitazawa Y, Lutjen-Drecoll E, Stjernschantz J, Weinreb RN, eds. Uveoscleral OUtflow: Biology and Clinical Aspects. London: Mosby-Wolfe; 1998:57–72

44. Ocklind A. Effect of latanoprost on the extracellular matrix of the ciliary muscle. A study on cultured cells and tissue sections. Exp Eye Res 1998; 67:179–191

45. Sharif NA, Kelly CR, Crider JY, Williams GW, Xu SX. Ocular hypotensive FP prostaglandin (PG) analogs: PG receptor subtype binding affinities and selectivities, and agonist potencies at FP and other PG receptors in cultured cells. J Ocul Pharmacol Ther 2003;19:501–515

46. Friström B, Nilsson SE. Interaction of PhXA41, a new prostaglandin analogue, with pilocarpine. A study on patients with elevated intraocular pressure. Arch Ophthalmol 1993;111:662–665

47. Yücel YH, Johnston MG, Ly T, et al. Identification of lymphatics in the ciliary body of the human eye: a novel "uveolymphatic" outflow pathway. Exp Eye Res 2009;89:810–819

48. Tam AL, Gupta N, Zhang Z, Yücel YH. Latanoprost stimulates ocular lymphatic drainage: an in vivo nanotracer study. Transl Vis Sci Technol 2013; 2:3

49. Bill A. Scanning electron microscopic studies of the canal of Schlemm. Exp Eye Res 1970;10:214–218

50. Streilein JW, Niederkorn JY. Induction of anterior chamber-associated immune deviation requires an intact, functional spleen. J Exp Med 1981; 153:1058–1067

51. Gooch N, Molokhia SA, Condie R, et al. Ocular drug delivery for glaucoma management. Pharmaceutics 2012;4:197–211

52. Nguyen P, Huang AS, Yiu SC. Nanobiotechnology in the management of glaucoma. Open Journal of Ophthalmology. 2013;3:127–133

53. Weinreb RN, Ong T, Scassellati Sforzolini B, Vittitow JL, Singh K, Kaufman PL. A randomised, controlled comparison of latanoprostene bunod and latanoprost 0.005% in the treatment of ocular hypertension and open angle glaucoma: the VOYAGER study. Br J Ophthalmol 2014; Dec:8

54. Shaffer RN, Weiss DI. Concerning cyclodialysis and hypotony. Arch Ophthalmol 1962;68:25–31

55. Suguro K, Toris CB, Pederson JE. Uveoscleral outflow following cyclodialysis in the monkey eye using a fluorescent tracer. Invest Ophthalmol Vis Sci 1985;26:810–813

56. Francis BA, Singh K, Lin SC, et al. Novel glaucoma procedures: a report by the American Academy of Ophthalmology. Ophthalmology 2011;118:1466–1480

10 What Is the Suprachoroidal Space and Can It Scar?

Don S. Minckler

Uveoscleral outflow (uveoscleral bulk flow) has been long recognized in rabbits, cats, and by Anders Bill in some monkeys as early as 1962.[1] This "unconventional" flow, perhaps accounting for 25 to 57% of total aqueous outflow in healthy subjects, is pressure independent at normal intraocular pressure (IOP) and is thought to include seepage into the ciliary muscle, through the sclera, and into the choroidal space vessels. Current researchers, however, doubt the preeminence of percolation through the sclera.[2]

Aqueous flow into and absorption by choroidal vessels is of current interest due to ongoing experimentation with suprachoroidal shunt devices such as the CyPass Micro-Stent® (Transcend Medical, Menlo Park, CA), a 6.35-mm-long polyimide tube with an internal diameter of 300 μm and an outer diameter of 510 μm with built-in stabilizing rings. In a preliminary 6-month clinical study, it proved to be a remarkably uncomplicated minimally invasive filtering option, with IOP lowering from a baseline of 30.5 to 19.9 (N = 52).[3] A larger 12-month clinical study of CyPass as an adjunct to cataract surgery found a 14% IOP reduction from baseline and a 49 to 75% reduction in medications without any problematic hypotony.[4] The compartment into which such devices can be placed is anatomically limited to the suprachoroidal space between the most external layers of the choroidal veins and the lamina fusca anterior to vortex vein ampullae and their extensions through the sclera to the superior and inferior orbital veins. Aqueous drainage, in theory, could occur throughout the entire suprachoroid, ideally as a micrometer-thin low-pressure fluid layer. Prolonged high-pressure flow would seem likely to precipitate at least transient choroidal effusion, undesirable inflammation, and vision compromise, none of which were encountered in the CyPass studies.[3,4] Preplacement evaluation of the space available for safe device insertion requires careful indirect ophthalmoscopy and ideally high-resolution ultrasound and care to avoid vortex vein ampullae in the suprachoroid, which rarely enlarge as varices.[5] Vortex veins, five to eight in number, and typically more numerous nasally, lie 15.5 to 16.5 mm posterior and nasal from the lateral rectus insertion in the superior temporal quadrant and ~ 3 mm posterior to the globe equator.[6] As with orbital drainage devices, the superior temporal quadrant would seem the most favorable quadrant for suprachoroidal device placement.

The microanatomy of the suprachoroidal space into which shunting devices might be safely placed and aqueous drained has been detailed by Torczynski[7] as a transition zone between the choroid and the sclera. Hemorrhagic and nonhemorrhagic equatorial choroidal effusions triggered by hypotony-induced vortex vein congestion, from which most eyes recover spontaneously, probably begin with transudation from the choriocapillaris and choroidal veins, with progressive edema of the loose intervening tissues and eventual coalescence and expansion of the suprachoroidal space. Clinically, such effusions are well known to occasionally enlarge the suprachoroidal space to dimensions that obliterate the vitreous cavity with apposition between opposite retinal surfaces. The connective tissue fibers connecting the sclera to the ciliary body and choroid anteriorly are longer and run more tangentially than those connecting the sclera and the choroid posteriorly. This arrangement favors expansion of the anterior and equatorial suprachoroid by extravasated fluid during hypotony.[8] Inseparable sheets of melanocytes form the lamina fusca, the innermost layer of the sclera that becomes the external barrier to such effusions. Sheets of melanocytes, which can be dissected from the outer choroidal veins, form a loose boundary along the major external veins.[7]

Importantly, with regard to potential suprachoroidal scar formation, detailed morphological studies including transmission electron microscopy and immunohistochemistry have demonstrated that fibroblasts and myofibroblasts are present throughout all layers of the choroid, no doubt readily available to respond to trauma, surgical manipulation, and any foreign body by scar formation.[9] Cells here retain the capacity to proliferate and migrate, which could affect the patency of indwelling drainage devices. That the choroid can generate remarkable inflammation, both granulomatous and nongranulomatous, is obvious as uveitis remains a hugely important clinical problem.

The suprachoroidal space and sclera contain occasional ganglion cell collections, possibly important to blood flow regulation. Posteriorly nonmyelinated and myelinated nerves extending from the ciliary ganglion within short posterior ciliary nerves, including sensory, motor, and sympathetic fibers, extend into the choroid.[7] The long posterior ciliary nerves and arteries pass obliquely through 3- to 7-mm scleral canals beginning posterior to the equator. The nerve branches lose myelin when entering the suprachoroid from where they provide innervation to the sclera and throughout the whole thickness of the choroid.

The arterial supply to the anterior suprachoroid is derived from anterior ciliary arteries entering the sclera and choroid from the rectus muscles and the long posterior ciliary arteries, branches of the ophthalmic artery, to the iris circle plexus. In vivo choroidal circulation studies have indicated that posterior ciliary arteries have segmental flow and behave as end-arteries. Watershed zones between the various arterial and venous choroidal vasculatures explain focal choroidal ischemic lesions.[10]

Experience with orbital glaucoma drainage devices, highly relevant to utilizing foreign materials to create a filtering bleb in any ocular compartment, has clearly established the importance of the inevitable barrier capsule around the equatorial plate as the limiting factor in the efficacy of IOP control when utilizing polymethylmethacrylate, silicon-rubber, or polypropylene.[11] With currently popular orbital drainage devices, the space-preserving plate is necessary for any bleb formation. Its efficacy of function without a space-preserving element to provoke a capsule and bleb remains to be seen in long-term studies with less reactive materials such as polyimide, from which the CyPass device is made.

Studies have confirmed the long-held impression that the choroid can behave as erectile tissue and that it is dynamic at least in its thickness as monitored by *optical coherence tomography* (OCT) and ultrasound.[12,13]

Aqueous drainage devices utilizing the suprachoroidal space will face challenges similar to those of orbital glaucoma drainage devices, and possibly even more complex challenges due to crowded anatomy and inflammatory potential. Also, their designs will have to accommodate the micro-movement and dynamic nature of the space, and be minimally inflammatory.

References

1. Duke-Elder S. System of Ophthalmology, Vol. IV: The Physiology of the Eye and of Vision. London: Henry Kimpton; 1968:127

2. Toris CB. Aqueous humor dynamics and intraocular pressure elevation. In: Shaarawy TM, Sherwood MB, Hitchings RA, Crowston JG, eds. Glaucoma, vol 1, 2nd ed. New York: Elsevier, Saunders; 2015:51

3. Ianchulev T, Ahmed I, Hoeh H, Rau M, DeJuan E. Minimally invasive ab-interno suprachoroidal device (CyPass) for IOP control in open-angle glaucoma. Poster presented at the annual meeting of the American Academy of Ophthalmology, Chicago, October 16–19, 2010

4. Hoeh H, Vold SD, Ahmed IK, et al. Initial clinical experience with the CyPass Micro-Stent: safety and surgical outcomes of a novel supraciliary microstent. J Glaucoma 2016;25:106–112

5. Hu Y, Wang S, Dong Y, et al. Imaging features of varix of the vortex vein ampulla: a small case series. J Clinic Experiment Ophthalmol 2011;2:173

6. Lim MC, Bateman JB, Glasgow BJ. Vortex vein exit sites scleral coordinates. Ophthalmol 1995;102:942–946

7. Torczynski E. Choroid and suprachoroid. In: Jakobiec FA, ed. Ocular Anatomy, Embryology, and Teratology. Philadelphia: Harper and Row; 1982: 553–585

8. Moses RA. Detachment of ciliary body—anatomical and physical considerations. Invest Ophthalmol 1965;4:935–941

9. Flügel-Koch C, May CA, Lütjen-Drecoll E. Presence of a contractile cell network in the human choroid. Ophthalmologica 1996;210:296–302

10. Hayreh SS. In vivo choroidal circulation and its watershed zones. Eye (Lond) 1990;4(Pt 2):273–289

11. Dempster AG, Molteno AC, Bevin TH, Thompson AM. Otago glaucoma surgery outcome study: electron microscopy of capsules around Molteno implants. Invest Ophthalmol Vis Sci 2011;52:8300–8309

12. Hogan MJ, Alvarado JA, Weddell J. Histology of the Human Eye. Philadelphia: Saunders; 1971:320

13. Ulaş F, Doğan U, Duran B, Keleş A, Ağca S, Celebi S. Choroidal thickness changes during the menstrual cycle. Curr Eye Res 2013;38:1172–1181

11 Suprachoroidal Drainage—Centenarian Progress: An Inventor's Perspective

Minas Theodore Coroneo

At the start of my ophthalmology training in the early 1980s, two of the three formative events occurred that contributed to my invention of a modern suprachoroidal stent.

As a junior trainee in Australia, I often served weekend, night-shift, and on-call duty, and thus saw many trauma cases. At the time, the sport of indoor cricket had become popular in Sydney, and it led to so many eye trauma cases that I accumulated enough cases to write my first ophthalmologic publication.[1] A case of traumatic cyclodialysis made an impression; the low pressure was difficult to manage at a time when treatment options for glaucoma were relatively limited. I noted that cyclodialysis and the suprachoroidal space are a low-resistance pathway—if only it could be controlled. One of the cases in the cricket eye injury literature had been described by Arthur D'Ombrain,[2] an Australian ophthalmologist, the first to recognize traumatic glaucoma.[3] I also attended a basic science course in New Zealand where I met Professor A.C. Molteno, the inventor of the Molteno glaucoma drainage devices and subsequently learned to implant these devices.

Recognizing that the trabecular meshwork was likely to be the most sophisticated biological valve that had ever evolved, I went on to complete my doctorate on the electrophysiology of trabecular meshwork cells,[4] confirming that there was more than one cell type in the angle, and that a population of trabecular meshwork cells was excitable and likely contractile.

I saw glaucoma as a "dismal" subspecialty; despite technically perfect surgery, operations failed, patients' vision often deteriorated, and the well-known treatment limitations and paradoxes led me to realize that I did not wish to be a glaucoma subspecialist. I continued research on central issues in glaucoma and developed an in vitro model for pressure-induced apoptotic cell death and means by which it could be blocked via TRAAK channels, which are pressure-sensitive cell membrane channels.[5,6]

Carrying out challenging cataract surgery in the Australian outback provided the stimulus for my first invention in ophthalmology—the use of trypan blue as a capsular and ocular dye. The first United States patents for VisionBlue were issued in 2002,[7,8] and the product entered the market.[9] This invention steered me toward cataract and refractive surgery and I became interested in how surgical techniques like phacoemulsification had revolutionized anterior segment surgery and how it even provided a safe intervention for narrow-angle glaucoma.[10] It dawned on me that glaucoma needed an equivalent to "phaco" to create a similar revolution for glaucoma management. The case of traumatic hypotony resurfaced just at the time when the first intraocular lens that could be rolled into a cylinder less than 1 mm in diameter, the ThinOptX (Abingdon, VA) intraocular lens (IOL), was developed in 2002.[11]

My interest in ultraviolet light and the focusing of peripheral light by the anterior eye[12] resulted in the development of a dysphotopsia-free intraocular lens[13,14] and so I had a keen interest in intraocular lens technology. Whereas most people saw an IOL, all I could think of was that the optic could be "repurposed, that is, connected to a tube and inserted atraumatically through a small side-port incision, transcamerally, into the suprachoroidal space. I obtained ThinOptX lenses, glued fine tubing to them (**Fig. 11.1**), and performed a series of experiments in perfused porcine eyes. A U.S patent was issued[15] in 2007.

In reviewing this area of research, it was apparent that following Leopold Heine's[16] landmark paper in 1905, describing cyclodialysis as a new operation for treating elevated intraocular pressure in uncontrolled glaucoma, many attempts have been made to take advantage of the suprachoroidal pathway to treat glaucoma. The combination of improved biomaterials and surgical implant techniques, which largely evolved from advances in cataract surgery, has resulted in relatively minimally invasive, atraumatic implantation of micro-stents into both the angle and the suprachoroidal space. The technology was licensed to Transcend Medical (Menlo Park, CA) in September 2006, and the Cypass ("ciliary bypass") micro-stent was developed. I was employed by this company as a consultant and contributed to both the design evolution and the development of the surgical technique. Recently, it has been reported that the implantation of this micro-stent effectively lowers intraocular pressure in > 80% of patients at 1 year.[17] In cases of suprachoroidal implantation, it appears that finally, a century after Heine's work, a controlled cyclodialysis had been achieved. In a small way, with my contribution to the potential "phaco-like" transformation of glaucoma surgery, it is hoped the outlook and practice in this area will be less dismal.

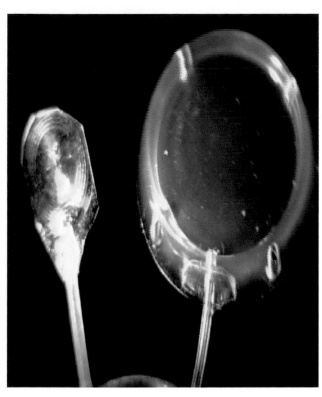

Fig. 11.1 Prototype suprachoroidal micro-stent manufactured from the optic of ThinOptX intraocular lens (IOL) with a fine tube attached *(left)*. One-plate Molteno glaucoma drainage device for comparison *(right)*.

Financial Disclosure

Minas Theodore Coroneo is the inventor of core patents for the Cypass suprachoroidal drainage device.

References

1. Coroneo MT. An eye for cricket. Ocular injuries in indoor cricketers. Med J Aust 1985;142:469–471

2. D'Ombrain A. Traumatic monocular chronic glaucoma. Trans Ophthalmol Soc Aust 1945;5:116–120

3. Tumbocon JA, Latina MA. Angle recession glaucoma. Int Ophthalmol Clin 2002;42:69–78

4. Coroneo MT, Korbmacher C, Flügel C, Stiemer B, Lütjen-Drecoll E, Wiederholt M. Electrical and morphological evidence for heterogeneous populations of cultured bovine trabecular meshwork cells. Exp Eye Res 1991; 52:375–388

5. Agar A, Li S, Agarwal N, Coroneo MT, Hill MA. Retinal ganglion cell line apoptosis induced by hydrostatic pressure. Brain Res 2006;1086:191–200

6. Coroneo MT, inventor. Methods for preventing pressure induced apoptotic neural cell death. Australian patent 2006236018. October 1, 2009

7. Coroneo MT, inventor. Methods for visualizing the anterior lens capsule of the human eye. US patent 6 367 480. April 9, 2002

8. Coroneo MT, inventor. Ophthalmic methods and uses. US patient 6 372 449. April 16, 2002

9. Coroneo M. Retrospective on staining with trypan blue. Cataract & Refractive Surgery Today. 2005;5:49–51

10. Roberts TV, Francis IC, Lertusumitkul S, Kappagoda MB, Coroneo MT. Primary phacoemulsification for uncontrolled angle-closure glaucoma. J Cataract Refract Surg 2000;26:1012–1016

11. Callahan WB, Callahan JS, inventors. Deformable intraocular corrective lens. US patent 6 096 077. August 1, 2000

12. Coroneo M. Ultraviolet radiation and the anterior eye. Eye Contact Lens 2011;37:214–224

13. Coroneo MT, Pham T, Kwok LS. Off-axis edge glare in pseudophakic dysphotopsia. J Cataract Refract Surg 2003;29:1969–1973

14. Coroneo MT, inventor. Treatment of photic disturbances in the eye. US patent 7 217 289. May 15, 2007

15. Coroneo MT, inventor. Ocular pressure regulation. US patent 7 291 125. November 6, 2007

16. Heine L. Die Cyclodialyse, eine neue glaukomoperation. Dtsch Med Wochenschr 1905;3:824–826

17. García-Feijoo J, Rau M, Grisanti S, et al. Supraciliary micro-stent implantation for open-angle glaucoma failing topical therapy: 1-year results of a multicenter study. Am J Ophthalmol 2015;159:1075–1081

12 Do Prostaglandins Make Uveoscleral Outflow More Pressure Dependent?

B'Ann T. Gabelt and Paul L. Kaufman

The question of pressure-dependency is important because it reflects the eye's capacity to adjust aqueous drainage in response to changes in eye pressure. Under normal conditions, the uveoscleral outflow pathway likely can make only small magnitude adjustments in outflow in response to different eye pressures. Before addressing the question of whether prostaglandins make uveoscleral outflow more pressure dependent, one must first determine if uveoscleral outflow is pressure dependent at all.

Some arguments are based on the belief that the driving force for uveoscleral flow is provided by the difference in pressure between the anterior chamber and the suprachoroidal space, which in the monkey is ~ 4 mm Hg. Within the intraocular pressure (IOP) range of ~ 10 to 40 mm Hg, a change in IOP is reflected by an equal change in pressure in the suprachoroidal space, thereby maintaining the pressure difference at a constant value.[1] In contrast to the pressure-dependent flow from the anterior chamber across the trabecular meshwork into Schlemm's canal, drainage via the uveoscleral pathway is virtually independent of pressure at IOP levels greater than 7 to 10 mm Hg.[2] Under normal circumstances, uveoscleral facility[2] in the monkey is ≤ 0.02 μL/min/mm Hg, and thus is a negligible component (< 6%) of trabecular outflow facility, which in the cited study was 0.307 μL/min/mm Hg.

However, under certain conditions, other investigators found uveoscleral outflow to be more pressure-sensitive than described by Bill.[2] Uveoscleral facility in monkeys has been shown to increase following the induction of inflammation by bovine serum injection into the vitreous cavity. Uveoscleral facility in control eyes ranged from 0.047 to 0.052 μL/min/mm Hg as determined from fluoresceinated dextran infusion at 15 mm Hg for 30 minutes. In inflamed eyes, uveoscleral facility increased two- to five-fold depending on the size of the tracer.[3] Cyclodialysis was also shown to increase uveoscleral facility in monkeys from 0.01 μL/min/mm Hg in control eyes to 0.07 μL/min/mm Hg in cyclodialysis eyes. The latter studies utilized fluoresceinated dextrans of 70,000 mw (molecular weight) and pressures of either 4 mm Hg or 35 mm Hg for 30 minutes.[4] Inflammation produced with both of these techniques likely resulted in the release of prostaglandins. Therefore, it is reasonable to hypothesize that uveoscleral outflow may become more sensitive to pressure following prostaglandin treatment.

We conducted studies using the isotope dilution technique[5] to measure uveoscleral outflow following unilateral topical prostaglandin F_2 (PGF$_{2\alpha}$)-isopropylester (PGF$_{2\alpha}$-IE) treatment of 2 μg twice daily for 4 or 5 days in cynomolgus monkeys as confirmation that the technique could detect changes in uveoscleral outflow, as requested for another study.[6] Because the IOP in most of the monkeys decreased below episcleral venous pressure during the isotope studies, a modification of the technique was made to also include data collection done with the pressure in both eyes elevated to ~ 16 mm Hg by flow from an external reservoir during

the same experiment. These studies were not optimized for the determination of uveoscleral facility, but some suggestive results were derived from them. Given all of the assumptions, uveoscleral facility in PGF$_{2\alpha}$-IE–treated eyes was calculated to be 0.18 ± 0.04 μL/min/mm Hg (mean ± standard error of the mean) compared with control eye values of 0.04 ± 0.01 μL/min/mm Hg (ratio 5.88 ± 1.50, $p < 0.02$, $n = 7$). Trabecular facility was decreased in treated compared with control eyes (ratio 0.22 ± 0.03, $n = 6$, $p < 0.001$), whereas the total outflow facility was unchanged **(Fig. 12.1)**.

These data suggest that PGF$_{2\alpha}$-IE may increase uveoscleral facility and that more definitive studies are warranted. Also these data suggest that following PGF$_{2\alpha}$-IE treatment, more fluid can be removed from the eye via the uveoscleral pathway as compared with the trabecular pathway in response to pressure.

The only study attempting to address this question has been that of Toris et al[7] in cats following treatment with PGA$_2$. In this study, PGA$_2$ decreased IOP by increasing uveoscleral outflow (measured directly by the isotope accumulation techniques) and trabecular outflow facility but not uveoscleral facility or total facility. It is difficult to explain how total facility can remain unchanged while trabecular facility increases. Also, this increase in trabecular facility in cats after PGA$_2$ is different from what has been found in monkeys after PGF$_{2\alpha}$-IE.[8]

In 2002–2003 there was renewed discussion about whether PGs can increase uveoscleral facility.[9] Becker and Neufeld[9] questioned how an increase in uveoscleral outflow can decrease IOP if uveoscleral outflow is pressure independent. They suggested modification of the Goldmann equation to contain a uveoscleral facility term:

$$F = C_{trab}(IOP - P_{ev}) + C_u(IOP - P_{eo})$$

$$C_{tot} = C_{trab} + C_u$$

where F = flow; C_{trab} = trabecular meshwork outflow facility; C_u = uveoscleral outflow facility; P_{ev} = episcleral venous pressure; P_{eo} = extraocular pressure. In a small way, with my contribution to the potential "phaco-like" transformation of glaucoma surgery, it is hoped the outlook and practice in this area will be less dismal.

Kaufman[10] agreed with Becker and Neufeld and went one step further to include a facility term for pseudofacility (Cps), the pressure-dependence of aqueous humor formation, so that

$$C_{tot} = C_{trab} + C_u + C_{ps}$$

Camras[11] disagreed with Becker and Neufeld, arguing that the predominant mechanism of action of most prostaglandins in most species was through a pressure-independent mechanism. However, he acknowledged more work was needed. Yablonski[12] also disagreed with Becker and Neufeld, stating his belief that the final pathway of uveoscleral flow is into the uveal blood rather

Flow vs intraocular pressure (IOP) calculated from various types of facility data after PGF$_{2\alpha}$-IE b.i.d. treatment for 4 days

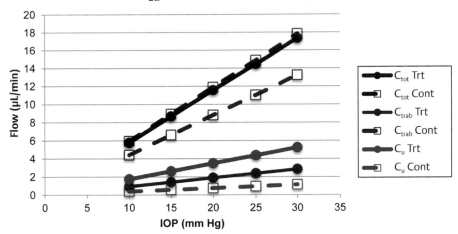

Fig. 12.1 Total, trabecular, and uveoscleral outflow facilities after PGF$_{2\alpha}$ treatment in monkeys. Keeping in mind the many assumptions used in generating these data, as explained in the text, one can see that total outflow facility measured by two-level constant pressure perfusion (C_{tot}) in control eyes (Cont) and treated eyes (Trt) is nearly identical (*black solid line* and *dashed line*, respectively). Similar to Bill's[24] graph, uveoscleral facility (C_u) in control eyes (*red dashed line*) changes very little with pressure. However, in treated eyes, uveoscleral facility (*solid red line*) increases and trabecular facility (C_{trab}, *blue solid line*) decreases, suggesting the resistance to flow is now much less in the uveoscleral pathway than through the trabecular pathway and that the resistance is now more pressure sensitive. Pseudofacility, different measurement techniques and timing, as well as assumptions made to generate these data may account for the differences in total outflow facility and trabecular facility in control eyes.

than across the sclera. Also he believed that the flux of protein across the sclera reported in Bill's[13] studies was primarily by diffusion. However, our studies demonstrated that the proportion of tracer in the periocular tissue of primate eyes treated for 4 days with PGF$_{2\alpha}$-IE was so large compared with control eyes, that posteriorly draining aqueous must have exited the eye transsclerally rather than being reabsorbed by uveal blood vessels.[14]

How can prostaglandins increase uveoscleral facility? Topical application of PGF$_{2\alpha}$,[15] as well as latanoprost,[16] reduces the content of several collagens in the ciliary muscle of monkeys. Increased content of several matrix metalloproteinases have also been recorded in human ciliary muscle cells exposed to PGF$_{2\alpha}$ or latanoprost[16–18] and in the ciliary muscle of monkey eyes treated with PGF$_{2\alpha}$ in vivo.[19] Factors other than reduction of collagen may well be involved. Stjernschantz et al[20] reported changes in the shape of ciliary muscle cells exposed to latanoprost with alterations in the localization of the cytoskeleton proteins actin and vinculin. The latter changes likely also occur in the trabecular meshwork and could theoretically account for some of the increases in total outflow facility that have been reported.[8,21,22] Changes in scleral collagens could also significantly alter scleral permeability.[23]

In conclusion, it is apparent that the various data sets in the literature scatter enough so that there is ambiguity and lack of consensus of exactly what is happening with prostaglandin treatment. In our view, uveoscleral outflow increases, trabecular outflow decreases, total outflow must remain the same, outflow always must equal inflow, and they both remain relatively constant, so that resistance, IOP, and episcleral venous pressure must adjust themselves in some manner to achieve this balance. Our data suggest that uveoscleral outflow becomes the primary outflow pathway, and in essence "takes over" from the trabecular meshwork, by virtue of tissue remodeling. In this process, uveoscleral outflow also becomes more pressure-dependent, resulting in nearly an order-of-magnitude increase from its very low resting value. There is even less data on episcleral venous

pressure, and it could be that the post-PGF$_{2\alpha}$ values for uveoscleral outflow facility might approach those for trabecular outflow facility, especially if the latter are abnormally low as in primary open-angle glaucoma (POAG). That does not mean that uveoscleral outflow becomes entirely pressure-dependent, but rather that it is more pressure-dependent than at rest. Thus, although we do not understand all of it, we posit that its characteristics are at least in part changed along the lines we have indicated, and that this is part of an elaborate mechanism by which fluid drainage from the eye is regulated under both normal and abnormal conditions. Aqueous humor dynamics regulation in the eye involves a very complex multipurpose, multitissue, multicontrol hydraulic system, much like water supply and distribution systems in large cities. We are still learning all the attributes of our little urban system in the eye, so that everyone there gets what they need and we cope with the occasional tsunami reasonably well.

References

1. Emi K, Pederson JE, Toris CB. Hydrostatic pressure of the suprachoroidal space. Invest Ophthalmol Vis Sci 1989;30:233–238

2. Bill A. Conventional and uveo-scleral drainage of aqueous humour in the cynomolgus monkey (Macaca irus) at normal and high intraocular pressures. Exp Eye Res 1966;5:45–54

3. Toris CB, Gregerson DS, Pederson JE. Uveoscleral outflow using different-sized fluorescent tracers in normal and inflamed eyes. Exp Eye Res 1987;45:525–532

4. Toris CB, Pederson JE. Effect of intraocular pressure on uveoscleral outflow following cyclodialysis in the monkey eye. Invest Ophthalmol Vis Sci 1985;26:1745–1749

5. Sperber GO, Bill A. A method for near-continuous determination of aqueous humor flow; effects of anaesthetics, temperature and indomethacin. Exp Eye Res 1984;39:435–453

6. Takagi Y, Nakajima T, Shimazaki A, et al. Pharmacological characteristics of AFP-168 (tafluprost), a new prostanoid FP receptor agonist, as an ocular hypotensive drug. Exp Eye Res 2004;78:767–776

7. Toris CB, Yablonski ME, Wang YL, Hayashi M. Prostaglandin A2 increases uveoscleral outflow and trabecular outflow facility in the cat. Exp Eye Res 1995;61:649–657

8. Gabelt BT, Kaufman PL. The effect of prostaglandin F2 alpha on trabecular outflow facility in cynomolgus monkeys. Exp Eye Res 1990;51:87–91

9. Becker B, Neufeld AH. Pressure dependence of uveoscleral outflow. J Glaucoma 2002;11:464

10. Kaufman PL. Letter to the editor. J Glaucoma 2003;12:89

11. Camras CB. Letter to the editor. J Glaucoma 2003;12:92–93

12. Yablonski ME. Letter to the editor. J Glaucoma 2003;12:90–92

13. Bill A. Movement of albumin and dextran through the sclera. Arch Ophthalmol 1965;74:248–252

14. Gabelt BT, Kaufman PL. Prostaglandin F2 alpha increases uveoscleral outflow in the cynomolgus monkey. Exp Eye Res 1989;49:389–402

15. Sagara T, Gaton DD, Lindsey JD, Gabelt BT, Kaufman PL, Weinreb RN. Topical prostaglandin F2alpha treatment reduces collagen types I, III, and IV in the monkey uveoscleral outflow pathway. Arch Ophthalmol 1999;117:794–801

16. Ocklind A. Effect of latanoprost on the extracellular matrix of the ciliary muscle. A study on cultured cells and tissue sections. Exp Eye Res 1998;67:179–191

17. Lindsey JD, Kashiwagi K, Boyle D, Kashiwagi F, Firestein GS, Weinreb RN. Prostaglandins increase proMMP-1 and proMMP-3 secretion by human ciliary smooth muscle cells. Curr Eye Res 1996;15:869–875

18. Weinreb RN, Kashiwagi K, Kashiwagi F, Tsukahara S, Lindsey JD. Prostaglandins increase matrix metalloproteinase release from human ciliary smooth muscle cells. Invest Ophthalmol Vis Sci 1997;38:2772–2780

19. Gaton DD, Sagara T, Lindsey JD, Gabelt BT, Kaufman PL, Weinreb RN. Increased matrix metalloproteinases 1, 2, and 3 in the monkey uveoscleral outflow pathway after topical prostaglandin F(2 alpha)-isopropyl ester treatment. Arch Ophthalmol 2001;119:1165–1170

20. Stjernschantz J, Selén G, Ocklind A, Resul B. Effects of latanoprost and related prostaglandin analogues. In: Alm A, Weinreb RN, eds. Uveoscleral Outflow. Biology and Clinical Aspects. London: Mosby-Wolfe Medical Communications; 1998:57–72

21. Lee PY, Podos SM, Severin C. Effect of prostaglandin F2 alpha on aqueous humor dynamics of rabbit, cat, and monkey. Invest Ophthalmol Vis Sci 1984;25:1087–1093

22. Alm A, Villumsen J. PhXA34, a new potent ocular hypotensive drug. A study on dose-response relationship and on aqueous humor dynamics in healthy volunteers. Arch Ophthalmol 1991;109:1564–1568

23. Weinreb RN. Enhancement of scleral macromolecular permeability with prostaglandins. Trans Am Ophthalmol Soc 2001;99:319–343

24. Bill A. Uveoscleral drainage of aqueous humor. In: Bito LZ, Stjernschantz J, eds. The Ocular Effects of Prostaglandins and Other Eicosanoids. New York: Alan R. Liss; 1989:417

IC Aqueous Production

13 Structure and Mechanisms of Aqueous Production

Sruthi Sampathkumar and Carol B. Toris

Aqueous humor, its production and drainage (**Fig. 13.1**), are essential for maintaining the normal functions of various avascular structures in the ocular anterior segment. A transparent filtrate of the plasma, the aqueous humor provides nutrition to and removes products of metabolism from the lens, cornea, anterior vitreous, and trabecular meshwork. It maintains an optically clear medium to optimize visual function, exerts hydrostatic pressure to maintain the shape of the eyeball, and aids in the circulation of inflammatory cells and distribution of pharmacological compounds.

Suppressing aqueous humor production is a technique to treat glaucoma by lowering the intraocular pressure (IOP). Classes of drugs approved for this purpose include carbonic anhydrase inhibitors, β-adrenergic antagonists, and α_2-adrenergic agonists. Other classes under investigation are forskolin, cannabinoid receptor agonists, serotonin, and angiotensin II. These drugs must be dosed several times per day to maintain IOP at a healthy level. Tachyphylaxis, side effects, and lack of patient compliance have limited the IOP efficacy of these drugs. Cyclodestructive procedures slow aqueous production without chronic drug use. By destroying tissues involved in aqueous humor secretion, IOP can be reduced, potentially around the clock. The minimally invasive modern cycloablative procedures are endoscopic cyclophotocoagulation (ECP), ECP plus, and high-intensity focused ultrasound (HIFU). All of these procedures are discussed in this chapter. It is hard to rule out the possibility that the new IOP-lowering drugs and procedures targeting the trabecular meshwork (TM) will also affect aqueous humor production, as the TM and ciliary processes lie in close proximity. This chapter provides an overview of aqueous humor production and describes various interventions that may affect the aqueous production rate.

Anatomic Considerations

The ciliary body (**Fig. 13.2**) is a small circumferential musculoepithelial structure with a double-layered epithelium overlying the stromal elements and neurovascular structures. The anterior part (pars plicata) has processes extending into the posterior chamber. The posterior region (pars plana) is relatively flat, avascular, and lacks these processes. The double-layered epithelium consists of pigmented epithelial cells toward the stroma and non-pigmented epithelial cells toward the posterior chamber. These layers are oriented apex to apex, forming a specialized unit for aqueous humor secretion[1] (**Fig. 13.3**). The ciliary body is supplied by anterior ciliary and long posterior ciliary arteries. The ophthalmic artery branches off into seven muscular arteries that supply the extraocular muscles and continues as the anterior ciliary arteries. These form the intermuscular circle in the ciliary muscle and minor arterial circle in the iris. Two long posterior ciliary arteries (medial and lateral) arise from the ophthalmic artery; they travel forward in the choroid to form the major arterial circle that supplies the ciliary processes and end in the minor arterial circle of the iris. Four vortex veins drain the ciliary body into the superior and inferior ophthalmic veins. The capillaries of the ciliary processes are leaky, allowing passage of proteins and solutes into the ciliary stroma for aqueous production. Not all substances in the ciliary stroma enter the aqueous humor due to the presence of tight junctions between the nonpigmented ciliary epithelial cells. This and the tight junctions of the iris capillaries form part of the blood–aqueous barrier.

Physiology of Aqueous Humor Production

The production of aqueous humor is a continuous and active process requiring energy. The constituents of the aqueous humor must pass through the ciliary capillary wall, ciliary stroma, and epithelial bilayer before reaching the posterior chamber. The nonpigmented epithelium (NPE) forms part of the blood–aqueous barrier and offers the most resistance to the secretion of aqueous humor. The formation and secretion of aqueous humor into the posterior chamber takes place in the following stages[2]:

1. Convective delivery of ions, proteins, and water by the ciliary circulation
2. Diffusion and ultrafiltration from the capillaries into the stroma driven by oncotic pressure, hydrostatic pressure, and a concentration gradient
3. Active ionic transport into the basolateral spaces between the nonpigmented epithelial cells followed by water movement into the posterior chamber

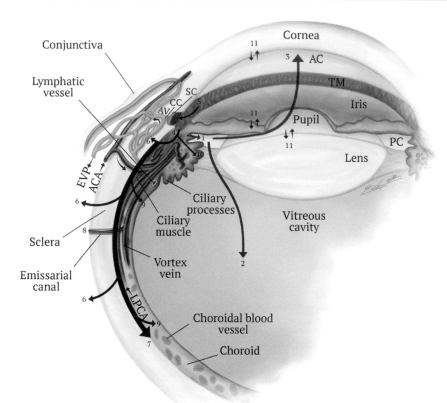

Conjunctiva

Lymphatic vessel

Sclera

Emissarial canal

Cornea

AC

TM

Iris

Pupil

PC

Lens

Vitreous cavity

Ciliary processes

Ciliary muscle

Vortex vein

Choroidal blood vessel

Choroid

Fig. 13.1 Production and circulation of aqueous humor. Aqueous humor that is secreted into the posterior chamber (1) flows across the vitreous cavity (2) or through the pupil into the anterior chamber (3). Fluid circulates around the anterior chamber and eventually drains into the anterior chamber angle (4). Aqueous humor drains from the anterior chamber angle via two routes: the trabecular meshwork, Schlemm's canal, collector channels, and episcleral veins (5); or the uveoscleral outflow route. The latter route starts with the ciliary muscle. From there, fluid may flow in many directions, including across the sclera (6), within the supraciliary and suprachoroidal spaces (7), through emissarial canals and vortex veins (8), into uveal vessels (9) and possibly into ciliary processes (10), where it could be secreted again. Lymphatic vessels, recently identified in the uvea, also may contribute to ocular fluid dynamics. The exchange of fluid in and out of the cornea and lens (11) does not contribute to aqueous flow. AC, anterior chamber; ACA, anterior ciliary artery; AV, aqueous vein; CC, collector channel; EVP, episcleral venous plexus; LPCA, long posterior ciliary artery; PC, posterior chamber; SC, Schlemm's canal; TM, trabecular meshwork.

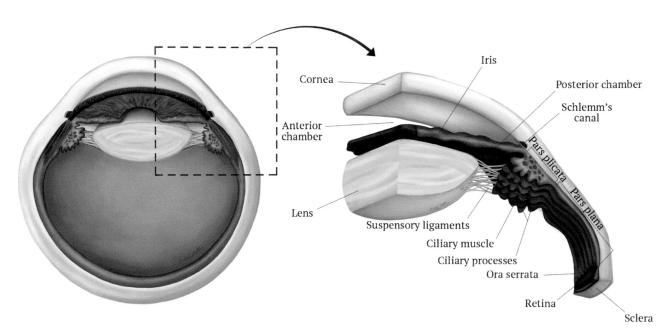

Iris

Cornea

Anterior chamber

Lens

Posterior chamber

Schlemm's canal

Pars plicata

Pars plana

Suspensory ligaments

Ciliary muscle

Ciliary processes

Ora serrata

Retina

Sclera

Fig. 13.2 The ciliary body comprises the pars plicata anteriorly and pars plana posteriorly. The ciliary processes are part of the highly vascular pars plicata and are involved in aqueous humor secretion into the posterior chamber. The pars plana is less vascular and as such is the site of entry for intraocular surgery.

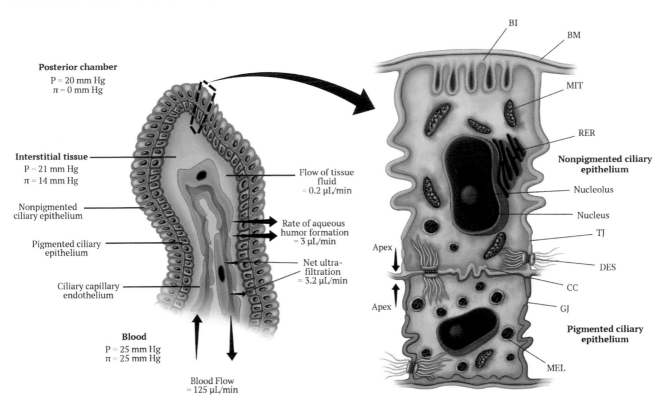

Fig. 13.3 Ciliary epithelium as a syncytium. The ciliary processes have a double-layered epithelium. The apices of the nonpigmented epithelium and pigmented epithelium face each other. The ciliary stroma has a rich vascular network with leaky endothelium. The nonpigmented epithelium is rich in mitochondria, which provide energy for aqueous humor secretion. It has rough endoplasmic reticulum and a few pigment granules. The pigmented epithelium has several melanosomes and pigment granules with a few mi-tochondria. Tight junctions are present between the apices of the nonpigmented epithelial cells to prevent entry of interstitial fluid into the posterior chamber. BI, basal infoldings; BM, basement membrane; CC, ciliary channels; DES, desmosomes; FE, fenestrated capillary endothelium; GJ, gap junction; MEL, melanosome; MIL, mitochondria; RER, rough endoplasmic reticulum; TJ, tight junction.

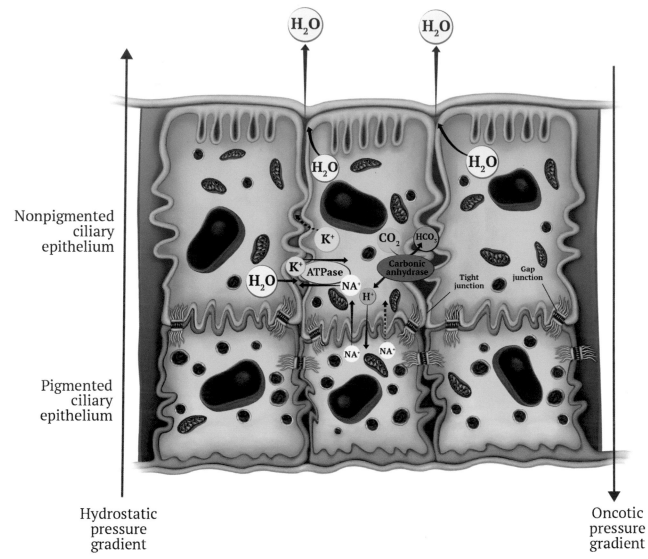

Fig. 13.4 Overview of aqueous humor formation. Aqueous humor is formed from blood plasma by the continuous and active transport of ions from the nonpigmented ciliary epithelium (NPE) cells into the interstitial clefts. The ions in the interstitial clefts establish an osmotic gradient that draws in water. Various solute pumps are involved in the transport, with Na-K adenosine triphosphatase (ATPase) playing a major role. Apical tight junctions in the NPE cells facilitate movement of water into the posterior chamber.

The formation and secretion of aqueous humor **(Fig. 13.4)** cannot be measured directly. However, its movement from the posterior chamber into the anterior chamber is calculated by various methods as the aqueous flow rate.[3] Over the past few decades, fluorophotometry has become the gold standard for measuring aqueous flow. The rate of aqueous flow is less than the rate of aqueous humor secretion because some of it enters the vitreous cavity or is absorbed by the ciliary body, lens, or iris, and is lost to measurement.

Variations in Rate of Aqueous Flow

Aging

The anterior chamber depth and volume diminish and aqueous humor production slows with age.[4] Several key studies reporting an age-related slowing of aqueous flow are summarized in

Table 13.1. On average, the aqueous flow decreases by 0.0015 to 0.003 µL/min/year. This correlates with a 2 to 3.5% reduction every decade after 10 years of age.[5–7] In people over 60 years of age, this decline accelerates to 0.025 µL/min with each year of life or 1 to 2% reduction every year.[8] However, sample size and the age of the volunteers may lead to different conclusions.[9]

The exact mechanism by which aqueous humor flow decreases with age has been the focus of numerous studies. Light microscopic observations[11] show age-related changes in the NPE, stromal blood vessels, and ciliary muscle fibers. The basement membrane of the NPE is thicker in the eyes of subjects between 60 and 70 years of age than in the eyes of subjects younger than 50 years of age. Age-related accumulation of lipofuscin, lysosomes, and lipids occurs in NPE cells. Accumulation of extracellular matrix in the stroma along with thickening of the endothelial basement membrane might impair the supply of nutrients and oxygen to ciliary epithelial cells, thereby reducing aqueous humor formation.[12] It is speculated that other factors, such as neural and hormonal autoregulation, NPE cell count, cel-

Table 13.1 Effect of Aging on Aqueous Flow in Ocular Normotensive Healthy Humans

Reference	Method	Mean age (years)	n	Fa (µL/min)	% Reduction
Toris et al, 1999[5]	Fluorophotometry	25.5 ± 2.4	51	2.9 ± 0.9	3.5% per decade
		66.3 ± 4.6	53	2.4 ± 0.6	
Diestelhorst and Kriegistein, 1992[7]	Fluorophotometry	26.5 ± 3.8	148	2.21 ± 1	2.5% per decade
		65.5 ± 10.5	75	1.89 ± 1.1	
Brubaker et al, 1981[6]	Fluorophotometry	20 - 29	132	2.88 ± 0.67	2.4% per decade
		60 - 69	35	2.49 ± 0.61	
Gaasterland et al, 1978[9]	Tonography	20.8	33	0.92 ± 0.04	
		61.8	18	0.81 ± 0.04*	
Becker, 1954[10]	Tonography	<40	244 eyes	2.0 ± 0.82	
		>60	318 eyes	1.2 ± 0.60	

Abbreviation: Fa, aqueous flow.
*No significant difference.

lular and organelle functioning, and response to cell signaling molecules, might also change as one ages.

Intraocular Pressure

The rate of aqueous humor secretion and flow is relatively insensitive to changes in IOP. When healthy subjects are tilted to a head-down position for 30 minutes to 8 hours, the IOP increases rapidly, remains elevated while in the head-down position, and returns to normal a few minutes after returning to a head-up position. Fluorophotometric aqueous flow remains unchanged despite the short-term variations in IOP associated with body position.[13] Even with chronic IOP elevation, such as in exfoliation syndrome, primary open-angle glaucoma (POAG), and ocular hypertension (OHT),[14–17] the aqueous flow remains relatively constant. Increasing the outflow facility to lower the IOP does not change aqueous production.[18,19] In abnormal reductions of IOP (ocular hypotony), one can find reductions in aqueous flow especially when the hypotony is related to inflammation such as iridocyclitis. When the hypotony is related to injury, such as cyclodialysis cleft, aqueous flow remains normal. Clearly, aqueous humor production is not the regulatory mechanism controlling IOP.

Twenty-Four Hour Rhythms of Aqueous Humor Formation

The aqueous flow shows a predictable rhythm over a 24-hour period (**Table 13.2**). The daytime aqueous flow is 2 to 4 µL/min and at night it slows by almost 50% in healthy volunteers.[5,20] This 24-hour rhythm is maintained in all age groups despite an age-associated decline in aqueous humor production.[21,22] Daytime aqueous flow is normal in OHT and POAG.[23,24] The nocturnal decrease of aqueous flow is present in OHT, but in POAG there is some evidence that the aqueous flow is not decreased as much as in healthy age-matched control subjects.[16,25]

Various hypotheses as to what regulates this 24-hour rhythm of IOP and aqueous flow have been proposed. Downregulation of β-adrenergic activity during sleep might contribute to the nighttime slowing of aqueous flow. This is supported by the finding that β-adrenergic antagonists do not lower IOP at night.[29] Adrenergic agonists such as epinephrine, norepinephrine, isoproterenol, and terbutaline affect aqueous flow but not

in a consistent manner. Patients with Horner's syndrome[30] (oculosympathetic palsy) or bilateral adrenalectomy[31] have no variations in the diurnal or nocturnal aqueous flow when compared with healthy subjects. Corticosteroids, melatonin, cyclic adenosine monophosphate (cAMP), adenosine, arginine-vasopressin, and dopamine have some effect on the daily variations in aqueous flow. Apparently, a complex interaction between the neurohormonal milieu and specialized cells in the ciliary body and suprachiasmatic nucleus determine the aqueous flow rate at any given time.

Aqueous Humor Formation in Pathological States

The major contributing factor to elevated IOP is increased resistance to aqueous outflow through the trabecular meshwork. Studies of various glaucomatous conditions and associated systemic predispositions indicate that aqueous flow is not a contributory factor to the pathology (**Table 13.3**). In a glaucomatocyclitic crisis, aqueous flow measured before the availability of fluorophotometers showed varied results. The presence of flare and cells in the anterior chamber during attacks interferes with fluorescein detection and might have been the reason behind an apparent delay in fluorescein clearance with fluorophotometry. The acute attacks in this condition are not associated with increased aqueous flow rates.[32,33] Aqueous flow is low in eyes of monkeys with experimental iridocyclitis.[34] In addition to enhanced uveoscleral outflow, a low aqueous flow might explain the occurrence of ocular hypotony in patients with long-standing uveitis.[35]

Topography of Aqueous Humor Formation

To aid in conceptualizing aqueous humor formation and calculating secretion rate, the formation of aqueous humor is assumed to be uniform over the entire surface of the ciliary epithelium. However, regional differences in expression of proteins such as Na-K adenosine triphosphatase (ATPase) in the human ciliary processes,[47] and a preferential secretion by the posterior ciliary epithelium and absorption by the anterior ciliary epithelium in rabbits, support the idea that there might be topographic

Table 13.2 Daytime and Nighttime Variation in Aqueous Humor Flow by Fluorophotometry

Reference	Subjects	n	Diurnal Flow (µL/min)	Nocturnal Flow (µL/min)	% Reduction
Vanlandingham et al, 1998[26]	Healthy adults Mean age = 27 years	25	2.97 ± 0.64	1.28 ± 0.30	56
Sit et al, 2008[22]	Healthy adults Mean age = 29 years	34	2.26 ± 0.73	1.12 ± 0.75	50
Liu et al, 2011[27]	Healthy adults Mean age = 57 years	30	2.05 ± 0.87	1.04 ± 0.42	49
Nau et al, 2013[21]	Healthy adults Mean age = 59 years	21	2.48 ± 0.96	1.27 ± 0.63	48
Larsson et al, 1995[16]	Healthy Adults Mean age = 63 years	20	2.39 ± 0.59	1.02 ± 0.27	57
Ziai et al, 1993[24]	Ocular hypertension	20	3.0 ± 0.9	1.1 ± 0.4	63
Fan et al, 2011[23]	Ocular hypertension Mean age = 59 years	30	2.13 ± 0.71	1.11 ± 0.38	48
Toris et al, 2007[25]	Ocular hypertension and POAG Mean age = 62 years	24	2.37 ± 0.11	1.78 ± 0.1	25
Larsson et al, 1995[16]	POAG Mean age = 63 years	20	2.7 ± 0.62	1.29 ± 0.55	52
Larsson et al, 1993[28]	Low tension glaucoma Mean age = 71 years	10	2.48 ± 0.61	1.24 ± 0.45	50

Abbreviation: POAG, primary open-angle glaucoma.

variations in aqueous humor secretion.[48] It is tempting to hypothesize that the topographic variations in aqueous production may be associated with segmental flow of aqueous humor through the trabecular meshwork.

Modifying Aqueous Humor Flow

Pharmacological Modification of Aqueous Flow

Slowing aqueous humor production is an effective way to lower IOP. This is accomplished by carbonic anhydrase inhibitors (CAIs) and β-adrenergic antagonists. Depending on the duration of treatment, α-adrenergic agonists have a combined effect on production and drainage.

Carbonic anhydrase inhibitors are sulfonamide drugs that have been used systemically for decades to lower IOP. Inhibition of the carbonic anhydrase enzyme in ciliary epithelium blocks the active transport of sodium, chloride, and bicarbonate into the posterior chamber, thereby slowing the osmotic movement of water and hence reducing aqueous humor formation. The newer topical CAIs are less efficacious than oral CAIs but have fewer side effects and are additive when combined with IOP-lowering drugs of other classes.[49]

β-adrenergic antagonists inhibit the synthesis of cAMP in the ciliary epithelium to reduce aqueous humor formation. Long-term therapy is associated with tachyphylaxis and "drift," wherein almost 50% of patients treated with β-blockers as monotherapy will require addition of a different class of drug to maintain the target IOP.[50]

Epinephrine stimulates both α- and β-adrenergic receptors. Ciliary muscle contraction with improvement in trabecular outflow facility is thought to be the primary IOP-lowering mechanism. Reduction in aqueous flow secondary to vasoconstriction has been documented by several studies, but the effect has not been consistent. The final rate of aqueous flow with epinephrine treatment is likely to entail the combined activation of several different adrenergic receptors at any one time. However, epinephrine is no longer commercially available for ocular use in the United States. Dipivefrin hydrochloride, a prodrug of epinephrine, has the same IOP-lowering effect with a better adverse effect profile. This class of drug is rarely prescribed today because of better options from which to choose.

Apraclonidine is an α₂-adrenergic agonist with some α₁ activity. IOP reduction is secondary to vasoconstriction and decreases in aqueous flow. With continued use, it increases trabecular outflow facility and lowers episcleral venous pressure.[51] With time the IOP effect diminishes and side effects intensify. This has limited its usefulness to less than 1 month of treatment.

Brimonidine is a highly selective α₂-agonist that reduces aqueous flow due to ciliary vasoconstriction. This effect is lost within 1 month of use, after which an increase in uveoscleral outflow is the main IOP-lowering mechanism.[52]

Several new classes of aqueous flow suppressants are under investigation for potential glaucoma therapy. Forskolin increases intracellular cAMP, thereby reducing aqueous humor production.[53] Cannabinoid derivatives act on the CB1 receptor, the main cannabinoid receptor expressed in the inflow and outflow pathways. The main hypotensive effect is thought to be increased outflow facility secondary to Schlemm's canal dilation. Because

Table 13.3 Aqueous Flow Rate in Pathological States

Disorder	IOP	Fa	Reference
OHT	↑	↔	17,24
POAG	↑	↔ day, ↑ night	16
Normal tension glaucoma	↔	↔	28
Pigment dispersion syndrome with normal IOP	↔	↔	36,37
Pigment dispersion syndrome with OHT	↑	↔	36,37
Exfoliation syndrome with normal IOP	↔	↔	14,38
Exfoliation syndrome with OHT	↑	↔	14
Glaucomatocyclitic crisis	↑	↑	39–41
		↔	32,33,42
Myotonic dystrophy	↓	↔	43
Diabetes mellitus, type 1	↔	↓	44,45
Cystic fibrosis	↔	↔	46

Abbreviations: Fa, aqueous flow; IOP, intraocular pressure; OHT, ocular hypertension; POAG, primary open-angle glaucoma.
Source: Modified from Toris CB. Aqueous humor dynamics and intraocular pressure elevation. In: Shaarawy TM, ed. Glaucoma, 2nd ed. New York: Elsevier Limited; 2014:47–56; Table 62. Reprinted with permission.
Note: Arrows indicate values greater than (↑), unchanged from (↔) or less than (↓) healthy age-matched controls.

the receptors are present in the uveal tract, cannabinoids might also modulate aqueous flow and uveoscleral outflow.[54] Serotonergic compounds and angiotensin II have a combined agonist-antagonist action and target multiple sites. They are thought to lower IOP by either increasing uveoscleral outflow or reducing aqueous flow. Their derivatives act preferentially on select receptor subtypes resulting in the observed effects. **Table 13.4** lists the pharmacological agents that reduce aqueous humor formation.

Cilio-Ablative Microinvasive Glaucoma Procedures

Numerous factors greatly impact the medical management of glaucoma, including patients' failure to follow dosing instructions, the high cost of treatment, and loss of IOP efficacy with chronic dosing. To circumvent these problems, nonpharmacological and surgical methods have been developed to lower the IOP. Some of these procedures ablate the ciliary epithelium and reduce formation of aqueous humor to reach the IOP goal.

Destruction of the ciliary epithelium and associated blood vessels (ciliodestruction) is primarily reserved for advanced cases of glaucoma. Various types of energy including heat (cyclodiathermy), cold (cyclocryotherapy), or lasers (xenon, argon, neodymium:yttrium-aluminum-garnet [Nd-YAG]), and diode; or laser cyclophotocoagulation) are delivered to the ciliary body from outside (transscleral) or within (endoscopy) the globe.

Table 13.4 Medical Strategies for Reducing Aqueous Humor Production

Current medical strategies

Carbonic anhydrase inhibitors

- Dorzolamide (Trusopt)
- Brinzolamide (Azopt)
- Acetazolamide* (Diamox)
- Methazolamide* (Neptazane)

β-blockers

- Timolol (Betimol, Timoptic, Istalol)
- Carteolol (Ocupress)
- Metipranolol (OptiPranolol)
- Levobunolol (Betagan, AKBeta)
- Betaxolol (Betoptic)
- Nipradilol

Sympathomimetic agents

- Brimonidine (Alphagan, Alphagan P)
- Apraclonidine (Iopidine)
- Dipivefrine (Propine)
- Epinephrine (Epifrin, Gluacon)

Fixed-dose combinations

- Dorzolamide/timolol (Cosopt, Cosopt PF)
- Brimonidine/timolol (Combigan)
- Brinzolamide/brimonidine (Simbrinza)

Future medical strategies

- Forskolin
- Cannabinoids
- Serotonin
- Angiotensin II

*Oral medication.

In the 1980s, transscleral cyclophotocoagulation (TSCPC) was developed using laser energy to destroy the ciliary epithelia. This procedure is fraught with unpredictability, as well as complications such as inflammation and phthisis. Less invasive and targeted procedures have been developed recently to reduce aqueous humor formation. These procedures are discussed below.

Endocyclophotocoagulation

Endocyclophotocoagulation (ECP) overcomes many of the limitations of TSCPC.[55] It uses a single endoscopic microprobe containing an 810-nm diode laser with a 175-W xenon light source,

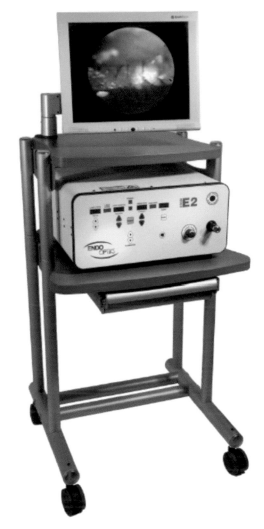

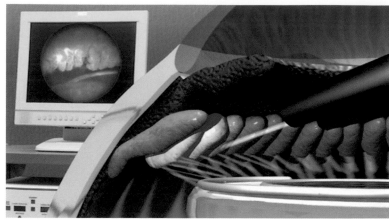

Fig. 13.5 Endoscopic cyclophotocoagulation (ECP). **(a)** The laser console and monitor for visualizing the procedure. The endoscopy probe is connected to the console by three separate cables, one each for the diode laser, video camera, and xenon light source. A foot pedal controls laser delivery. **(b)** During anterior ECP, the probe enters through a clear corneal incision. The probe tip is positioned just beneath the pupillary border, and laser energy is applied to the ciliary processes. The treatment distance is usually 2 mm for treating six ciliary processes. With treatment, the ciliary processes whiten and contract.

a helium neon laser aiming beam, and video imaging (EndoOptiks, Little Silver, NJ; **Fig. 13.5**). The ciliary body can be visualized directly and ablated through a clear corneal incision; hence, it is also called "anterior ECP." The pigment in the ciliary epithelial layer preferentially absorbs this wavelength of energy, making ECP a highly targeted therapy. The most common indication for ECP has been mild to moderate POAG in combination with phacoemulsification.

The IOP-lowering effects of ECP can range from 3.9 to 28.3 mm Hg (18 to 68%) with a mean final IOP of 15.6 mm Hg. Coagulative necrosis of the ciliary epithelium secondary to diode laser burns with reduction in aqueous humor secretion seems to be the main mechanism.[56] These burns also extend into the stroma causing hyalinization and atrophy of the ciliary processes.[57] Rabbits treated with either TSCPC or ECP had acute occlusive vasculopathy. The ECP group showed some areas of reperfusion over time.[58] Direct injury to the ciliary epithelium and indirect injury from ischemia appear to reduce aqueous humor formation. Tissue disruption may also increase uveoscleral outflow and further lower IOP. This effect is more likely to occur with TSCPC than with ECP.

ECP Plus

ECP Plus **(Fig. 13.6)** targets the ciliary body through a pars plana approach. Under direct visualization, the anterior and posterior ciliary processes, together with the anterior 1 to 2 mm of the pars plana, are ablated. Eyes with uncontrolled glaucoma that have failed multiple glaucoma procedures like trabeculectomy, aqueous shunt, transscleral cyclophotocoagulation, and anterior ECP benefit from ECP plus. A long-term study found an IOP reduction of 78% by the end of 12 and 24 months, a 77% reduction in the mean number of glaucoma medications and an adverse-effect profile similar to that for anterior ECP.[59] The treatment is thought to disrupt vascular elements involved in aqueous humor production. Photocoagulation of the pars plana in addition to the anterior and posterior ciliary processes seems to destroy more of the blood vessels and ciliary epithelium. Disruption of the epithelial layers and part of the stroma might open up interstitial spaces to increased uveoscleral drainage. Local prostaglandin release might also play a role in increasing outflow through the uveoscleral route. The role of pars plana epithelium in aqueous humor production is questionable.

High-Intensity Focused Ultrasound

High-intensity focused ultrasound (HIFU) uses ultrasound-generated heat to disrupt the ciliary epithelium, reduce aqueous humor formation, and lower IOP. The commercially available EyeOP1 system (EyeTechCare, Rillieux la Pape, France; **Fig. 13.7**) has been approved by Conformité Européene (CE Mark) for treatment of refractory glaucoma. The transducer in the system

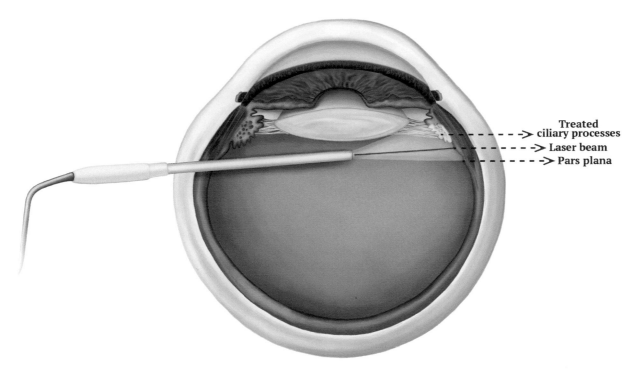

Fig. 13.6 ECP plus. The pars plana approach for ECP is used in pseudophakic/aphakic eyes that have undergone multiple unsuccessful glaucoma procedures. The ciliary processes and the anterior 1 to 2 mm of the pars plana is treated with laser energy.

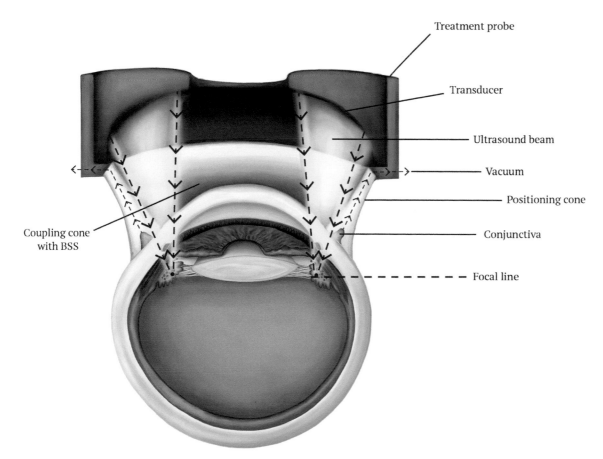

Fig. 13.7 High-intensity focused ultrasound (HIFU). The coupling cone is centered on the eyeball. The treatment probe is ring shaped and has six piezoelectric transducers that deliver highly focused therapeutic ultrasound. The treatment probe is placed over the coupling cone and the cavity is filled with buffered saline solution (BSS). The ultrasound beam has its focal point on the ciliary body. At the focal point, the ultrasound energy coagulates target tissue by controlled hyperthermia.

contains piezoelectric units that convert electrical energy into vibrations and finally to therapeutic high-intensity focused ultrasound. At the target point, these waves generate heat and cause coagulative necrosis without damaging the surrounding tissues. The concept underlying HIFU is ultrasound circular cyclocoagulation (UC³). It involves the use of a circular treatment probe with six separate miniaturized 21-MHz ultrasound microtransducers to simultaneously treat the entire ciliary body. The ultrasound energy can be titrated and duration of treatment varied to reach the desired IOP.

The first clinical pilot study on HIFU was completed in 2011 on 12 human eyes with refractory glaucoma. IOP was significantly reduced from a mean preoperative value of 37.9 ± 10.7 mm Hg to a mean postoperative value of 24.7 ± 8.5 mm Hg at 6 months. Four patients with prior corneal abnormalities developed postoperative superficial punctate keratitis and central superficial corneal ulceration, No major complications occurred during and after treatment.[60] EyeMUST is an ongoing, large multicenter clinical trial in Europe to assess the outcome of HIFU in a large population of patients.

Fluid in the suprachoroidal space and reduced IOP have been found in eight of 12 eyes treated with HIFU.[60] A study on rabbits found the tissues of the drainage pathway to be free of cellular debris and inflammatory cells. Necrosis in the ciliary epithelium extended into the deeper layers. With time, there was regeneration of a single nonsecretory layer of epithelium. Focal disruption of the blood vessels was present in treated areas of the ciliary body and pars plana. No damage was noticed in the adjacent untreated areas. Most interestingly, fluid-filled spaces between the ciliary body and sclera were present in the treated sectors and persisted for as long as 6 months. Scleral thinning occurred as a late event in almost all treated sectors.[61]

Ciliary epithelial necrosis and involution of the ciliary processes reduce the surface area for aqueous humor secretion. However, this may not be the only mechanism of IOP reduction. Detection of suprachoroidal fluid provides indirect evidence that uveoscleral outflow might be increased. This could be secondary to the release of endogenous prostaglandins and the formation of drainage tracks between thinned areas of the ciliary body.

Other Directed Ultrasonic Devices

Two new IOP-lowering sonic and ultrasonic instruments are currently under development for potential clinical use. A deep wave trabeculoplasty (DWT) device from OcuTherix (Stillwater, MN) applies low-amplitude and sonic-range frequency mechanical oscillations to the perilimbal region beneath which lies the trabecular meshwork.[62] The Therapeutic Ultrasound for Glaucoma (TUG, Eyesonix, Long Beach, CA) device emits a low-frequency ultrasonic energy (20,000 to 100,000 Hz) to the perilimbal region.[63] Several mechanisms have been proposed by which these devices lower the IOP. Local hyperthermia leads to release of small heat shock proteins and beneficial cytokines, resulting in initiation of a response in the TM that reduces IOP. The ultrasound causes stretch and relaxation of the TM, which aids in dislodgment of debris trapped in this tissue. The above processes are thought to reduce tissue resistance and improve outflow facility. The effects of ultrasound procedures on the ciliary body and ciliary processes are not known but it is possible that these nearby structures are altered by the treatment.

Future Considerations

Aqueous humor has the important function of nourishing the ocular anterior segment structures and removing metabolites while leaving the visual pathway clear. The blood–aqueous barrier, tight junctions on the iris epithelium, and anterior movement of aqueous humor through the pupil decreases the amount of proteins and metabolites entering the posterior chamber. Hence, the composition of aqueous humor in the posterior chamber, where it is first formed, is different from that in the anterior chamber angle near the trabecular meshwork. The reason for this compartmentalization and the impact of long-term reduction in aqueous humor formation from physical or pharmacological treatments are important avenues for further research.

Fluorophotometric measurement of aqueous flow into the anterior chamber is the current gold standard for estimating aqueous humor production despite several limitations. It should be emphasized that aqueous flow does not equal aqueous humor production, as some aqueous humor diffuses into the ciliary body, vitreous cavity, lens, and iris stroma, and is not detected by the measurement. Some ocular surgeries, such as phacoemulsification, alter the aqueous flow patterns and invalidate some of the assumptions in the methods. Patients with a history of ocular surgery are usually excluded from fluorophotometry studies, leaving a gap in our knowledge of how such surgeries affect aqueous humor dynamics. Designing techniques to directly measure aqueous humor production rather than aqueous flow will help fill these gaps, provide directions for advancing glaucoma therapy, and clarifying the role of aqueous humor production in health and disease.

References

1. Tamm ER, Lütjen-Drecoll E. Ciliary body. Microsc Res Tech 1996;33:390–439

2. Kiel JW, Hollingsworth M, Rao R, Chen M, Reitsamer HA. Ciliary blood flow and aqueous humor production. Prog Retin Eye Res 2011;30:1–17

3. Gabelt BT, Kaufman PL. Production and flow of aqueous humor. In: Levin LA, Nilsson SFE, Ver Hoeve J, Wu SM, Kaufman PL, Alm A, eds. Adler's Physiology of the Eye, 11th ed. Edinburgh: Elsevier; 2011:274

4. Fontana ST, Brubaker RF. Volume and depth of the anterior chamber in the normal aging human eye. Arch Ophthalmol 1980;98:1803–1808

5. Toris CB, Yablonski ME, Wang YL, Camras CB. Aqueous humor dynamics in the aging human eye. Am J Ophthalmol 1999;127:407–412

6. Brubaker RF, Nagataki S, Townsend DJ, Burns RR, Higgins RG, Wentworth W. The effect of age on aqueous humor formation in man. Ophthalmology 1981;88:283–288

7. Diestelhorst M, Kriegistein GK. Does aqueous humor secretion decrease with age? Int Ophthalmol 1992;16:305–309

8. Becker B. The decline in aqueous secretion and outflow facility with age. Am J Ophthalmol 1958;46(5 Part 1):731–736

9. Gaasterland D, Kupfer C, Milton R, Ross K, McCain L, MacLellan H. Studies of aqueous humour dynamics in man. VI. Effect of age upon parameters of intraocular pressure in normal human eyes. Exp Eye Res 1978;26:651–656

10. Becker B. Decrease in intraocular pressure in man by a carbonic anhydrase inhibitor, Diamox: a preliminary report. Am J Ophthalmol 1954;37:13–15

11. Okuyama M, Okisaka S, Kadota Y. [Histological analysis of aging ciliary body]. Nippon Ganka Gakkai Zasshi 1993;97:1265–1273

12. Schlötzer-Schrehardt U, Wirtz PM, Müller HG, Lang GK, Naumann GO. [Morphometric analysis of age-dependent changes in the human ciliary body]. Fortschr Ophthalmol 1990;87:59–68

13. Carlson KH, McLaren JW, Topper JE, Brubaker RF. Effect of body position on intraocular pressure and aqueous flow. Invest Ophthalmol Vis Sci 1987;28:1346–1352

14. Johnson TV, Fan S, Camras CB, Toris CB. Aqueous humor dynamics in exfoliation syndrome. Arch Ophthalmol 2008;126:914–920

15. Beneyto Martin P, Fernández Vila PC, Pérez Martinez TM, Aliseda Peréz D. A fluorophotometric study on the aqueous humor dynamics in primary open angle glaucoma. Int Ophthalmol 1992;16:311–314

16. Larsson LI, Rettig ES, Brubaker RF. Aqueous flow in open-angle glaucoma. Arch Ophthalmol 1995;113:283–286

17. Toris CB, Koepsell SA, Yablonski ME, Camras CB. Aqueous humor dynamics in ocular hypertensive patients. J Glaucoma 2002;11:253–258

18. Brubaker RF, Liesegang TJ. Effect of trabecular photocoagulation on the aqueous humor dynamics of the human eye. Am J Ophthalmol 1983; 96:139–147

19. Yablonski ME, Cook DJ, Gray J. A fluorophotometric study of the effect of argon laser trabeculoplasty on aqueous humor dynamics. Am J Ophthalmol 1985;99:579–582

20. Reiss GR, Lee DA, Topper JE, Brubaker RF. Aqueous humor flow during sleep. Invest Ophthalmol Vis Sci 1984;25:776–778

21. Nau CB, Malihi M, McLaren JW, Hodge DO, Sit AJ. Circadian variation of aqueous humor dynamics in older healthy adults. Invest Ophthalmol Vis Sci 2013;54:7623–7629

22. Sit AJ, Nau CB, McLaren JW, Johnson DH, Hodge D. Circadian variation of aqueous dynamics in young healthy adults. Invest Ophthalmol Vis Sci 2008;49:1473–1479

23. Fan S, Hejkal JJ, Gulati V, Galata S, Camras CB, Toris CB. Aqueous humor dynamics during the day and night in volunteers with ocular hypertension. Arch Ophthalmol 2011;129:1162–1166

24. Ziai N, Dolan JW, Kacere RD, Brubaker RF. The effects on aqueous dynamics of PhXA41, a new prostaglandin F2 alpha analogue, after topical application in normal and ocular hypertensive human eyes. Arch Ophthalmol 1993;111:1351–1358

25. Toris CB, Zhan G, Fan S, et al. Effects of travoprost on aqueous humor dynamics in patients with elevated intraocular pressure. J Glaucoma 2007;16:189–195

26. Vanlandingham BD, Maus TL, Brubaker RF. The effect of dorzolamide on aqueous humor dynamics in normal human subjects during sleep. Ophthalmology 1998;105:1537–1540

27. Liu H, Fan S, Gulati V, et al. Aqueous humor dynamics during the day and night in healthy mature volunteers. Arch Ophthalmol 2011;129:269–275

28. Larsson LI, Rettig ES, Sheridan PT, Brubaker RF. Aqueous humor dynamics in low-tension glaucoma. Am J Ophthalmol 1993;116:590–593

29. Gulati V, Fan S, Zhao M, Maslonka MA, Gangahar C, Toris CB. Diurnal and nocturnal variations in aqueous humor dynamics of patients with ocular hypertension undergoing medical therapy. Arch Ophthalmol 2012;130:677–684

30. Larson RS, Brubaker RF. Isoproterenol stimulates aqueous flow in humans with Horner's syndrome. Invest Ophthalmol Vis Sci 1988;29:621–625

31. Maus TL, Young WF Jr, Brubaker RF. Aqueous flow in humans after adrenalectomy. Invest Ophthalmol Vis Sci 1994;35:3325–3331

32. Grant WM. Clinical measurements of aqueous outflow. Am J Ophthalmol 1951;34:1603–1605

33. Mansheim BJ. Aqueous outflow measurements by continuous tonometry in some unusual forms of glaucoma. AMA Arch Opthalmol 1953;50:580–587

34. Toris CB, Pederson JE. Aqueous humor dynamics in experimental iridocyclitis. Invest Ophthalmol Vis Sci 1987;28:477–481

35. Johnson D, Liesegang TJ, Brubaker RF. Aqueous humor dynamics in Fuchs' uveitis syndrome. Am J Ophthalmol 1983;95:783–787

36. Brown JD, Brubaker RF. A study of the relation between intraocular pressure and aqueous humor flow in the pigment dispersion syndrome. Ophthalmology 1989;96:1468–1470

37. Toris CB, Haecker NR, Teasley LA, Zhan G, Gulati V, Camras CB. Aqueous humor dynamics in pigment dispersion syndrome. Arch Ophthalmol 2010;128:1115–1118

38. Gharagozloo NZ, Baker RH, Brubaker RF. Aqueous dynamics in exfoliation syndrome. Am J Ophthalmol 1992;114:473–478

39. Spivey BE, Armaly MF. Tonographic findings in glaucomatocyclitic crises. Am J Ophthalmol 1963;55:47–51

40. Sugar HS. Heterochromia iridis with special consideration of its relation to cyclitic disease. Am J Ophthalmol 1965;60:1–18

41. Nagataki S, Mishima S. Aqueous humor dynamics in glaucomato-cyclitic crisis. Invest Ophthalmol 1976;15:365–370

42. Hart CT, Weatherill JR. Gonioscopy and tonography in glaucomatocyclitic crises. Br J Ophthalmol 1968;52:682–687

43. Khan AR, Brubaker RF. Aqueous humor flow and flare in patients with myotonic dystrophy. Invest Ophthalmol Vis Sci 1993;34:3131–3139

44. Larsson LI, Pach JM, Brubaker RF. Aqueous humor dynamics in patients with diabetes mellitus. Am J Ophthalmol 1995;120:362–367

45. Lane JT, Toris CB, Nakhle SN, Chacko DM, Wang YL, Yablonski ME. Acute effects of insulin on aqueous humor flow in patients with type 1 diabetes. Am J Ophthalmol 2001;132:321–327

46. McCannel CA, Scanlon PD, Thibodeau S, Brubaker RF. A study of aqueous humor formation in patients with cystic fibrosis. Invest Ophthalmol Vis Sci 1992;33:160–164

47. Ghosh S, Hernando N, Martín-Alonso JM, Martin-Vasallo P, Coca-Prados M. Expression of multiple Na+,K(+)-ATPase genes reveals a gradient of isoforms along the nonpigmented ciliary epithelium: functional implications in aqueous humor secretion. J Cell Physiol 1991;149:184–194

48. McLaughlin CW, Zellhuber-McMillan S, Macknight AD, Civan MM. Electron microprobe analysis of rabbit ciliary epithelium indicates enhanced secretion posteriorly and enhanced absorption anteriorly. Am J Physiol Cell Physiol 2007;293:C1455–C1466

49. Toris CB, Zhan GL, Yablonski ME, Camras CB. Effects on aqueous flow of dorzolamide combined with either timolol or acetazolamide. J Glaucoma 2004;13:210–215

50. Marquis RE, Whitson JT. Management of glaucoma: focus on pharmacological therapy. Drugs Aging 2005;22:1–21

51. Toris CB, Tafoya ME, Camras CB, Yablonski ME. Effects of apraclonidine on aqueous humor dynamics in human eyes. Ophthalmology 1995;102:456–461

52. Toris CB, Gleason ML, Camras CB, Yablonski ME. Effects of brimonidine on aqueous humor dynamics in human eyes. Arch Ophthalmol 1995;113:1514–1517

53. Wagh VD, Patil PN, Surana SJ, Wagh KV. Forskolin: upcoming antiglaucoma molecule. J Postgrad Med 2012;58:199–202

54. Hudson BD, Beazley M, Szczesniak AM, Straiker A, Kelly ME. Indirect sympatholytic actions at β-adrenoceptors account for the ocular hypotensive actions of cannabinoid receptor agonists. J Pharmacol Exp Ther 2011;339:757–767

55. Kaplowitz K, Kuei A, Klenofsky B, Abazari A, Honkanen R. The use of endoscopic cyclophotocoagulation for moderate to advanced glaucoma. Acta Ophthalmol (Copenh) 2015;93:395–401

56. Assia EI, Hennis HL, Stewart WC, Legler UF, Carlson AN, Apple DJ. A comparison of neodymium: yttrium aluminum garnet and diode laser transscleral cyclophotocoagulation and cyclocryotherapy. Invest Ophthalmol Vis Sci 1991;32:2774–2778

57. Cavens VJ, Gemensky-Metzler AJ, Wilkie DA, Weisbrode SE, Lehman AM. The long-term effects of semiconductor diode laser transscleral cyclophotocoagulation on the normal equine eye and intraocular pressure(a). Vet Ophthalmol 2012;15:369–375

58. Lin SC, Chen MJ, Lin MS, Howes E, Stamper RL. Vascular effects on ciliary tissue from endoscopic versus trans-scleral cyclophotocoagulation. Br J Ophthalmol 2006;90:496–500

59. Tan JC, Francis BA, Noecker R, Uram M, Dustin L, Chopra V. Endoscopic cyclophotocoagulation and pars plana ablation (ECP-plus) to treat refractory glaucoma. J Glaucoma 2016;25:e117–e122

60. Aptel F, Charrel T, Lafon C, et al. Miniaturized high-intensity focused ultrasound device in patients with glaucoma: a clinical pilot study. Invest Ophthalmol Vis Sci 2011;52:8747–8753

61. Aptel F, Béglé A, Razavi A, et al. Short- and long-term effects on the ciliary body and the aqueous outflow pathways of high-intensity focused ultrasound cyclocoagulation. Ultrasound Med Biol 2014;40:2096–2106

62. Krader CG, Kahook M. DWT shows promise for reducing IOP. Ophthalmology Times 2014; Jan 15

63. Schwartz D, Samples J, Korosteleva O. Therapeutic ultrasound for glaucoma: clinical use of a low-frequency low-power ultrasound device for lowering intraocular pressure. J Ther Ultrasound 2014;2:15

14 How Does Cyclodestruction Affect Diurnal Intraocular Pressure Variation?

Peng Lei and Joseph Caprioli

It is well accepted that intraocular pressure (IOP) fluctuates through the 24-hour light/dark cycle. Some argue that IOP peaks in the morning because of the morning rise in cortisol,[1] whereas others assert that IOP peaks in the evening due to the supine position during sleep.[2] IOP fluctuations may explain why some patients continue to experience visual field decline despite seemingly adequate IOP control during clinic appointments. Some studies have found that the range of IOP fluctuation is greater in patients with glaucoma versus normal subjects,[3] and that it may even be an independent risk factor for glaucoma progression.[4]

Several studies have looked at the effect of medical, laser, and surgical therapies on IOP fluctuation. Over a 24-hour period, prostaglandins appear superior to timolol, brimonidine, and dorzolamide in decreasing IOP.[5] Timolol showed good diurnal IOP reduction but poor nocturnal IOP reduction.[6] Both argon laser trabeculoplasty (ALT)[7] and selective laser trabeculoplasty (SLT)[8] effectively decrease mean IOP and the range of IOP. Interestingly, in some cases in which SLT did not achieve significant IOP reduction during clinic hours, nocturnal IOPs were diminished after laser treatment.[9] Compared with medical therapy, surgical therapy with trabeculectomy may be more successful in blunting IOP fluctuation.[10,11]

Studies that measure IOP fluctuation have several limitations. Due to the logistical difficulties, they typically have small sample sizes, IOPs may be measured for only 8 to 20 hours during a 24-hour period, or IOPs may be measured every 2 to 6 hours instead of every hour. Also, study protocols may differ in how IOP measurements are made (sleep center versus home monitoring), in what body position nocturnal IOPs are measured (supine versus sitting), or how much time elapses between awakening and IOP measurement. It has been suggested that there may be a transient IOP spike immediately after awakening.[12] Current study models for 24-hour IOP measurement in humans are not physiological because of the lack of a truly continuous IOP monitoring system.

To date, there are no published studies that have addressed the effect of cryotherapy, transscleral cyclophotocoagulation, or endocyclophotocoagulation on IOP fluctuations. It is possible that by decreasing the mean IOP, there will be a reduction in the range of IOP fluctuations.[12] However, whether there will be a reduction in the latter that is independent of the former is unclear. Current studies seem to suggest that therapies aimed at increasing aqueous outflow, such as prostaglandins, ALT/SLT, and trabeculectomy, have a greater effect on IOP fluctuations. Cyclodestructive procedures, which decrease aqueous production, may be similar to timolol, whose effect is greatest during diurnal IOP and least during nocturnal IOP.

References

1. Weitzman ED, Henkind P, Leitman M, Hellman L. Correlative 24-hour relationships between intraocular pressure and plasma cortisol in normal subjects and patients with glaucoma. Br J Ophthalmol 1975;59:566–572

2. Liu JH, Kripke DF, Hoffman RE, et al. Nocturnal elevation of intraocular pressure in young adults. Invest Ophthalmol Vis Sci 1998;39:2707–2712

3. Drance SM. Diurnal variation of intraocular pressure in treated glaucoma. Arch Ophthalmol 1963;70:302–311

4. Nouri-Mahdavi K, Hoffman D, Coleman AL, et al; Advanced Glaucoma Intervention Study. Predictive factors for glaucomatous visual field progression in the Advanced Glaucoma Intervention Study. Ophthalmology 2004;111:1627–1635

5. Stewart WC, Konstas AG, Nelson LA, Kruft B. Meta-analysis of 24-hour intraocular pressure studies evaluating the efficacy of glaucoma medicines. Ophthalmology 2008;115:1117–1122.e1

6. Liu JH, Kripke DF, Weinreb RN. Comparison of the nocturnal effects of once-daily timolol and latanoprost on intraocular pressure. Am J Ophthalmol 2004;138:389–395

7. Agarwal HC, Sihota R, Das C, Dada T. Role of argon laser trabeculoplasty as primary and secondary therapy in open angle glaucoma in Indian patients. Br J Ophthalmol 2002;86:733–736

8. Guzey M, Arslan O, Tamcelik N, Satici A. Effects of frequency-doubled Nd:YAG laser trabeculoplasty on diurnal intraocular pressure variations in primary open-angle glaucoma. Ophthalmologica 1999;213:214–218

9. Lee AC, Mosaed S, Weinreb RN, Kripke DF, Liu JH. Effect of laser trabeculoplasty on nocturnal intraocular pressure in medically treated glaucoma patients. Ophthalmology 2007;114:666–670

10. Medeiros FA, Pinheiro A, Moura FC, Leal BC, Susanna R Jr. Intraocular pressure fluctuations in medical versus surgically treated glaucomatous patients. J Ocul Pharmacol Ther 2002;18:489–498

11. Konstas AG, Topouzis F, Leliopoulou O, et al. 24-hour intraocular pressure control with maximum medical therapy compared with surgery in patients with advanced open-angle glaucoma. Ophthalmology 2006;113:761–5.e1

12. Wilensky JT. The role of diurnal pressure measurements in the management of open angle glaucoma. Curr Opin Ophthalmol 2004;15:90–92

15 How Does Cyclodestruction Affect the Blood–Aqueous Barrier?

Chi-Hsin Hsu and Shan C. Lin

In the past, cyclodestruction was performed by various methods, including surgical excision, diathermy, cryotherapy, and laser. Nowadays, laser cyclophotocoagulation (CPC) is the principal method for reducing aqueous inflow.[1] However, all of these treatments cause a certain level of damage to the nonpigmented layer of the ciliary epithelium, which forms the blood–aqueous barrier (BAB), and thus might break down the immune privilege status within the eye.

Transscleral diode cyclophotocoagulation (TCP) is a popular choice because of its relatively good tolerance and efficacy, which may be due to its theoretical advantages of effective penetration and selective absorption by the pigmented tissue of the ciliary body. A newer method to directly photocoagulate the ciliary processes within the eye using direct endoscopic visualization, known as endoscopic diode cyclophotocoagulation (ECP), is increasingly used to treat refractory glaucoma in eyes with relatively intact central visual acuity.[2]

Transscleral diode cyclophotocoagulation has been shown to induce significant damage (including coagulative necrosis) to the pars plicata and surrounding tissues, including the sclera, iris, and pars plana.[3] However, during ECP treatment, typically only the raised processes are treated without affecting the "valleys" between processes, which could control the damage so that it is more specific and localized. Furthermore, laser energy is applied to each process just until shrinkage and whitening occur, which may avoid excessive energy (when the process explodes or "pops" with bubble formation), leading to excessive inflammation and further breakdown of the BAB.[1]

However, there have not been any studies to assess how these cyclophotocoagulative procedures affect the functional BAB, but indirect evidence enables us to speculate based on histological and clinical findings. Our group at University of California, San Francisco (UCSF) studied the acute and late effects of TCP and ECP on the histology and ciliary blood flow in rabbits.[4] Endoscopic fluorescein angiography (EFA) was used to assess blood flow within the treated ciliary processes at each of the following time points: immediate, 1 day, 1 week, and 1 month after laser. Both TCP and ECP resulted in severely reduced or nonexistent blood flow at the immediate, 1 day, and 1 week time points. At 1 month, the treatment spots in TCP eyes remained severely underperfused with a similarly depressed intensity of fluorescence (36% of control levels), but ECP eyes demonstrated partial reperfusion of the ciliary processes with the intensity increased to 80% of control levels. The histopathology of both ECP- and TCP-treated eyes showed substantial shrinkage, coagulative necrosis, and disorganization of the architecture of the ciliary processes at 1 day, with loss of epithelium and shrinkage and avascularity of the stroma. By 1 month after ECP, the histopa-thology of the treated eyes still showed disorganized, disrupted, and scarred stromal tissue and absence of normal epithelial architecture, with a few showing continuing exudative response. However, deeper ciliary vessels appeared patent, and consistent with the physiological reperfusion seen with EFA. In contrast, we found that TCP caused severe disruption of the ciliary processes and iris root up to 1 month after treatment. Pantcheva et al[5] observed acute histological changes in human autopsy eyes after ECP and diode TCP, and also greater tissue disruption seen with TCP as compared with ECP, although both treatments caused nonpigmented epithelial damage, which means breakdown of the BAB happened in both groups.

When the BAB is broken, we speculate that the risk of sympathetic ophthalmia (SO) might increase. Studies showed that the incidence of SO following treatment with CPC was only 0.001 to 0.07%.[6,7] However, all 12 cases that have been reported were all post-TCP treatment, and there have been no ECP-related cases.[6,7] In addition, if the postcorneal transplanted eye is no longer immune privileged, we would expect the graft failure rate to be higher after CPC. One study compared the graft failure rate among trabeculectomy, glaucoma drainage device surgery, and CPC for treating intractable glaucoma after penetrating keratoplasty.[8] The results showed that the graft failure rate was higher in the TCP group than the other two groups, which indirectly supports the notion of disruption of the BAB by CPC. However, no ECP-induced corneal graft failure cases have been reported yet.

Huang et al[9] assessed the effect of CPC on survival of corneal grafts and found that nonspecific anterior chamber inflammation and corneal endothelial cell density reduction 6 months after treatment were significantly less in the ECP than the TCP group. These findings indirectly suggest that TCP compromises the BAB more than ECP does. However, the lack of ECP-related cases may simply be due to the fact that it is a relatively new procedure.

In contrast, others may speculate that despite disruption of the BAB in both procedures, the negative impact of breakdown of the barrier may be less in ECP-treated eyes due to reperfusion of the ciliary processes. Paradoxically, sustained ciliary avascularity in post-TCP eyes may indirectly limit immune responses that lead to corneal graft failure.

In conclusion, because ECP seems to selectively target the ciliary epithelium without markedly altering other structures or causing damage as severe as TCP, we speculate that the severity of BAB breakdown should be less in ECP. However, it is still unclear how cyclophotocoagulation affects the BAB chronically. Future prospective trials using laser flare photometry, which is the only objective and quantitative method for reliably measuring intraocular inflammation, with long-term posttreatment follow-up may be required to better answer this question.

References

1. Lin S. Endoscopic cyclophotocoagulation. Br J Ophthalmol 2002;86:1434–1438

2. Ishida K. Update on results and complications of cyclophotocoagulation. Curr Opin Ophthalmol 2013;24:102–110

3. Lin SC. Endoscopic and transscleral cyclophotocoagulation for the treatment of refractory glaucoma. J Glaucoma 2008;17:238–247

4. Lin SC, Chen MJ, Lin MS, Howes E, Stamper RL. Vascular effects on ciliary tissue from endoscopic versus trans-scleral cyclophotocoagulation. Br J Ophthalmol 2006;90:496–500

5. Pantcheva MB, Kahook MY, Schuman JS, Noecker RJ. Comparison of acute structural and histopathological changes in human autopsy eyes after endoscopic cyclophotocoagulation and trans-scleral cyclophotocoagulation. Br J Ophthalmol 2007;91:248–252

6. Albahlal A, Al Dhibi H, Al Shahwan S, Khandekar R, Edward DP. Sympathetic ophthalmia following diode laser cyclophotocoagulation. Br J Ophthalmol 2014;98:1101–1106

7. Edwards TL, McKelvie P, Walland MJ. Sympathetic ophthalmia after diode laser cyclophotocoagulation: now an issue in informed consent. Can J Ophthalmol 2014;49:e102–e104

8. Ayyala RS, Pieroth L, Vinals AF, et al. Comparison of mitomycin C trabeculectomy, glaucoma drainage device implantation, and laser neodymium: YAG cyclophotocoagulation in the management of intractable glaucoma after penetrating keratoplasty. Ophthalmology 1998;105:1550–1556

9. Huang T, Wang YJ, Chen JQ, Yu MB, Jin CJ, Wang T. [Effect of endocyclophotocoagulation on survival of corneal grafts]. Zhonghua Yan Ke Za Zhi 2007;43:313–318

16 What Roles Do Posterior Ciliary Processes and Pars Plana Play in Aqueous Formation?

Handan Akil, Brian A. Francis, James C. Tan, and Robert Noecker

Glaucoma is the most common cause of irreversible blindness worldwide.[1] Although the pathophysiology of glaucoma is multifactorial, the treatment strategy essentially depends on lowering the intraocular pressure (IOP). This is accomplished either by increasing aqueous outflow or decreasing aqueous production. Aqueous humor is secreted by ciliary processes of the ciliary body pars plicata region.[2] Aqueous then exits the eye through the trabecular meshwork or the uveoscleral outflow pathways. Because the ciliary body produces aqueous humor, it is a major target of medical and surgical interventions for glaucoma. The ciliary processes are not uniform in structure and function along their anteroposterior length, and if they are to be treated, there may be value in selectively targeting treatment to different regions of the processes.

The aqueous humor is a clear fluid filling the anterior and posterior chambers of the eye. It is one of the fundamental components of the eye's optical system in providing a transparent and colorless medium between the cornea and the lens. Additionally, it provides nutrition, removes excretory products from metabolism, transports neurotransmitters, stabilizes the ocular structure, and contributes to homeostasis of the avascular ocular tissues such as the posterior cornea, trabecular meshwork, lens, and anterior vitreous. The aqueous humor also permits inflammatory cells and mediators to circulate in the eye in pathological conditions, and drugs to be distributed to different ocular structures.[3,4]

The ciliary body is an annular structure on the inner wall of the globe, positioned just behind the posterior surface of the iris. On cross section, its shape is that of a right-angled triangle, ~ 6 mm in length. The base of the ciliary body is home to the ciliary muscle, the contraction and relaxation of which causes the lens to become thicker or thinner for near or distance vision. The ciliary body is highly vascular and supplied by the anterior ciliary and long posterior ciliary vessels anastomosing as a major arterial circle in the ciliary body.[5,6] The surface of the ciliary body is elaborated into a series of ridges named ciliary processes.[7] The ciliary processes start anteriorly where they are contiguous with the posterior iris, and taper posteriorly to merge into the pars plana. Anterior and posterior ciliary processes are not separate structures but refer, respectively, to the part of the process lying in front of the equator of the lens and to the part lying behind it.

The ciliary processes consist of a central core of loose connective tissue stroma covered by a specialized double-layered epithelium of nonpigmented ciliary epithelia (NPCE) and pigmented ciliary epithelia (PCE). The ciliary epithelium extends from just posterior to the iris, where it is a highly convoluted structure termed the pars plicata, toward the retina, where the ciliary epithelium flattens and becomes the pars plana.[2] The NPCE is a monolayer of columnar cells located internally facing the posterior chamber in direct contact with aqueous, and the PCE is a monolayer of cuboidal cells containing numerous melanin granules located more externally facing the ciliary body stroma. The two monolayers interact with each other along their apical surfaces and rest on basement membranes along their basal surfaces. The NPCE and PCE work in concert during aqueous formation.[8] Tight junctions between NPCE cells form a barrier between vascularized and avascular ocular tissues that is extremely important for maintaining optical transparency of the anterior segment.[7]

It is assumed that elaboration of the ciliary body into ridges in the form of ciliary processes is a strategy to pack more capillaries into the tissue to serve the ciliary epithelial cells, optimize aqueous production, and nourish avascular tissues of the anterior segment.[7] Studies in rabbits show that blood supply to different regions of the ciliary body and processes occurs through separate vascular territories.[9] Although interspecies ciliary body anatomic variation is seen,[9] it represents a conceptual framework for more selectively treating the tissue.[10] Vascular territories may be divided as those supplying (1) anterior iridial ciliary processes, (2) prelenticular major ciliary processes, and (3) postlenticular minor ciliary processes between posterior extensions of the major ciliary processes. These morphologically separate vascular territories also respond differently to pharmacological probing, indicating region-specific vascular supply and vasoregulation of the ciliary processes along their anterior-posterior axis.[11] The pars plana has a vascular network of its own that anastomoses with the peripheral choriocapillaris.

The nonpigmented epithelial layer of the ciliary body secretes aqueous humor and regulates transepithelial transfer of solutes from the stroma to the posterior chamber, establishing an osmotic gradient, with water moving in response to that gradient. Main mechanisms involved in aqueous humor formation are diffusion, ultrafiltration, and active secretion. The first two processes are passive and do not require cellular energy.[12] Diffusion and ultrafiltration are responsible for the accumulation of plasma ultrafiltrate in the stroma, behind tight junctions of the nonpigmented epithelium.[13] Active secretion, the major contributor to aqueous formation, occurs by driving selective transcellular movement of molecules across the blood–aqueous barrier's concentration gradient, mediated by protein transporters in the epithelial membrane,[14] especially Na^+-K^+–activated adenosine triphosphatase (ATPase).[15] The aqueous humor resembles blood plasma in composition with some exceptions: a much higher concentration of ascorbic acid, lactate, and bicarbonate, and a much lower concentration of glucose and protein in aqueous humor compared with plasma.[16]

Morphologically, epithelia of the anterior and posterior nonpigmented ciliary processes appear similar,[17] but they apparently fulfill different functions as secretion across the ciliary epithelium is not uniform. A degree of aqueous processing and absorption occurs in the anterior processes facilitated by Na$^+$ absorption through Na$^+$ channels and Na$^+$/H$^+$ exchange.[18] This means that net secretion is weighted toward the posterior region of ciliary processes. The anterior-posterior regional difference provides novel possibilities for regulating net aqueous secretion[18,19] by selective therapy. For example, selective stimulation of reabsorption by the anterior epithelium might provide a novel approach for reducing the net rate of aqueous formation and intraocular pressure.

Histological studies demonstrate that expression of proteins and biologically active peptides shows regional selectivity across the ciliary epithelium.[20] One example is the higher expression of certain Na$^+$-K$^+$–activated ATPase isoforms in NPE cells of the anterior than of the posterior ciliary processes of young calves.[15] Another example is the preferential localization of Na$^+$-K$^+$-2Cl$^-$ cotransporters to the basolateral edge of PCE cells in the anterior processes of young calves.[21] The possibility has been raised that such regional differences have functional implications,[21] and that the rate of aqueous humor formation is not uniform over the ciliary epithelial surface. However, small size, structural complexity, and difficult in vivo access to the ciliary epithelium have impeded progress in experimentally testing that proposition.

Better understanding regional variations in the role of ciliary epithelium in aqueous humor secretion is important in developing new strategies for managing glaucoma. Medical strategies may involve agents that suppress aqueous secretion posteriorly and stimulate reabsorption anteriorly. Surgical strategies could selectively target highly secretory regions of the ciliary body. Recently, endoscopic-guided techniques such as endoscopic cyclophotocoagulation (ECP) that lower the IOP by targeted ciliary body ablation have gained popularity. Clinically, they have shown effective IOP lowering with a good safety profile in treating uncontrolled and refractory forms of glaucoma.[22]

In a recent study, the clinical outcomes of ECP by a pars plana approach with treatment of the pars plana and posterior ciliary processes (ECP plus) was reported.[10] It was concluded that IOP lowering was relatively sustained after treatment with ECP plus in eyes with refractory glaucoma in which maximally tolerated medical treatment and multiple glaucoma surgeries had failed to control IOP. The authors postulated that extensive photocoagulation of the secretory ciliary epithelium from the pars plicata to the pars plana resulted in markedly reduced aqueous humor production. Additionally, this ECP approach affected the regional blood supply and vascular territories of the ciliary body, causing more profound aqueous suppression that may have been accompanied by increased aqueous escape through the pars plana to the uveoscleral outflow route. Selective targeting of posterior ciliary processes, a primary site for secretion, while sparing anterior reabsorption sites[18] may have been a further reason.

Reducing the rate of aqueous humor formation is an important strategy for lowering IOP in glaucoma. Regional differences of the ciliary epithelium regulating net aqueous humor inflow should be evaluated to provide novel medical and surgical approaches for managing glaucoma.

References

1. Resnikoff S, Pascolini D, Etya'ale D, et al. Global data on visual impairment in the year 2002. Bull World Health Organ 2004;82:844–851

2. Lutjen-Drecoll E. Functional morphology of the ciliary epithelium. In: Lutjen-Drecoll E, ed. Basic Aspects of Glaucoma Research. New York: F.K. Schattauer; 1982;69–87

3. Hogan MH, Alvarado JA, Weddell JE. The limbus. In: Hogan MH, Alvarado JA, Weddell JE, eds. Histology of the Human Eye. Philadelphia: WB Saunders; 1971

4. Sires B. Orbital and ocular anatomy. In: Wright KW, ed. Textbook of Ophthalmology. Baltimore: Williams & Wilkins; 1997

5. Aiello AL, Tran VT, Rao NA. Postnatal development of the ciliary body and pars plana. A morphometric study in childhood. Arch Ophthalmol 1992; 110:802–805

6. Goel M, Picciani RG, Lee RK, Bhattacharya SK. Aqueous humor dynamics: a review. Open Ophthalmol J 2010;4:52–59

7. Delamere NA. Ciliary Body and Ciliary Epithelium. Adv Organ Biol 2005; 10:127–148

8. Francis BA, Kwon J, Fellman R, et al. Endoscopic ophthalmic surgery of the anterior segment. Surv Ophthalmol 2014;59:217–231

9. Morrison JC, DeFrank MP, Van Buskirk EM. Comparative microvascular anatomy of mammalian ciliary processes. Invest Ophthalmol Vis Sci 1987;28:1325–1340

10. Tan JC, Francis BA, Noecker R, Uram M, Dustin L, Chopra V. Endoscopic cyclophotocoagulation and pars plana ablation (ECP-plus) to treat refractory glaucoma. J Glaucoma 2016;25:e117–e122

11. Funk R, Rohen JW. SEM studies on the functional morphology of the rabbit ciliary process vasculature. Exp Eye Res 1987;45:579–595

12. Millar C, Kaufman PL. Aqueous humor: secretion and dynamics. In: Tasman W, Jaeger EA, eds. Duane's Foundations of Clinical Ophthalmology. Philadelphia: Lippincott-Raven; 1995

13. Gabelt BT, Kaufman PL. Aqueous humor hydrodynamics. In: Hart WM, ed. Adler's Physiology of the Eye, 9th ed. St. Louis: Mosby; 2003

14. Yamaguchi Y, Watanabe T, Hirakata A, Hida T. Localization and ontogeny of aquaporin-1 and -4 expression in iris and ciliary epithelial cells in rats. Cell Tissue Res 2006;325:101–109

15. Coca-Prados M, Sanchez-Torres J. Molecular approaches to the study of the Na+-K+-ATPase and chloride channels in the ocular ciliary epithelium. In: Civan MM, ed. The Eye's Aqueous Humor. San Diego: Academic Press; 1998:25–53

16. Kinsey VE. The chemical composition and the osmotic pressure of the aqueous humor and plasma of the rabbit. J Gen Physiol 1951;34:389–402

17. Oyster CW. The Human Eye: Structure and Function. Sunderland, MA: Sinauer Associates; 1999

18. McLaughlin CW, Zellhuber-McMillan S, Macknight AD, Civan MM. Electron microprobe analysis of rabbit ciliary epithelium indicates enhanced secretion posteriorly and enhanced absorption anteriorly. Am J Physiol Cell Physiol 2007;293:C1455–C1466

19. McLaughlin CW, Zellhuber-McMillan S, Peart D, Purves RD, Macknight AD, Civan MM. Regional differences in ciliary epithelial cell transport properties. J Membr Biol 2001;182:213–222

20. Ghosh S, Hernando N, Martín-Alonso JM, Martin-Vasallo P, Coca-Prados M. Expression of multiple Na+,K(+)-ATPase genes reveals a gradient of isoforms along the nonpigmented ciliary epithelium: functional implications in aqueous humor secretion. J Cell Physiol 1991;149:184–194

21. Dunn JJ, Lytle C, Crook RB. Immunolocalization of the Na-K-Cl cotransporter in bovine ciliary epithelium. Invest Ophthalmol Vis Sci 2001;42:343–353

22. Francis BA, Berke SJ, Dustin L, Noecker R. Endoscopic cyclophotocoagulation combined with phacoemulsification versus phacoemulsification alone in medically controlled glaucoma. J Cataract Refract Surg 2014;40:1313–1321

ID Subconjunctival Filtration

17 Structure and Mechanisms of Subconjunctival Outflow

Tony Wells and Michael A. Coote

Why Include Subconjunctival Filtration in a Book About Alternative Glaucoma Surgery Approaches?

Glaucoma surgery has been the concern of ophthalmologists for over a century. It is widely recognized that glaucoma surgery is imperfect, and as glaucoma surgeons we strive to improve it. Existing techniques are refined in new versions of the surgery (e.g., "trabeculectomy 9.15"), as new approaches and devices become available.

But new approaches and devices need a context. The current standards of modern trabeculectomy are adjunctive antimetabolite surgery and glaucoma drainage device (GDD) surgery. Both types of surgery entail drainage of the aqueous humor to the sub-Tenon's space or subconjunctival space as their chief function. Both types of surgery entail drainage of the aqueous humor to the sub-Tenon's space or subconjunctival space as their chief function. Both types have been well studied and their advantages and disadvantages described.

New approaches seek to address the acknowledged deficiencies in existing strategies, often with sophisticated work-arounds. New approaches to glaucoma surgery are judged by whether they have improved efficacy without increasing the financial costs. As described in the next section, glaucoma filtration to the subconjunctival space initially had some disadvantages, but it has been refined over the years so that the risks and complications have been minimized. New approaches must prove themselves to be at least as good as established surgeries. Trabeculectomy, which is now widely acknowledged to be superior to full-thickness surgery, took more than 15 years to become a standard of care.

There are many challenges in developing new approaches to glaucoma surgery, such as the considerable financial costs of procedures, the high learning curves for new procedures, and the smaller numbers of procedures performed as more patients are treated with the improving nonsurgical options. An effect of fewer glaucoma patients needing surgery is that surgeons will have less experience, which is further diluted if each surgeon performs multiple techniques. As each procedure is performed less frequently, it also becomes increasingly difficult to acquire enough data to meaningfully assess the surgical outcomes. If a surgeon is performing a particular procedure fewer than 30 times a year, an 80% success rate is practically indistinguishable from a 90% success rate. Surgeons will then be guided by a perception that a certain procedure generally has a good outcome but that in some patients the procedure fails or causes problems.

A Brief History of Approaches to Subconjunctival Filtration

Intraocular pressure (IOP) rises because the resistance to aqueous outflow rises. Increasing outflow from the eye either by restoring trabecular function or by bypassing the meshwork has been the aim of glaucoma surgeons for over 150 years.

The first effective glaucoma surgery is attributed to Albrecht von Graefe, who in 1857 reported curing acute glaucoma with an iridectomy. He went on to report that one in five eyes developed a cyst or a scar at the site of the incision; he considered such a cyst to be of little consequence other than a cause of irritation and possible infection. Von Graefe generally recommended excising blebs if they formed. Only a decade later, Louis de Wecker took an opposite view, and reported that blebs had value in lowering the IOP; he recommended performing a formal sclerostomy (with iridectomy) to increase the likelihood of a bleb forming.

It is worth noting that these procedures were done before topical anesthesia or tonometry was available. It was not until the early 20th century that better surgical strategies, techniques, facilities, and instrumentation led to refinements in the surgical principles and approaches.

In the early 20th century, iridencleisis was widely performed. The iris incarceration in the sclerostomy increased the likelihood of continued patency, and prevented the iris from obstructing the sclerostomy. The importance of a patent sclerostomy was understood by the midpoint of the 20th century, but all the operations at that time were full-thickness procedures, culminating in Harold Scheie's procedure **(Fig. 17.1)**, which was routinely performed from the late 1950s until the late 1960s, when trabeculectomy with a guarding flap was described by Sugar in 1961 and later by Cairns in 1968.

Cairns originally proposed that a trabeculectomy would enable aqueous humor to enter the exposed end of Schlemm's canal. Soon after his original description, it was deduced that the dominant mechanism of pressure lowering was actually external filtration. In spite of this, the term *trabeculectomy* persisted, and the operation proved safer and more predictable than full-thickness procedures, but it entailed a higher failure rate due to scarring of the trapdoor and subconjunctival space.

Both trabeculectomy and nonpenetrating glaucoma surgery (e.g., deep sclerectomy) were developed to eliminate the filtration bleb. But it has been demonstrated that both are best at controlling IOP when subconjunctival drainage is present. The current state-of-the-art glaucoma surgery still requires glaucoma surgeons to be "blebologists."

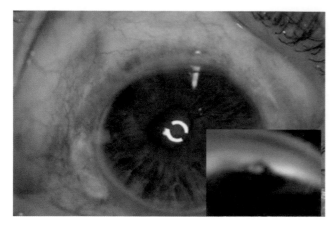

Fig. 17.1 Scheie's procedure. A patient with congenital glaucoma was operated on 52 years ago with a modified Scheie's procedure. The patient's intraocular pressure (IOP) is 10 mm Hg 52 years postprocedure with no medications. Iris incarceration, which was a variation based on the iridencleisis procedure, can be seen on this gonio photo.

Seminal trials in the use of 5-fluorouracil (5-FU) and later mitomycin C (MMC) as wound-modulating agents improved the success rate of trabeculectomy and enabled surgeons to improve the postoperative healing.

Although implants to shunt aqueous subconjunctivally were trialed as far back as 1912 with Emil Zorab's silk seton,[1] the first modern glaucoma drainage device was developed by Tony Molteno, then in South Africa, which he reported in the *British Journal of Ophthalmology* in 1969 and in simultaneous papers showing animal experimentation and the first human results.[2,3] The original Molteno implant was the first to have a tube and plate design, with the plate acting as a spacer to enable fluid to percolate into the subconjunctival tissue and be absorbed. Subsequent iterations and changes in the design of tubes have led to some improvements, but the basic design of a channel for egress and a plate for distribution and absorption remains unchanged.

More recently, the focus has returned to the trabecular space and Schlemm's canal, with the development of so-called minimally invasive glaucoma surgery with its range of procedures and implants, which offer bypasses or manipulations of portions of the outflow pathway. Significant challenges exist if manipulation of the existing pathways is to result in resuscitation of normal outflow. Although the principal pathology appears to be in the trabecular meshwork or juxtacanalicular tissue, downstream collapse of Schlemm's canal and collecting ducts frustrates our attempt to perform what Cairns envisaged in his original paper in the late 1960s.

Subconjunctival filtration is still the method with the longest track record of use and of proven success in achieving sustained and significant IOP lowering. It is a clinically versatile procedure by the surgeon even in the postoperative phase.

How Successful Is Modern Subconjunctival-Drainage Glaucoma Surgery?

In the 1990s, two major randomized controlled trials, the Collaborative Initial Glaucoma Treatment Study (CIGTS)[4] and the Advanced Glaucoma Intervention Study (AGIS),[5] included surgical treatment arms involving trabeculectomy. Although surgical techniques have since evolved to improve success and decrease adverse outcomes, these studies are still considered the benchmark data from that era. Trabeculectomy precipitated cataract formation in many patients, but it offered an unqualified (no adjunctive medications or further surgery) IOP control success rate of ~ 80%. Although postsurgery complication rates were up to 50%, almost all complications resolved without intervention and seemed not to compromise the outcome.

The decades of refinement in both GDD and trabeculectomy surgery have delivered progressive improvements in outcomes. A patient who undergoes one of these procedures has a very good chance, after a couple of months of intensive management, of long-term controlled IOP on fewer or no glaucoma medications (**Fig. 17.2**). Landers et al[6] published 20-year trabeculectomy follow-up data in 2012 that demonstrated that 60% of trabeculectomy eyes maintained IOP control with no topical medication. Several older studies also show good success rates at 10 years, on the order of ~ 70%.[7-10]

Yet in the Tube Versus Trabeculectomy (TVT) study,[11] trabeculectomy had a 5-year success rate of only 50%, reflecting about a 10% failure rate per year. The GDD failure rate was about half of that, 5% per year. The reason for the discrepancy in trabeculectomy success rates is not clear, but possible explanations include the following: (1) newer medications, in particular prostaglandin analogues, are successfully treating less recalcitrant eyes without the need for surgery, so that surgeons are operating on only

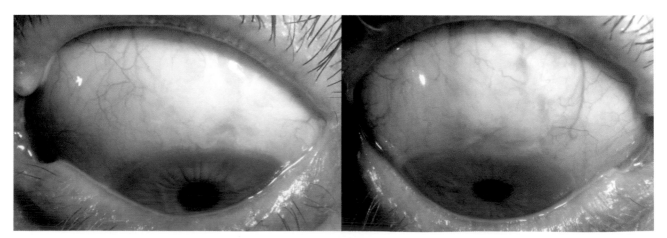

Fig. 17.2 Bilateral trabeculectomy procedures performed 37 years ago. Currently, IOP is 10 mm Hg in the right eye and 11 mm Hg in the left eye. A trabeculectomy's effects are maintained for many years in some eyes. These blebs have good morphology and function.

severe cases; (2) newer medications are delaying surgery in all eyes, so that the cumulative dosage of medications and conjunctival propensity to scar is greater; (3) newer medications may change conjunctival physiology or fibroblast activation, predisposing patients to more aggressive scaring.

There are many reports on glaucoma surgical outcomes in the literature, but few of the studies are of high quality. The majority of older reports were limited by being small or retrospective studies or by having inconsistent reporting, population issues, publication bias, variations in surgical technique, lack of masking, or variable success criteria, or were performed simultaneously with other surgery (e.g., cataract). Since the publication of the Guidelines on Design and Reporting of Glaucoma Surgical Trials produced by the World Glaucoma Association, which delineate excellent research standards, publication quality has increased.

The TVT[11] was a high-quality randomized controlled trial (RCT) that provided some of our best information on success rates for alternative procedures for subconjunctival drainage. There has been criticism that the reported complication rates are higher than previous rates; this may in part reflect the better documentation of issues in a competitive RCT that might not otherwise be recorded in routine clinical practice and therefore missed in retrospective studies. With more recent advances in surgical techniques and postoperative care, for example via the Moorfields Safer Surgery System,[12] more current studies may start to report improved outcomes.

Recently, Kirwan et al[13] published a series of 428 procedures with more than 2 years of follow-up. This was a multicenter study pooling data from nine glaucoma units with fellowship-trained glaucoma specialists who followed a broadly similar surgical approach, including fornix-based conjunctival flap, adjustable or releasable sutures, and antimetabolite use. A subgroup analysis used inclusion and assessment criteria based on the TVT study; the unqualified success rate (without IOP-lowering medications) was 85%, with qualified success rates (including use of IOP-lowering medications) of 92%. In three patients, vision decreased by three or more Snellen lines (one of these patients had declined treatment for hypotony maculopathy); 31% had cataract surgery subsequently; bleb leaks were identified in 13.6%, with 95% of these in the first weeks after surgery; 7.2% of cases had an IOP reading of less than 5 mm Hg between 6 months and the final postsurgery visit. These results depended on relatively intensive postsurgical management, with 27% having subconjunctival 5-FU injections, 16% requiring bleb needling, and 5% receiving additional sutures. Perhaps the most interesting aspect of the study was the low rate of postoperative complications related to scleral flap construction and suturing. Shallow anterior chamber was seen in 0.9%, with none flat, and choroidal detachment was seen in 5%. By comparison, CIGTS and AGIS reported shallow anterior chambers in 13 to 15% of patients after trabeculectomy.

Introduction of the Ex-Press glaucoma implant (Alcon Laboratories, Fort Worth, TX) without flow restriction faced the same difficulties as early glaucoma implants and unguarded full-thickness surgery. It was intended to drain directly under the conjunctiva, but it had a high incidence of hypotony[14,15] (see discussion of cystic blebs and full-thickness drainage, below), which is expected of shunts that freely drain aqueous to the subconjunctival space without any flow restriction. The obvious modification to the Ex-Press implantation, placing it under a scleral flap, was quickly adopted. Comparative studies between trabeculectomy and trabeculectomy with an Ex-Press implant placed beneath the scleral flap have shown short-term advantages, especially better early anterior chamber (AC) and IOP control, but no benefit in long-term outcomes. Kirwan et al's[13] results suggest that with due care to flap construction and adjustable/

releasable suture use, addition of an expensive implant may not bring enough additional value, although we may yet see further technique refinement, just as we have with trabeculectomy and GDD surgery.

Established GDD implants such as the Baerveldt, Molteno, and Ahmed implants were thought to entail higher risks of complications than trabeculectomy, but this has been challenged by the TVT study. At 3 years the serious complication rate was very similar, and GDDs narrowly outperformed trabeculectomy at 5 years.[11] An issue that has yet to be fully explored is the possibility of late corneal decompensation from GDD-induced endothelial trauma. Another issue is that the implants may be less cost-effective than trabeculectomy.[16]

Direct comparisons between IOP outcomes of different GDD implants and comparisons of GDD with trabeculectomy are challenging. Plate size is a major determinant of IOP control after tube implant surgery, but the relationship is not consistent, and it is not clear how it translates to subconjunctival filtration without a plate, except perhaps for the commonly held notion that the larger the area of filtration, the lower the IOP. Despite the TVT results, many surgeons expect IOP after trabeculectomy to be lower than after tube surgery. An IOP in the single digits is relatively uncommon after GDD implantation, but it is not uncommon after successful trabeculectomy. The effect of bleb management in the early months after trabeculectomy is relatively undocumented. There is likely to be enormous variability in the surgical approach among glaucoma surgeons and little information on outcomes arising from such variations.

Subconjunctival filtration with or without a GDD makes for quite different blebs due to several factors: shifting of the region of subconjunctival filtration away from the limbus, fibrosis due to a foreign body response or implant micromovements, and a plate that sets bleb space dimensions that may limit the area of aqueous absorption into the periocular tissues and orbital lymphatic drainage. Some glaucoma surgeons prefer to avoid IOP-lowering medications with a functioning trabeculectomy bleb because reducing flow and collapsing the bleb may decrease its drainage function and compromise the long-term outcomes.

Conjunctival Bleb Morphology

Bleb Types and Implications for Subconjunctival Drainage and IOP

Blebs around GDDs are easiest to delineate, as the plate determines the bleb area. A fibrous capsule determines resistance to flow, and typically little subconjunctival flow occurs outside this area once the bleb is established. These are the easiest blebs to study from a biomechanical perspective because variability is small and zones are typically well defined. There is consensus that increasing plate (bleb) size leads to a lower IOP,[17] but the relationship is not always observed.[18]

Trabeculectomy blebs are much more variable, but are described parsimoniously as one of only a few variants—diffuse, cystic, and encapsulated—with the latter often being an indication for postsurgical management. The range of possible appearances and implications are far wider than this coarse grading would suggest. For example, a significant prognostic factor for long-term bleb and trabeculectomy survival is the conjunctival vascularity surrounding the central elevated area, which is not even addressed in the classic variants above.[19] Bleb grading systems, such as the Moorfields Bleb Grading System (www.blebs.net) can capture these systems for advanced clinical or research use.

Diffuse blebs are the most desirable **(Fig. 17.3)**. They are usually associated with good IOP control and a low risk of bleb-related infection, discomfort, or failure. It is thought that such

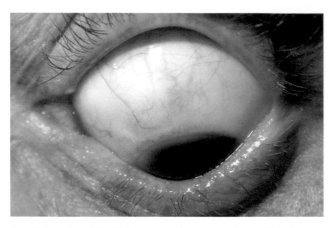

Fig. 17.3 Diffuse bleb. This is optimal bleb morphology, with little or no risk of bleb infection or dysesthesia. The IOP in this eye is 11 mm Hg on no medications, more than 5 years after trabeculectomy with mitomycin C (MMC). Although using a large MMC treatment area and a scleral flap that is significantly larger than the sclerostomy can increase the likelihood of this result, reliably achieving this outcome is difficult.

blebs facilitate fluid drainage by having a sufficiently large although relatively unscarred area by which aqueous may escape the bleb. Possible routes of aqueous drainage from the subconjunctival space are the vascular or lymphatic systems of the conjunctiva–Tenon's complex or a transconjunctival route into the tears. The exact mechanisms and destination(s) of subconjunctival aqueous drainage remain unclear and warrant further study.

Diffuse blebs may extend circumferentially, causing an appearance of chemosis or sporadic subconjunctival bleeds,[20] which are concerning for the patient but self-limiting and benign. At a microscopic level, the blebs have a subconjunctival space contiguous with the anterior chamber via a fistula, covered by a noncondensed Tenon's capsule beneath the conjunctiva.

Cystic blebs (**Fig. 17.4**) are common, much less desirable, thin-walled, demarcated, and avascular. The mechanisms by

which they occur are poorly understood. Although antimetabolites are frequently implicated, these bleb types were common with full-thickness surgery prior to antimetabolite use. Therefore, surgical site construction and local effects, in particular aqueous jets from full-thickness drainage and the effects on tissue remodeling,[21,22] have a significant impact. These blebs may cause discomfort and predispose to potentially devastating bleb-related ocular infections that are, fortunately, quite uncommon, considering how common it is to see thin-walled avascular blebs. Cystic blebs often have quite low IOPs, which is helpful for glaucoma control but carries the potential for pathology if they leak or become infected.

Encysted blebs (**Fig. 17.5**) are defined as being thick-walled and demarcated, typically with a raised IOP. They pose particular management issues but tend to occur only within a brief timeframe after surgery; most have morphed into either diffuse or cystic blebs either spontaneously or as a result of treatment within a few months of surgery.

Microcysts

Microcysts (**Fig. 17.6**) are commonly seen in functioning blebs and are often not evenly distributed throughout the entire bleb area, probably reflecting regional transmural flow variations. They represent conjunctival epithelial and subepithelial edema. The visible cysts are extracellular fluid collections indicating tissue saturation with aqueous. Such collections may increase the diffusion distance and metabolic stress of the tissue. The interstitial fluid needs to be absorbed into a functioning capillary system via oncotic drivers across the capillary walls. The clinical sign of microcysts suggests reasonable egress of aqueous from the eye, porosity of the subconjunctival tissue, and favorable filtration predictive of long-term surgical success,[23] albeit with some tissue stress from chronic interstitial edema.

A caveat is that not all well-functioning blebs have visible microcysts, and microcysts may be present when the bleb is functioning poorly with high IOP. Microcysts demonstrate transconjunctival filtration and subconjunctival flow, but on their own they are not evidence of bleb function commensurate with adequately reduced IOP.

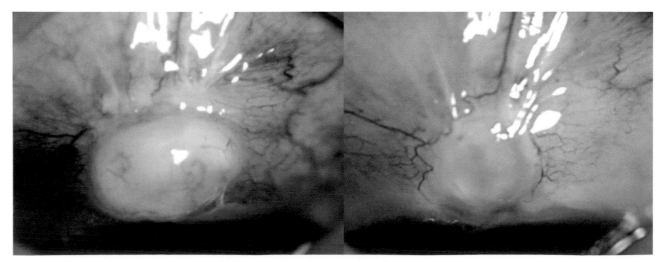

a · b

Fig. 17.4 Avascular, demarcated (often referred to as cystic bleb) in development: at 4 months **(a)** and at 1 year **(b)**. These blebs often have good IOPs but are at risk for most of the undesirable bleb-related complications. Bleb morphology is not static, as is often assumed; despite good bleb grading systems developed more than 10 years ago, and 30 years of studying trabeculectomy surgery, there is no failsafe way of avoiding these complications.

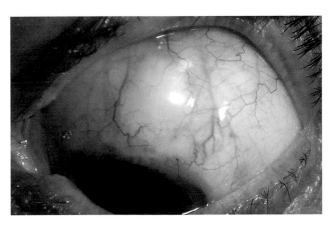

Fig. 17.5 Encysted bleb. A dome-shaped cap of Tenon's tissue has formed over the scleral flap, causing IOP to be 20 mm Hg. These blebs are usually amenable to medical management but occasionally require injected antifibrosis medications or needling procedures.

Bleb Function

The bleb is the single most important determinant of the long-term success of trabeculectomy. Remodeling of the sclerostomy and scleral flap area occurs several weeks after surgery and results in establishment of a fistula between the anterior chamber and the sub-Tenon's space through which aqueous flows. In the vast majority of cases, resistance to aqueous outflow—the inverse of outflow facility—and IOP are determined not by the fistula but by characteristics of the sub-Tenon–episcleral fascia interface, here referred to as the bleb tissues.

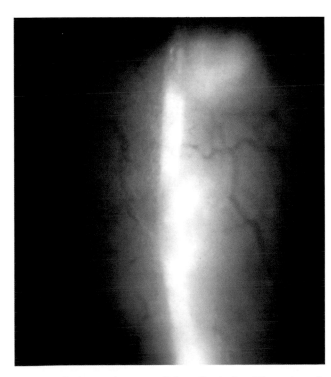

Fig. 17.6 A microcyst is seen on slit-lamp illumination. Microcysts are in the epithelium and subepithelial tissues and represent extracellular edema, which is often interpreted as evidence of successful subconjunctival filtration.

Modeling Blebs and Their Stressors

A hydraulic engineering assessment of glaucoma surgery identifies three main areas: egress of aqueous from the eye through the wall of the eye and its distribution underneath the flap; lateral traverse flow resistance and the porosity of the subconjunctival tissue; and absorption of aqueous from the bleb and surrounding tissues. Failure of any of these three areas will impact surgery-induced outflow facility and IOP control. We will focus on subconjunctival tissue porosity and lateral flow resistance. Engineering modeling of blebs **(Fig. 17.7)**[24] identified lateral flow resistance (and thus bleb wall porosity) as key determinants of outflow resistance and factors most likely to change over time.[25] Lateral flow resistance determines the physical appearance of the bleb and the IOP, although the two are not always as tightly linked as we might like.

Too high a resistance of the bleb tissues to lateral flow within the subconjunctival space induces high stress in the bleb wall and creates or increases encystment and failure of the drainage procedure. Too low a resistance leads to hypotony and encircling blebs. Having just the right amount of lateral flow resistance is associated with a bleb that has form, structure, and boundaries commensurate with maintaining reduced, therapeutic IOP.

It is possible to transfer that resistance to a GDD, but the device needs to take into account tissue changes over time, and the ultimate surgically induced outflow facility is the sum total of resistance resulting from the device, the tissues, and their interaction. This is why many surgeons implanting GDDs adopt resistance systems, ranging from absorbable external tube ligatures to intraluminal stents and valved implants for the early implantation phase. Later, a process of conjunctiva–Tenon complex scarring, encapsulation, and remodeling around the GDD plate sets the subconjunctival outflow resistance and IOP.

Resistance in the subconjunctival space is determined by bleb tissue porosity. The tissue porosity may vary with the direction of flow in the subconjunctival space, and, unscarred conjunctiva mostly have a low level of resistance to circumferential flow. Bleb tissue porosity is determined mostly by extracellular matrix elements.[26] In the subconjunctival tissue, this includes the laying down of collagen and glycosaminoglycans, which play clinically relevant roles in determining bleb tissue porosity and outflow function. Modeling studies suggest that ongoing loss of bleb tissue porosity further aggravates the loss of bleb function, leading to greater transluminal pressure and higher shear stresses in areas of the bleb that are still retaining good porosity.[27,28] This in turn may lead to further reduction in bleb wall porosity and higher IOP.

Understanding the stresses on the tissues and managing and manipulating the conditions influencing lateral flow resistance and bleb tissue porosity are key tasks for the glaucoma surgeon during the intraoperative the postoperative periods.

Bleb Complications

Trabeculectomy bleb complications may be subdivided into two groups: blebs that predispose to failure via scarring, such as primary bleb failure and encapsulation; and blebs that risk infection and hypotony or cause discomfort, often in association with having a thin wall. The latter are typically of greater concern, but judicious use of antimetabolites and needling-revision procedures often solves or helps prevent these issues.

Thin-walled or cystic blebs that may leak and risk becoming infected are the most concerning long-term complication. There is a 30% risk of severe consequences if bleb-related endophthalmitis occurs. Fortunately, these are uncommon, with the risk of bleb-related infection on the order of 1 to 2% at 10 years.[29] Of

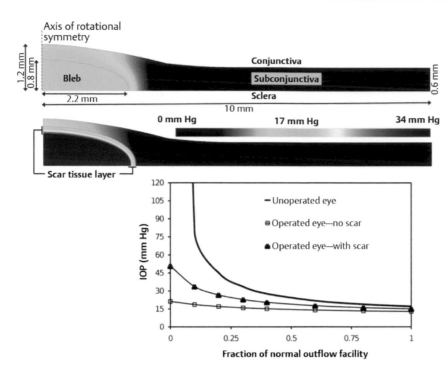

Fig. 17.7 Modeling of bleb capsule porosity and with low and high resistance in the Tenon's cyst wall. The lowest graph maps the IOP to the native outflow facility without operation, with operation and scar, and operation without scar. Note that postoperative IOP is determined by the total of native facility and surgically induced facility of outflow, and that IOP rises nonlinearly with loss of outflow in the unoperated eye. (From Gardiner BS, Smith DW, Coote M, Crowston JG. Computational modeling of fluid flow and intra-ocular pressure following glaucoma surgery. PLoS ONE 2010;5:13178. Open access.)

these cases, the majority are presentations of blebitis alone, with endophthalmitis implicated in about one third of them.[30] Antimetabolites are frequently implicated in causing thin-walled blebs, despite some evidence challenging this idea[31,32] and the fact that thin-walled blebs were uncommon in the pre-antimetabolite era. Improvements in trabeculectomy technique can be expected to decrease the risk of cystic bleb formation,[33] and may be judged more objectively using high-fidelity grading systems[34] that in turn provide opportunities to improve bleb outcomes.

Bleb complications after tube implant surgery are much less common than after trabeculectomy. Thinning and erosion of bleb tissue overlying a GDD implant may cause implant exposure, which in addition to exposing the intraocular space and causing hypotony also provides a possible route and nidus for infection that may necessitate removal of the implant.

We understand from clinical experience, published data, animal studies, and theoretic modeling that blebs function better in the absence of inflammation and with subconjunctival aqueous flow distributed over a larger area. It is quite likely that factors in aqueous from inflamed or primary open-angle glaucoma eyes compromise bleb function.[35] In encapsulated blebs, this is associated with increased subconjunctival tissue resistance in unevenly distributed zones, tissue compaction, and relative shear stress during fluid passage. Cells here respond by further increasing fibrous extracellular matrix deposition that decreases bleb tissue permeability.[36]

Manipulation of bleb morphology after trabeculectomy by needling is best described as an art, mainly because there is so little science to back it up, but its benefits in yielding improved IOP control are well documented[37,38] and are now better analyzed.[33] Anecdotally, needling may also be used to improve bleb morphology and reduce the risk of further bleb leaks by redirecting flow over a larger area and reducing intrableb pressure.

Conclusion

Over the past 40 years, continual refinements of glaucoma surgery predicated on subconjunctival drainage have yielded proce-

dures for efficaciously treating elevated IOP. They have become gold standard procedures, achieving good pressure control in the vast majority of patients with a very low risk of serious complications. Developing better ways to manipulate the subconjunctival outflow resistance of blebs will further optimize these surgeries. Additionally, new generation drainage devices with appropriate flow restriction (InnFocus microshunt, InnFocus Inc., Miami, FL) or that permit ab interno insertion (XEN gel stent, Aquesys Inc., Aliso Viejo, CA) by a minimally invasive approach are currently in clinical trials and may change the way we surgically shunt aqueous into the subconjunctival space. In the future, these improvements and innovations may result in more effective and efficient, safer, and better customizable treatments to meet patients' needs.

References

1. Zorab A. The reduction of tension in chronic glaucoma. Ophthalmoscope 1912;10:258–261

2. Molteno AC. New implant for drainage in glaucoma. Animal trial. Br J Ophthalmol 1969;53:161–168

3. Molteno AC. New implant for drainage in glaucoma. Clinical trial. Br J Ophthalmol 1969;53:606–615

4. Jampel HD, Musch DC, Gillespie BW, Lichter PR, Wright MM, Guire KE; Collaborative Initial Glaucoma Treatment Study Group. Perioperative complications of trabeculectomy in the Collaborative Initial Glaucoma Treatment Study (CIGTS). Am J Ophthalmol 2005;140:16–22

5. Advanced Glaucoma Intervention Study (AGIS). The Advanced Glaucoma Intervention Study (AGIS): 4. Comparison of treatment outcomes within race. Seven-year results. Ophthalmology 1998;105:1146–1164

6. Landers J, Martin K, Sarkies N, Bourne R, Watson P. A twenty-year follow-up study of trabeculectomy: risk factors and outcomes. Ophthalmology 2012;119:694–702

7. Wilensky JT, Chen TC. Long-term results of trabeculectomy in eyes that were initially successful. Trans Am Ophthalmol Soc 1996;94:147–159, discussion 160–164

8. Bevin TH, Molteno ACB, Herbison P. Otago Glaucoma Surgery Outcome Study: long-term results of 841 trabeculectomies. Clin Experiment Ophthalmol 2008;36:731–737

9. Akafo SK, Goulstine DB, Rosenthal AR. Long-term post trabeculectomy intraocular pressures. Acta Ophthalmol (Copenh) 1992;70:312–316

10. Popovic V, Sjöstrand J. Long-term outcome following trabeculectomy: I Retrospective analysis of intraocular pressure regulation and cataract formation. Acta Ophthalmol (Copenh) 1991;69:299–304

11. Gedde SJ, Schiffman JC, Feuer WJ, Herndon LW, Brandt JD, Budenz DL; Tube versus Trabeculectomy Study Group. Treatment outcomes in the Tube Versus Trabeculectomy (TVT) study after five years of follow-up. Am J Ophthalmol 2012;153:789–803.e2

12. Khaw PT, Chiang M, Shah P, Sii F, Lockwood A, Khalili A. Enhanced trabeculectomy: the Moorfields Safer Surgery System. Dev Ophthalmol 2012; 50:1–28

13. Kirwan JF, Lockwood AJ, Shah P, et al; Trabeculectomy Outcomes Group Audit Study Group. Trabeculectomy in the 21st century: a multicenter analysis. Ophthalmology 2013;120:2532–2539

14. Stewart RM, Diamond JG, Ashmore ED, Ayyala RS. Complications following ex-press glaucoma shunt implantation. Am J Ophthalmol 2005;140: 340–341

15. Wamsley S, Moster MR, Rai S, Alvim HS, Fontanarosa J. Results of the use of the Ex-PRESS miniature glaucoma implant in technically challenging, advanced glaucoma cases: a clinical pilot study. Am J Ophthalmol 2004; 138:1049–1051

16. Kaplan RI, De Moraes CG, Cioffi GA, Al-Aswad LA, Blumberg DM. Comparative cost-effectiveness of the Baerveldt implant, trabeculectomy with mitomycin, and medical treatment. JAMA Ophthalmol 2015;133:560–567

17. Gedde SJ, Panarelli JF, Banitt MR, Lee RK. Evidenced-based comparison of aqueous shunts. Curr Opin Ophthalmol 2013;24:87–95

18. Allan EJ, Khaimi MA, Jones JM, Ding K, Skuta GL. Long-term efficacy of the Baerveldt 250 mm2 compared with the Baerveldt 350 mm2 implant. Ophthalmology 2015;122:486–493

19. Wells AP, Ashraff NN, Hall RC, Purdie G. Comparison of two clinical Bleb grading systems. Ophthalmology 2006;113:77–83

20. Wells AP, Marks J, Khaw PT. Spontaneous inferior subconjunctival haemorrhages in association with circumferential drainage blebs. Eye (Lond) 2005;19:269–272

21. Shelton L, Rada JS. Effects of cyclic mechanical stretch on extracellular matrix synthesis by human scleral fibroblasts. Exp Eye Res 2007;84:314–322

22. Liu C, Feng P, Li X, Song J, Chen W. Expression of MMP-2, MT1-MMP, and TIMP-2 by cultured rabbit corneal fibroblasts under mechanical stretch. Exp Biol Med (Maywood) 2014;239:907–912

23. Wong MHY, Husain R, Ang BCH, et al. The Singapore 5-fluorouracil trial: intraocular pressure outcomes at 8 years. Ophthalmology 2013;120: 1127–1134

24. Gardiner BS, Smith DW, Coote M, Crowston JG. Computational modeling of fluid flow and intra-ocular pressure following glaucoma surgery. PLoS ONE 2010;5:13178

25. Nguyen DQ, Ross CM, Li YQ, et al. A model to measure fluid outflow in rabbit capsules post glaucoma implant surgery. Invest Ophthalmol Vis Sci 2012;53:6914–6919

26. Levick JR. Flow through interstitium and other fibrous matrices. Q J Exp Physiol 1987;72:409–437

27. Ross C, Pandav SS, Li YQ, et al. Determination of bleb capsule porosity with an experimental glaucoma drainage device and measurement system. JAMA Ophthalmol 2015;133:549–554

28. Yamamoto T, Kuwayama Y, Kano K, Sawada A, Shoji N; Study Group for the Japan Glaucoma Society Survey of Bleb-related Infection. Clinical features of bleb-related infection: a 5-year survey in Japan. Acta Ophthalmol (Copenh) 2013;91:619–624

29. Zahid S, Musch DC, Niziol LM, Lichter PR; Collaborative Initial Glaucoma Treatment Study Group. Risk of endophthalmitis and other long-term complications of trabeculectomy in the Collaborative Initial Glaucoma Treatment Study (CIGTS). Am J Ophthalmol 2013;155:674–680, 680.e1

30. Kim E-A, Law SK, Coleman AL, et al. Long-term bleb-related infections after trabeculectomy: incidence, risk factors, and influence of bleb revision. Am J Ophthalmol 2015;159:1082–1091

31. Vaziri K, Kishor K, Schwartz SG, et al. Incidence of bleb-associated endophthalmitis in the United States. Clin Ophthalmol 2015;9:317–322

32. Olayanju JA, Hassan MB, Hodge DO, Khanna CL. Trabeculectomy-related complications in Olmsted County, Minnesota, 1985 through 2010. JAMA Ophthalmol 2015;133:574–580

33. Rai P, Kotecha A, Kaltsos K, et al. Changing trends in the incidence of bleb-related infection in trabeculectomy. Br J Ophthalmol 2012;96:971–975

34. Wells T. Time, the great physician. Clin Experiment Ophthalmol 2014; 42:407–408

35. Yamanaka O, Saika S, Ikeda K, Miyazaki K, Kitano A, Ohnishi Y. Connective tissue growth factor modulates extracellular matrix production in human subconjunctival fibroblasts and their proliferation and migration in vitro. Jpn J Ophthalmol 2008;52:8–15

36. Swartz MA, Fleury ME. Interstitial flow and its effects in soft tissues. Annu Rev Biomed Eng 2007;9:229–256

37. Suzuki R, Susanna-Jr R. Early transconjunctival needling revision with 5-fluorouracil versus medical treatment in encapsulated blebs: a 12-month prospective study. Clinics (Sao Paulo) 2013;68:1376–1379

38. Tatham A, Sarodia U, Karwatowski W. 5-Fluorouracil augmented needle revision of trabeculectomy: does the location of outflow resistance make a difference? J Glaucoma 2013;22:463–467

18 Does Subconjunctival Filtration Affect Intraocular Pressure Fluctuation?

Grace M. Richter and Anne L. Coleman

Greater short-term and long-term fluctuation of intraocular pressure (IOP) have been linked to glaucomatous progression in several studies.[1-9] As such, it is important to understand the effects of various treatment modalities on circadian IOP fluctuation. Konstas et al,[10] in a prospective observational study, reported that post-trabeculectomy patients have reduced mean, peak, and range of IOP compared with baseline IOP-matched glaucoma patients on maximally tolerated medical therapy. Mansouri et al[11] and Medeiros et al[12] demonstrated reduced peak IOP in response to a water drinking test in post-trabeculectomy patients compared with medically treated patients. A limitation to these and similar studies[13] is that IOP is often measured at only a few time points in a 24-hour period, and usually with the subject in the sitting position. The sitting position results in a lower IOP than the habitual sleeping position,[14] and we do not fully know the effect of wakefulness on nocturnal IOP measurements. Most importantly, having only a few measurements in a day means that peak or trough IOP values may be missed.

Why would patients with subconjunctival filtration have reduced diurnal or nocturnal IOP fluctuation? These patients have a new nonphysiological route for aqueous outflow, a drainage pathway directly from the anterior chamber into the subconjunctival space. Liu et al[15-19] demonstrated that, for most patients, IOP is highest during sleep, as measured in the habitual position. However, because aqueous production also decreases significantly during this time period,[20-22] the elevation in nocturnal IOP is hypothesized to be due to changes in aqueous outflow. Sit et al[23] explored whether changes in outflow facility, episcleral venous pressure, or uveoscleral flow account for the higher nocturnal IOP. Based on their modeling results, they concluded that changes in episcleral venous pressure or uveoscleral flow were responsible for elevated nocturnal IOP. Assuming this is true, it follows that post-trabeculectomy patients would have reduced IOP fluctuation because trabeculectomies bypass the physiological outflow mechanisms responsible for the circadian variation of IOP.

Furthermore, the fact that post-trabeculectomy patients also withstand the water drinking test with less of an IOP spike[11] suggests that not only does subconjunctival filtration offer a circadian-independent mode of aqueous outflow, it also seems to provide a lower resistance pathway for dealing with aqueous loads compared with medically treated patients. This supports the idea that a post-trabeculectomy patient would be able to better withstand stressors from aqueous overproduction and thus would have reduced long-term fluctuation in IOP.

Clinical data have shown that patients with subconjunctival filtration have reduced IOP fluctuation[10-13] and that patients with reduced IOP fluctuation have reduced rates of glaucomatous progression.[1-9] The greatest limitation to understanding all of this lies in our extremely limited data points of IOP throughout any given day, a problem that new continuous monitoring technologies aim to address. If drinking a liter of water in 15 minutes can cause significant IOP elevations in unoperated glaucoma patients, what other activities and habits among them are causing IOP spikes that we have never detected in the clinic? Until we can advance from isolated snapshots of IOP to a continuous around-the-clock assessment, our understanding will be limited by our numerous assumptions about what is truly happening.

References

1. Bergeå B, Bodin L, Svedbergh B. Impact of intraocular pressure regulation on visual fields in open-angle glaucoma. Ophthalmology 1999;106:997–1004, discussion 1004–1005

2. Asrani S, Zeimer R, Wilensky J, Gieser D, Vitale S, Lindenmuth K. Large diurnal fluctuations in intraocular pressure are an independent risk factor for patients with glaucoma. J Glaucoma 2000;9:134–142

3. Nouri-Mahdavi K, Hoffman D, Coleman AL, et al; Advanced Glaucoma Intervention Study. Predictive factors for glaucomatous visual field progression in the Advanced Glaucoma Intervention Study. Ophthalmology 2004;111:1627–1635

4. Hong S, Seong GJ, Hong YJ. Long-term intraocular pressure fluctuation and progressive visual field deterioration in patients with glaucoma and low intraocular pressures after a triple procedure. Arch Ophthalmol 2007;125:1010–1013

5. Lee PP, Walt JW, Rosenblatt LC, Siegartel LR, Stern LS; Glaucoma Care Study Group. Association between intraocular pressure variation and glaucoma progression: data from a United States chart review. Am J Ophthalmol 2007;144:901–907

6. Caprioli J, Coleman AL. Intraocular pressure fluctuation a risk factor for visual field progression at low intraocular pressures in the advanced glaucoma intervention study. Ophthalmology 2008;115:1123–1129.e3

7. Fukuchi T, Yoshino T, Sawada H, et al. The relationship between the mean deviation slope and follow-up intraocular pressure in open-angle glaucoma patients. J Glaucoma 2013;22:689–697

8. Sakata R, Aihara M, Murata H, et al. Intraocular pressure change over a habitual 24-hour period after changing posture or drinking water and related factors in normal tension glaucoma. Invest Ophthalmol Vis Sci 2013;54:5313–5320

9. Grippo TM, Liu JH, Zebardast N, Arnold TB, Moore GH, Weinreb RN. Twenty-four-hour pattern of intraocular pressure in untreated patients with ocular hypertension. Invest Ophthalmol Vis Sci 2013;54:512–517

10. Konstas AG, Topouzis F, Leliopoulou O, et al. 24-hour intraocular pressure control with maximum medical therapy compared with surgery in patients with advanced open-angle glaucoma. Ophthalmology 2006;113:761–5.e1

11. Mansouri K, Orguel S, Mermoud A, et al. Quality of diurnal intraocular pressure control in primary open-angle patients treated with latanoprost compared with surgically treated glaucoma patients: a prospective trial. Br J Ophthalmol 2008;92:332–336

12. Medeiros FA, Pinheiro A, Moura FC, Leal BC, Susanna R Jr. Intraocular pressure fluctuations in medical versus surgically treated glaucomatous patients. J Ocul Pharmacol Ther 2002;18:489–498

13. Liang YB, Xie C, Meng HL, et al. Daytime fluctuation of intraocular pressure in patients with primary angle-closure glaucoma after trabeculectomy. J Glaucoma 2013;22:349–354

14. Tsukahara S, Sasaki T. Postural change of IOP in normal persons and in patients with primary wide open-angle glaucoma and low-tension glaucoma. Br J Ophthalmol 1984;68:389–392

15. Liu JH, Kripke DF, Hoffman RE, et al. Nocturnal elevation of intraocular pressure in young adults. Invest Ophthalmol Vis Sci 1998;39:2707–2712

16. Liu JH, Kripke DF, Twa MD, et al. Twenty-four-hour pattern of intraocular pressure in the aging population. Invest Ophthalmol Vis Sci 1999;40: 2912–2917

17. Liu JH, Kripke DF, Twa MD, et al. Twenty-four-hour pattern of intraocular pressure in young adults with moderate to severe myopia. Invest Ophthalmol Vis Sci 2002;43:2351–2355

18. Liu JH, Bouligny RP, Kripke DF, Weinreb RN. Nocturnal elevation of intraocular pressure is detectable in the sitting position. Invest Ophthalmol Vis Sci 2003;44:4439–4442

19. Liu JH, Zhang X, Kripke DF, Weinreb RN. Twenty-four-hour intraocular pressure pattern associated with early glaucomatous changes. Invest Ophthalmol Vis Sci 2003;44:1586–1590

20. Reiss GR, Lee DA, Topper JE, Brubaker RF. Aqueous humor flow during sleep. Invest Ophthalmol Vis Sci 1984;25:776–778

21. Larsson LI, Rettig ES, Sheridan PT, Brubaker RF. Aqueous humor dynamics in low-tension glaucoma. Am J Ophthalmol 1993;116:590–593

22. Larsson LI, Rettig ES, Brubaker RF. Aqueous flow in open-angle glaucoma. Arch Ophthalmol 1995;113:283–286

23. Sit AJ, Nau CB, McLaren JW, Johnson DH, Hodge D. Circadian variation of aqueous dynamics in young healthy adults. Invest Ophthalmol Vis Sci 2008;49:1473–1479

19 Benzalkonium Chloride and Outflow Resistance

Ridia Lim and Ivan Goldberg

Benzalkonium chloride (BAK), a quaternary ammonium detergent, has been the most common preservative in glaucoma drops. Increasing research interest in BAK and its effect on the ocular surface and conjunctiva has shown detrimental effects of BAK on corneal and conjunctival epithelial cells, trabecular meshwork cells, and corneal nerves.[1] BAK activates conjunctival fibroblasts, mobilizes inflammatory cells, damages goblet cells, and may enhance subconjunctival fibrosis.[2]

Glaucoma filtration surgery aims to optimize aqueous outflow. Chronic antiglaucoma medications may contribute to trabeculectomy failure,[3] as may BAK in a dose–response manner.[4]

Many glaucoma patients instill multiple antiglaucoma drops with inevitable additive BAK doses; each product with BAK has doses between 0.004% and 0.02%. By the time trabeculectomy surgery is indicated, we may have created an environment for surgical failure. Anecdotally, higher doses of mitomycin and greater numbers of 5-fluorouracil injections may be necessary for success, with attendant increases in complications.

Less toxic preservatives such as Purite, SofZia, and Polyquad have been used increasingly, along with unpreserved eyedrops. We need research to determine how these options affect trabeculectomy success.

In addition, excipients in preservative-free latanoprost have been shown to excite an inflammatory response.[5] The effects of excipients needs further study.

Given our current knowledge, what steps are available to a clinicians to reduce a BAK effect? BAK-containing drops should be minimized, especially long-term and particularly prior to surgery, if possible. Fluorometholone, instilled four-times daily for 1 month preoperatively, reduces conjunctival fibroblasts and inflammatory cells.[6] The following eyedrops contain BAK:

- Fluorometholone 0.1% (FML: BAK 0.004%, Flucon: BAK 0.01%)
- Ketorolac trometamol 0.5% (Acular: BAK 0.01%)
- Prednisolone acetate 1% (Prednefrin Forte: BAK 0.004%, Pred Forte: 0.006%)
- Dexamethasone 1 mg/mL 0.1% (Maxidex: BAK 0.01%)
- Homatropine 2% or 5% (BAK 0.1 mg/ml 0.01%)

The BAK load should be kept in mind; unpreserved formulations (such as dexamethasone 0.1% minims or prednisolone 1% minims) should be considered.

References

1. Anwar Z, Wellik SR, Galor A. Glaucoma therapy and ocular surface disease: current literature and recommendations. Curr Opin Ophthalmol 2013;24:136–143

2. Baudouin C, Labbé A, Liang H, Pauly A, Brignole-Baudouin F. Preservatives in eyedrops: the good, the bad and the ugly. Prog Retin Eye Res 2010;29: 312–334

3. Broadway DC, Grierson I, O'Brien C, Hitchings RA. Adverse effects of topical antiglaucoma medication. II. The outcome of filtration surgery. Arch Ophthalmol 1994;112:1446–1454

4. Boimer C, Birt CM. Preservative exposure and surgical outcomes in glaucoma patients: The PESO study. J Glaucoma 2013;22:730–735

5. Smedowski A, Paterno JJ, Toropainen E, Sinha D, Wylegala E, Kaarniranta K. Excipients of preservative-free latanoprost induced inflammatory response and cytotoxicity in immortalized human HCE-2 corneal epithelial cells. J Biochem Pharmacol Res 2014;2:175–184

6. Broadway DC, Grierson I, Stürmer J, Hitchings RA. Reversal of topical antiglaucoma medication effects on the conjunctiva. Arch Ophthalmol 1996;114:262–267

20 The Fibroblast and Glaucoma Surgery

John R. Samples and Paul A. Knepper

Current glaucoma surgery involves an incision in the conjunctiva and the meshwork such as by trabeculectomy or a draining device or a tube placed into the suprachoroidal space. Future possibilities include tubes or shunts placed into other spaces, such as Schlemm's canal or the suprachoroidal space.

The wound-healing response is an important determinant of the success of glaucoma surgery. It is a multistep process: First, platelets respond, fibrin is deposited, and clotting occurs. Second, inflammation removes the damaged tissues and cells, and platelet-derived growth factor (PDGF) released from α-granules facilitates tissue healing. Third, proliferation occurs, including angiogenesis and collagen deposition. Finally, remodeling occurs, with collagen and extracellular matrix responses.

Fibroblasts are the most common cells in connective tissues. The fibroblast is a type of cell that synthesizes collagen and other components of the extracellular matrix, the main structural framework (stroma) for tissues. Thus, fibroblasts play a critical role in wound healing. They are attracted to wounds by chemicals such as chemokines, cytokines, and inflammatory mediators released at the site of injury. We often tell patients that, under the microscope, these cells look like little snails that migrate to the site of a wound and create a scar; it is always important to point out that the snails that are depositing scar-making material are "made out of you," that is, of their own cells.

Fibroblasts likely exist in a variety of subtypes and may arrive at the wound in a pluripotent state. At present, there is limited information on how fibroblasts differentiate in the wound-healing process. Myofibroblasts, a fibroblast subtype, are found in fibrovascular membranes in the eye. They are widely distributed in some normal ocular tissues, in which they possibly evolved from quiescent fibroblasts.[1] The glaucoma surgeon may be vexed by the adherent membranes and peripheral anterior synechiae they instigate. With all of the glaucoma devices, irrespective of which spaces they connect, it is important that the devices be biocompatible to prevent them from attracting the cells that lead to scar formation. Strategies to enhance biocompatibility include the use of heparin coating, biocompatible hydrogels, and a variety of other bio-friendly materials.

The wounding response specifically associated with the placement of a stent or device through tissue and the subsequent release of small molecules and peptides is very complex and involves mediators in varying amounts. Laser treatment to almost any ocular tissue likely also evokes these wound-healing responses, as we have shown with interleukin-1β and tumor necrosis factor-α (TNF-α).[2] The notion that these cytokines are ubiquitous and seem to lack specificity is somewhat counterintuitive, as they likely have specific roles in each situation. These cytokines in the trabecular meshwork induce mitosis and alter the trabecular outflow pathways in a positive manner by secondary effects on matrix metalloproteinases. Most wound and inflammatory responses also evoke a macrophage response.

The macrophage-like response of trabecular cells is an often-overlooked quality. Fibroblasts interact with macrophages and may be removed by them. Although stem cells have successfully been used to regulate outflow in the meshwork, the therapeutic effect of their phagocytic response, once the cells have settled on trabecular beams, is yet to be fully considered.[3] Moreover, stimulation of trabecular cell phagocytic activity may be a means of modifying fibroblast-driven scarring in the eye.

Not much is known about the subtypes of fibroblasts and scar-forming cells in the eye and the degree to which a fibroblast derived from Tenon's capsule is different from a fibroblast from the conjunctiva. It is likely that these cells vary in their ability to respond to a variety of stimuli and have varying degrees of specialization.

Variation in response to chemotherapy among the cell types seems likely. Wound-healing responses in the eye have traditionally been addressed by antimetabolites such as 5-fluorouracil and mitomycin C. Attempts to manipulate growth factors associated with wound healing have not yet produced success. Yet there are many other molecular mechanisms that can modulate a response to wounding in glaucoma surgical therapy. A multitude of strategies now exist to address fibroblast behavior, including RNA interference therapy; antibodies against growth factors, such as new-generation anti–vascular endothelial growth factor (VEGF), anti-PDGF, and other anti–growth factor treatments; as well as numerous small molecule inhibitors. A better understanding of fibroblasts will likely take us far beyond the present use of corticosteroids to modulate wound healing in our surgeries.

Hyaluronic acid (HA) is just one of many key factors in the eye that may affect fibroblast motility, proliferation and cellular differentiation. CD44, the principal receptor for HA, is abnormal in its soluble form in the glaucoma eye and may offer one of many explanations of why scar formation and fibroblast proliferation may be abnormal in the glaucomatous eye.[4] Notably, the aqueous humor of primary open-angle glaucoma (POAG) has a higher content of low molecular weight HA (**Fig. 20.1**). Low molecular weight HA signals through the innate immune receptor complex CD44-Toll-4-MD-2 to cause an upregulated proinflammatory response. Significantly, low molecular weight HA effects can be blocked by the administration of naloxone, a toll-like receptor 4 antagonist.[5] The use of naloxone or other antagonist of the innate immune system may be a future consideration to prevent excessive wound-healing responses and improve outcomes of glaucoma surgery.

There are additional approaches to controlling fibroblasts. We are working on specific mixtures of collagen gels, with or without additional small molecules to repel fibroblasts from almost any active wound site (in development, Eyegenetix, Columbia, SC). Sustained release reservoirs embedded in the sclera may gradually elute wound-modifying peptides, antibodies, or

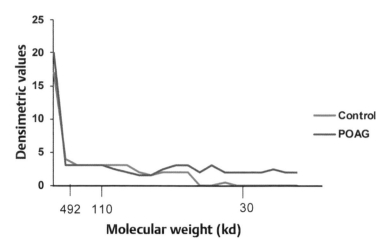

Fig. 20.1 Hyaluronic acid was isolated from aqueous humor samples of primary open-angle glaucoma (POAG) and age-matched controls, and the molecular weight of hyaluronic acid was determined using highly sensitive mini-slab 15% Tris/borate/ethylenediaminetetraacetic acid (EDTA) gels with pulsed electrophoresis and stained with 0.05% stains.

small molecules such as naloxone. These delivery devices have wide applicability to glaucoma and may also be used to administer neuroprotectants that are otherwise hard to deliver due to molecule size or other pharmacological properties (in development, Refocus, Fort Worth, TX). A better understanding of the interaction of lymphatic channels and fibroblast interactions may yield surprising results because lymphatics may play an important role in conjunctival filtration. Eventually these approaches and others are likely to make the present concerns about bleb failure and scarring at other wound sites a matter of historical interest. New approaches and methods for modulating fibroblasts appear annually at the American Society for Cell Biology conference. Additional insights may help with understanding healing elsewhere, including in the retina, vitreous, and cornea.

References

1. Minckler D. Neovascular glaucoma In: Schacknow P, Samples J, eds. The Glaucoma Book. New York: Springer; 2010:507

2. Bylsma SS, Samples JR, Acott TS, Van Buskirk EM. Trabecular cell division after argon laser trabeculoplasty. Arch Ophthalmol 1988;106:544–547

3. Kelley M. Trabecular stem cells. In: Knepper P, Samples J, eds. Glaucoma Research and Clinical Advances. Amsterdam: Kugler; 2015

4. Knepper PA, Nolan MJ, Yue BJT. Now the revolution in cell biology with affect glaucoma: biomarkers. In: Schacknow P, Samples J, eds. The Glaucoma Book. New York: Springer; 2010:933

5. Grybauskas A, Koga T, Kuprys PV, et al. ABCB1 transporter and innate immune Toll-like 4 receptor interaction in trabecular meshwork cells. Mol Vis 2015;21:201–212

21 Imminent Replacements for Trabeculectomy

Paul Palmberg

Minimally invasive glaucoma surgery (MIGS) may soon be obsolete, as operations that appear to be as safe and are far more effective should soon be available in the United States. MIGS was intended to achieve an adequate intraocular pressure (IOP) lowering while reducing the complications associated with the gold standard, mitomycin C (MMC) trabeculectomy. Although MIGS is a safe procedure, the IOP control it offers has been less than optimal, and it as not reduced the need for supplemental medications.

Fortunately, new filtering operations now in Food and Drug Administration (FDA) clinical trials have been shown in studies outside the United States to match the effectiveness of a MMC trabeculectomy without the risk of hypotony maculopathy, and with a greatly reduced risk of bleb leaks or infection.

Both the AqueSys XEN (AqueSys, Aliso Viejo, CA; **Figs. 21.1** and **21.2**) and the InnFocus MicroShunt (InnFocus, Miami, FL; **Figs. 21.3, 21.4, 21.5, 21.6**) replace the scleral flap of a trabeculectomy with a small-diameter tube that sets a predictable transscleral pressure gradient at normal aqueous flow. This was achieved by employing the Hagen-Poiseuille law to calculate the internal diameter needed to produce the desired pressure gradient from one end of the tube to the other at normal aqueous flow. (The pressure gradient is proportional to the length of the tube, the viscosity of the aqueous, and the rate of aqueous flow, and inversely proportional to the tube internal diameter to the fourth power.)[1] Indeed, neither device has produced persistent hypotony or hypotony maculopathy in any of several hundred cases in studies done outside the United States. At 2.5 μL/min

Ab-Interno Sub-Conjunctival Drainage

- IOP reduction achieved in minimally invasively procedure

- Bypasses the TM and scleral resistances

- Conjunctiva sparing: alternative surgical options remain

Gelatin Material is
Tissue Conforming

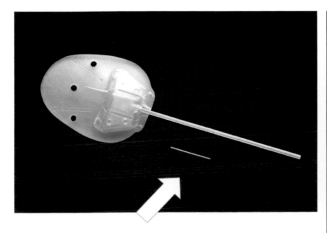
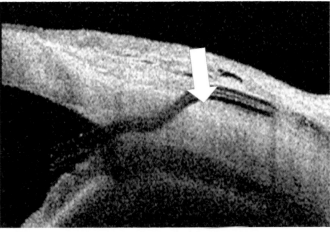

Fig. 21.1 The AqueSys XEN implant shown in relation to an Ahmed Implant **(a)** and an ultrasound biomicroscopy (UBM) image **(b)** showing the path of the flexible implant tube connecting the anterior chamber to the subconjunctival space. (AqueSys is not approved for sale in the United States; it has Investigational Device Exemption [IDE]-approved investigative status.) (© Copyright 2012. AqueSys and the AqueSys logo are registered trademarks of AqueSys, Inc.)

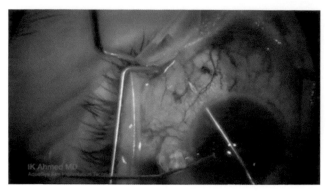

Fig. 21.2 Operative photo of the 27-g needle tip emerging under the conjunctiva 3 mm behind the superior nasal limbus, with the tip of the implant visible in the bevel just prior to delivering it ab interno. A portion of the inserter in which the needle is mounted is seen in the anterior chamber. The chamber is maintained with viscoelastic during the insertion, and is then rinsed. (AqueSys is not approved for sale in the United States; it has Investigational Device Exemption [IDE]-approved investigative status.) (© Copyright 2012. AqueSys and the AqueSys logo are registered trademarks of AqueSys, Inc.)

flow, the AqueSys XEN, with a 45- to 55-µm internal diameter and 6-mm length, sets a pressure gradient of ~ 7 mm Hg,[1] and the InnFocus MicroShunt, with a 62- to 70-µm internal diameter and 8.5-mm length sets a pressure gradient of ~ 6 mm Hg (in part due to hydrophobic effects). The AqueSys XEN is made of cross-linked porcine collagen, and the InnFocus MicroShunt is made of SIBS, a polystyrene plastic.

The two devices share the additional advantage of being placed through a 3-mm needle track in the sclera that avoids chamber shallowing during placement and therefore obviates the need for an iridectomy. The external portion of the tube extends

an additional 2 to 3 mm behind the limbus, so that aqueous drains quite posteriorly, producing diffuse blebs.

In addition to the difference in the material of which these devices are composed, the devices also differ in that the AqueSys XEN is inserted ab interno across the anterior chamber, thus also eliminating the conjunctival flap, and the InnFocus MicroShunt is inserted ab externo after making a fornix-based conjunctival flap. The XEN inserter has a 27-gauge needle mounted at the tip, in which is loaded the dry implant. After advancing the device through an inferior temporal corneal incision across the anterior chamber toward the superior nasal angle and penetrating to the scleral surface under the conjunctiva (**Fig. 21.2**), the surgeon advances a slider on the handle that, due to an ingenious dual cam, simultaneously extrudes the implant and withdraws the needle tip, leaving the implant in position, with ~ 1 mm in the anterior chamber, 2 to 3 mm in the scleral needle track, and 2 to 3 mm in the sub-Tenon's space. The InnFocus MicroShunt is placed through a 25-g needle track from the outside (**Fig. 21.4**), with 2 to 3 mm inside the anterior chamber, 2 to 3 mm in the scleral needle track, and 4 mm in the sub-Tenon's space.

Both devices depend on the use of MMC for their maximum effectiveness. The XEN is on the market in Europe and Canada, with MMC used optionally in the majority of cases as a preoperative subconjunctival injection of 10 to 30 µg. Data collection for the XEN FDA trial for refractory cases should be completed soon.

The InnFocus MicroShunt is using Mitosol on sponges in the U.S. trial, limited to the FDA-approved MMC dose of 0.2 mg/mL, although trials conducted outside the U.S. suggested that an MMC dose of 0.4 mg/mL yielded even better efficacy, without the risk of hypotony. The MicroShunt study has completed phase I, is scheduled to be completed in 2016–2017, and is a randomized trial of the MicroShunt versus a MMC trabeculectomy in primary cases.

The devices use different strategies for fixation to avoid migration. The XEN is inserted dry, and when in place it imbibes fluid and swells, causing it to fit tightly in the needle track. The

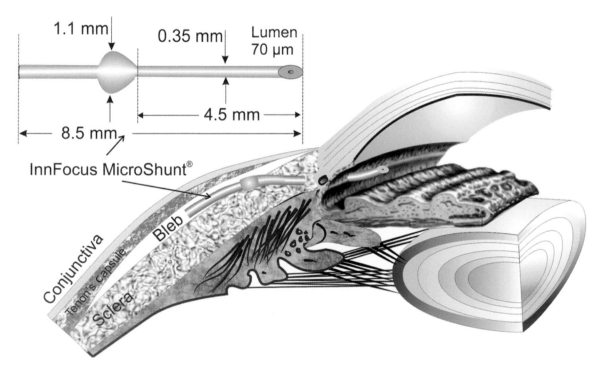

Fig. 21.3 Dimensions of the InnFocus MicroShunt® and diagram of its path from the anterior chamber to the sub-Tenon's capsule space.

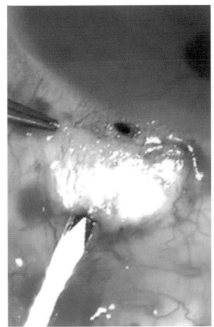

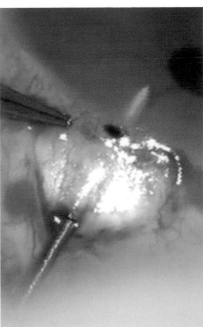

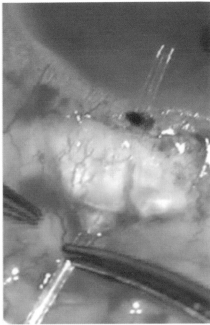

| Cut a 1 x 1 mm shallow pocket in sclera with MVR knife | Form 25 gauge needle tract through pocket and under limbus | Thread MicroShunt through needle tract and wedge fins in pocket |

Fig. 21.4 InnFocus MicroShunt® placement. **(a)** Special knife makes a 2 × 1 mm pocket. **(b)** A 25-gauge needle track parallel to the iris plane. **(c)** The device held in forceps is being inserted ab externo the needle track. The fin of the tube, which will hold it in place at the pocket, is seen 3 mm from the posterior end of the device.

Ultra-stable backbone with no cleavable groups means no degradation and insignificant inflammation and tissue encapsulation

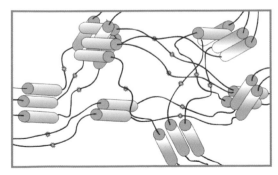

Morphology of SIBS showing rubbery strands (black lines) of polyisobutylene held together by glassy regions (cylinders) of polystyrene

Fig. 21.5 The structure of SIBS [poly(styrene-block-isobutylene-block-styrene], showing that it has only hydrophobic moieties on its surface, and no reactive or polar moieties, accounting for its favorable biocompatibility.

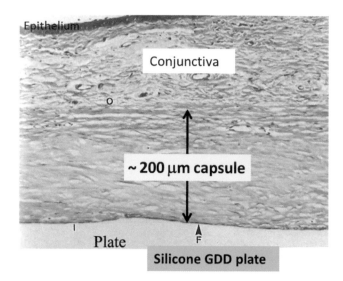

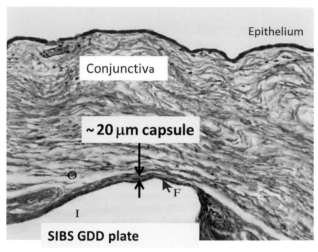

Encapsulation thickness is function of the polymer's biocompatibility

Fig. 21.6 Testing of the biocompatibility of a disk of SIBS relative to that of silicone rubber. A disk of each material was placed under the conjunctiva of a rabbit and then the tissue reaction was analyzed 3 months later. GDD, glaucoma drainage device. (Courtesy of Sander Dubovy, MD.)

MicroShunt has a small fin 3 mm from the exterior end that seats snuggly in a 1-mm triangular pocket at the exterior needle entry site. Neither device requires a patch graft to avoid tube erosion to the surface because they exit 3 mm behind the superior limbus, well behind the excursion of the upper lid, and indeed no tube exposures have occurred in that location.

The InnFocus MicroShunt trial is following corneal endothelial cell density and pachymetry in cases in which the device is placed and in the control MMC trabeculectomy group. In prior studies, neither devices has produced corneal decompensation, as have the Baerveldt, Ahmed, and Molteno aqueous drainage devices, in which the tube is made of silicone, nor do they produce blebs large enough to interfere with motility.

As an example of the outcomes reported with the devices, at the 2015 American Glaucoma Society conference, Ike Ahmed reported his results with the AqueSys XEN used with MMC, and I reported the results of trials performed in the Dominican Republic and in France.

Ahmed reported on 57 cases followed for an average of 12 months, in which the IOP was reduced from 27 to 12.5 mm Hg at 1 year and 13.1 mm Hg at 2 years, and the average number of medications was reduced from 3.5 to 0.5 at 1 year and 0.8 at 2 years; three patients required reoperation for failure, and there were no cases of persistent hypotony. Some 11% of eyes required a needling of a sheath of tissue from around the tube tip.[1]

I reported for Juan Battle (Dominican Republic) and Isabelle Riss (France) on 50 eyes that underwent either primary surgery (*N* = 32) or were performed with phacoemulsification (*N* = 18), in which the mean IOP was reduced from 23.5 to 10.7 mm Hg at 3 years (*N* = 22) and the average number of medications was reduced from 2.7 to 0.5. The success rate was 73% of patients off medications and 95% of patients with medications, and there were no cases of persistent hypotony or bleb infection.[2]

Thus, both devices yielded success rates comparable to or better than published series of trabeculectomy with MMC,[3] and with neither device was a case of hypotony maculopathy or a bleb infection encountered.

The materials used to produce the implants are important to their success. Both materials appear to incite less reaction than has been seen with silicone tubes, such as the Ahmed, Baer-

veldt, or Molteno. The cross-linked porcine collagen used in the AqueSys XEN has been tested in rabbits and was not degraded after 5 years, so, unlike Ologen, it does not dissolve. The SIBS polystyrene plastic used in the InnFocus MicroShunt is extremely inert, with no reactive groups on its surface (**Fig. 21.5**). (It has also been used in over 1 million heart stents during the past 12 years.) In testing performed by Jean-Marie Parel and Sander Dubovy at Bascom Palmer Eye Institute, a disk of silicone rubber placed under the conjunctiva of a rabbit after 3 months induced the formation of a 200-μm-thick capsule, whereas a disk of SIBS induced only a 20-μm-thick capsule (**Fig. 21.6**), corresponding to the rare occurrence of encapsulation of this tube in comparison to the usual encapsulation of the silicone tubes of other aqueous drainage devices.

Thus, we can say that replacements for an MMC trabeculectomy are almost here!

Financial Disclosure

Paul Palmberg is a consultant and medical monitor for InnFocus, Inc. for its FDA trial, and a consultant and trainer for AqueSys, Inc. He was a data and safety monitoring board (DSMB) member for an Aeon Astron trial. He is an unpaid consultant and trainer for Aurolab, India. He has been a consultant for Pfizer Asia. He owns no stock or options and has no patents in any of these companies.

References

1. Sheybani A, Reitsamer H, Ahmed IIK. Fluid dynamics of a novel micro-fistula Implant for the surgical treatment of glaucoma. Invest Ophthalmol Vis Sci 2015;56:4789–4795

2. Ahmed I, Shah M, Sheybani A. Use of a 45 um ab-interno subconjunctival gel stent with adjunctive mitomycin C for the treatment of uncontrolled open-angle glaucoma. American Glaucoma Society 2015 annual meeting abstracts, p. 87

3. Palmberg P, Batlle J. Two-center three-year follow up of a micro-lumen aqueous humor shunt. American Glaucoma Society 2015 annual meeting abstracts, p. 86

Section II Clinical Procedures

22   Phacoemulsification Cataract Extraction

Anjum Cheema and Kuldev Singh

Case Presentation

A 60-year-old woman with primary open-angle glaucoma (POAG) presents with worsening visual acuity in both eyes, particularly with disabling glare while driving. Best-corrected visual acuity is 20/40 in each eye, with glare testing resulting in worsening to 20/70 in both eyes. Intraocular pressure (IOP) on latanoprost and timolol both administered in both eyes once a day is 20 mm Hg in the right eye and 23 mm Hg in the left eye. Anterior segment biomicroscopic examination is significant for 2 to 3+ nuclear sclerosis of the lens with cortical spoking in both eyes. Funduscopic examination shows a cup-to-disk ratio of 0.6 in the right eye with an intact neuroretinal rim and 0.75 in the left eye with inferior thinning of the neuroretinal rim. Humphrey visual field (HVF) testing shows a normal examination in the right eye and an early superior arcuate defect in the left eye (**Fig. 22.1**). The patient is recommended to have phacoemulsification cataract extraction, beginning with the right eye. Postoperatively, visual acuity is improved to 20/20 after correction, with a dramatic improvement in glare testing. IOP is also improved to 15 mm Hg on latanoprost alone in the right eye and 17 mm Hg on latanoprost and timolol in the left eye at 1-year follow-up. Subsequent visual field testing has shown no demonstrable progression in either eye.

The Procedure

Cataract surgery is one of the most commonly performed surgeries in the United States, with 3 million procedures performed each year.[1] Since the introduction of phacoemulsification in 1967 by Charles Kelman, this technique has supplanted extracapsular cataract extraction in the Western world, having been used for more than 97% of all cataract surgeries performed in the United States since 2007.[2] Ultrasonic power delivered by an intraocular probe emulsifies and removes the nuclear portion of a cataract, allowing the use of small clear corneal incisions and obviating the need for large scleral incisions that require closure with sutures and violate the subconjunctival space. This preservation of the conjunctiva is of vital importance in patients with glaucoma.

Rationale Behind the Procedure

Because both cataract and glaucoma tend to increase in prevalence with age, it is quite common for glaucoma patients to have some degree of cataract formation. Cataractous lenses can affect both the ability to perform accurate surveillance for glaucomatous progression as well as impact the aqueous outflow. Funduscopic examinations of the optic nerve can become more difficult as the opacity from cataract worsens. Additionally, cataractous lenses have been shown to significantly impact both structural glaucoma tests such as optical coherence tomography (OCT) and functional tests such as automated static perimetry. For example, an increase in retinal nerve fiber layer (RNFL) thickness as well as signal strength as measured by spectral domain OCT can be seen after cataract surgery.[3] Similarly, a significant improvement in mean deviation on visual field testing can occur after cataract removal, partially resulting from elimination of lens-induced artifact.[4]

Performing early cataract surgery also offers several therapeutic advantages for glaucoma patients. It eliminates the future risk of one of the most common adverse effects of many glaucoma procedures—the development of a cataract. Approximately 20% of patients randomized to initial glaucoma surgery in the Collaborative Initial Glaucoma Treatment Study (CIGTS) required cataract extraction, with the leading cause of cataract formation being trabeculectomy.[5] As many as 50% of eyes develop a visually significant cataract within 5 years of trabeculectomy or tube shunt surgery.[6,7] Phacoemulsification prior to a glaucoma procedure, particularly trabeculectomy, is far preferable to phacoemulsification after establishment of a functioning bleb that is at risk following cataract removal. Husain et al,[8] in a study of 235 glaucoma patients who underwent trabeculectomy, found that the sooner cataract surgery was performed after trabeculectomy, the higher the likelihood of trabeculectomy failure. In this study, failure was defined as IOP greater than 21 mm Hg, and the hazard ratios for risk of trabeculectomy failure at 6 months, 1 year, and 2 years were 3.00, 1.73, and 1.32, respectively. Similarly, Sałaga-Pylak et al[9] retrospectively showed that eyes that underwent cataract extraction after trabeculectomy had a 20% lower success rate compared with those that did not require cataract extraction. Both bleb size and elevation were found to deteriorate after cataract surgery. Possible mechanisms of bleb failure after cataract surgery include increased permeability of the blood–aqueous barrier, leading to increased inflammation and subsequent bleb fibrosis.

Perhaps more importantly, as shown by numerous studies over the past few decades, cataract extraction leads to sustained reduction in IOP in patients with POAG) ocular hypertension, and primary angle-closure glaucoma (PACG). In 2002, Friedman et al[10] reported a 2 to 4 mm Hg reduction in IOP following cataract surgery in POAG eyes. Matsumara et al[11] prospectively showed an average IOP reduction of 1.5 mm Hg, 2.5 mm Hg, and 5.5 mm Hg in normal, controlled POAG (preoperative IOP < 21), and uncontrolled POAG (preoperative IOP ≥ 21) individuals, respectively, at 3 years following cataract surgery. There are also compelling data supporting cataract extraction as a means of lowering IOP in ocular hypertensive patients. Mansberger et al[12] analyzed data from the Ocular Hypertension Treatment Study (OHTS) and found that participants who underwent cataract extraction had an IOP reduction of 16.5% at 3 years.

Compared with POAG patients, PACG patients often can achieve greater IOP reduction after cataract surgery. In a comparison of PACG and POAG subjects 2 years after cataract surgery,

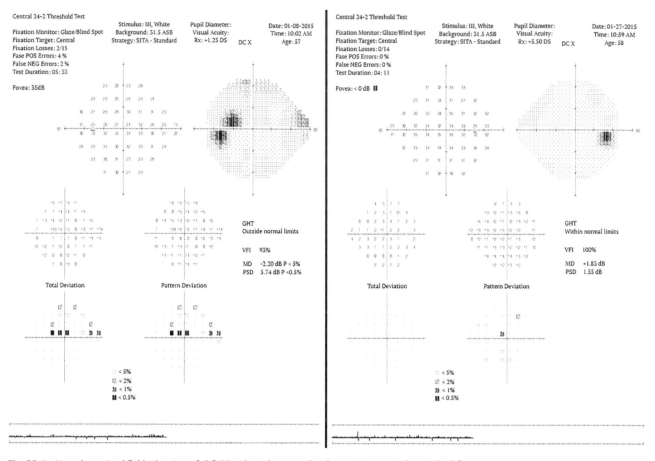

Fig. 22.1 Humphrey visual fields showing a full field in the right eye and early superior arcuate loss in the left eye.

Hayashi et al[13] found both a larger magnitude of IOP reduction (6.9 mm Hg vs 5.5 mm Hg, respectively) and less medication dependence (40% vs 19.1% medication free, respectively) in the former group.

Patient Selection

Patients with POAG, PACG, or ocular hypertension can potentially benefit from cataract surgery for both diagnostic and therapeutic purposes. To determine which patients may benefit the most, it is useful to explore the possible mechanisms resulting in IOP reduction after removal of a cataract.

In patients with PACG, cataract extraction relieves pupillary block, leading to deepening of the anterior chamber and improved access to the trabecular meshwork.[14] Euswas and Warrasak[15] found that the magnitude of IOP reduction was related to the degree of angle closure, as eyes with less than 270 degrees of peripheral anterior synechiae (PAS) experiencing a 3 mm Hg greater IOP reduction compared with eyes with less than 180 degrees of PAS.[15] Issa[16] developed a novel model to predict IOP reduction based on the ratio of preoperative IOP to anterior chamber depth (PD ratio). In general, the higher the preoperative IOP and the shallower the anterior chamber depth, the greater the IOP reduction following cataract extraction. Eyes with a PD ≥ 6.0 exhibited a mean IOP reduction of 4.90 mm Hg, whereas those with a PD < 6.0 had a more modest but still significant IOP reduction of 1.64 mm Hg.

In patients with POAG and ocular hypertension, the mechanism of IOP reduction after cataract surgery is less clear, and var-

ious hypotheses have been proposed. Kim et al[17] have theorized that high fluid flow during phacoemulsification may remove deposition of glycosaminoglycans in the trabecular meshwork. Tong and Miller[18] have postulated that microtrauma to the trabecular meshwork may produce an inflammatory effect akin to that seen after laser trabeculoplasty. Other proposed mechanisms include biochemical or blood–aqueous barrier alteration, ciliary body traction via posterior pressure on zonules intraoperatively leading to prevention of collapse of Schlemm's canal, and enhanced outflow due to stretching of the trabecular meshwork.[19–21] In terms of which POAG patients can expect the greatest IOP reduction, Poley[22] found that the greater the preoperative IOP, the greater the IOP reduction. Eyes with a preoperative IOP in the range of 23 to 31 mm Hg, 20 to 22 mm Hg, 18 to 19 mm Hg, and 15 to 17 mm Hg had IOP reductions of 6.5 mm Hg, 4.8 mm Hg, 2.5 mm Hg, and 1.6 mm Hg, respectively. Interestingly, eyes that had a preoperative IOP of 9 to 14 mm Hg did not have an IOP reduction, instead having a marginal increase in IOP of 0.2 mm Hg.

In summary, although cataract surgery is beneficial for the vast majority of glaucoma patients, those with the higher preoperative IOP, shallower anterior chamber, and narrower angle tend to have the greatest magnitude and longest duration of IOP reduction.

Surgical Technique

Surgeons must consider several issues regarding standard phacoemulsification when performing cataract surgery on glaucoma patients. In patients who have had prior glaucoma filtration surgery, the timing of cataract surgery is important. As mentioned previously, Husain et al[8] have demonstrated that there is a higher risk of trabeculectomy failure the sooner the cataract surgery is performed following the glaucoma procedure. Thus, cataract surgery should be delayed as long as possible following trabeculectomy without jeopardizing ocular health to decrease the risk of trabeculectomy failure.

There are some specific best practices with regard to cataract surgery in the glaucoma patient. Clear corneal incisions should be made whenever possible to avoid violating the conjunctival space, which is important to preserve for possible future glaucoma surgery. It is important to thoroughly remove all viscoelastic material at the conclusion of the procedure to reduce the risk of postoperative IOP spike. Consideration should be given to perioperative oral carbonic anhydrase inhibitors to further reduce this risk in select patients who are at risk of IOP spike-related glaucomatous damage in the early postoperative period. Alternatively, intracameral injection of miotic agent at the end of surgery can help prevent elevated IOP in addition to reversing the dilation.

As newer intraocular lenses (IOLs) are being developed, more options are available for optimal refractive correction with cataract surgery. However, patients with glaucoma may not be ideal candidates for certain types of implantable lenses. Multifocal IOLs are designed to provide multiple simultaneous images from different focal points onto the retina, relying on the fact that pupils constrict for near work and that different optical zones in the center and periphery of the IOL can be used for different tasks. Based on this design, however, there are some limitations, including unwanted photic phenomenon such as haloes or glare, but most importantly decreased contrast sensitivity. Because both multifocal IOLs and glaucomatous optic neuropathy decrease contrast sensitivity, glaucoma may be considered a relative contraindication for multifocal IOL placement. In contrast to multifocal IOLs, accommodating IOLs are monofocal and rely on replicating the physiological accommodating mechanism to provide near and intermediate vision.[23] Because they are monofocal IOLs, contrast sensitivity is not an issue. However, eyes with weakened zonules are likely to be poor candidates for accommodating IOLs because they also may have a compromised accommodative reflex. Toric IOLs are designed to correct for corneal astigmatism, and IOL stability is important, because rotation can result in loss of astigmatism correction, or when severe, result in induced astigmatism.[24] Thus, similar to accommodating IOLs, toric IOLs should be used with caution in patients with weakened zonules, as IOL decentration can compromise visual acuity.

Pseudoexfoliation, a common cause of secondary open-angle glaucoma, presents several potential intraoperative challenges, including small pupils, zonular instability with resultant difficulty completing a capsulorrhexis, posterior capsular laxity, and unstable capsular support for IOL placement, that require modification of surgical technique. Poor pupillary dilation may lead to a suboptimally sized capsulorrhexis, which in turn can make subsequent steps more difficult and increase the risk of further zonular compromise, vitreous loss, and postoperative capsular phimosis.[25] Various techniques and adjunctive surgical devices are available to facilitate a larger pupil, including mechanical stretching, pupil expansion rings, and iris retractors (**Figs. 22.2 and 22.3**). Surgeon preference dictates which technique to use in each case. In addition, staining of the anterior capsule with trypan blue can greatly improve visibility of the anterior capsule during capsulorrhexis (**Fig. 22.4**).

Zonular instability may present preoperatively as iris flutter, iridodonesis, phacodonesis, or frank lens subluxation and zonular dialysis. In other cases, though, it may only manifest intraoperatively with difficulty initiating a capsular tear, anterior capsular striae, and movement of the capsular bag during capsulorrhexis, posterior capsular laxity, and striae during cortical removal, or vitreous prolapse around an intact capsular bag. Fortunately, the use of intraoperative devices to improve capsular support can greatly enhance a surgeon's ability to safely complete cataract surgery. Capsular retractors are modified iris retractors designed

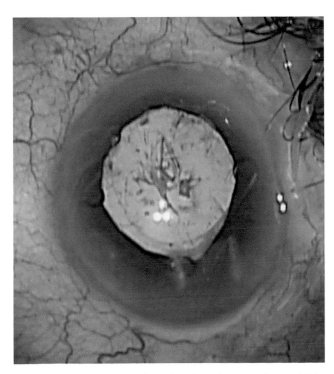

Fig. 22.2 A Malyugin ring has been placed to enhance pupillary mydriasis. All four islets can be seen hooking the iris.

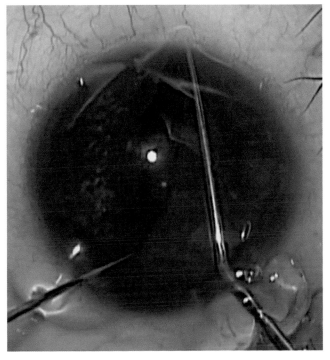

Fig. 22.3 Mechanical stretching can also be useful to achieve an adequate-sized pupil for cataract surgery.

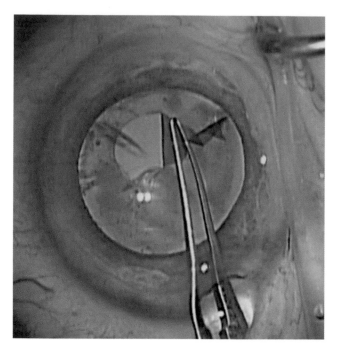

Fig. 22.4 Trypan blue has been used to stain the anterior capsule, greatly enhancing visibility during capsulorrhexis and subsequent steps of the procedure.

to be placed at the edge of a continuous curvilinear capsulorrhexis to provide adequate intraoperative support for the capsular bag during lens extraction **(Fig. 22.5)**. Placement of capsular tension rings or segments can provide both intraoperative and, perhaps more importantly, postoperative support to the capsular bag. An endocapsular tension ring (CTR) is a circular polymethylmethacrylate (PMMA) device that expands the capsular fornix and spreads zonular tension evenly among the remaining intact zonules **(Fig. 22.5)**. It is most useful in cases of mild zonulopathy, defined as an arc of no more than four hour positions on a clock face (≤ 120 degrees) of zonular loss.[25] A CTR can be placed at any time during surgery, but early placement may complicate cortical removal. An intact capsular bag and continuous curvilinear capsulorrhexis is required for placement of a CTR. With greater degrees of zonular loss, sutured devices such as a Cionni modified CTR (mCTR) or a capsule tension segment (CTS) are often useful.

Cortical removal may be difficult due to zonular compromise, and poor technique may exacerbate zonular loss. Adequate hydrodissection and possibly viscodissection to cleave cortical-capsular attachments are critical to reduce shearing forces on the zonules. Furthermore, tangential rather than radial cortical stripping can help to preserve zonular integrity.

Intraocular lens implantation is ideal if a well-centered, well-supported capsular bag is present. Placement of a CTR, mCTR, or CTS can help achieve this goal. If, however, the capsular bag has inadequate support, an IOL may need to be sutured to the iris or sclera, or placed in the anterior chamber. No strategy has been shown to be universally superior, so surgeons should proceed on a case-by-case basis.

Complications and Postoperative Management

Although cataract surgery is commonly a very safe procedure, care should be taken to avoid potential complications, particu-

larly in glaucoma patients. Moreover, postoperative management can be more complex in glaucoma patients compared with routine cases.

As mentioned earlier, there is a higher risk of trabeculectomy failure after cataract surgery, particularly if cataract surgery is performed soon after trabeculectomy.[8,9] Although the reason for trabeculectomy failure may be multifactorial, surgical and postsurgical inflammation likely play a large role in subsequent bleb fibrosis and failure. Careful and aggressive control of inflammation is imperative to decrease the risk of bleb failure. The postoperative management of cataract surgery in the presence of a preexisting trabeculectomy bleb should mimic that following trabeculectomy rather than standard cataract extraction. One may also consider revision of the trabeculectomy at the time of surgery to optimize bleb function. This can range from ab interno revision with a probe to break scleral flap adhesions, to bleb needling or full surgical bleb revision. A subconjunctival injection of 5-fluorouracil can be used if bleb revision is extensive.

Unlike the case with trabeculectomy surgery, cataract surgery after tube shunt surgery does not seem to carry the same risk of affecting IOP control. Erie et al[26] retrospectively reported no significant change from baseline IOP for a 21-month period after cataract surgery in patients with a Baerveldt tube shunt implant.

Spikes in IOP after cataract surgery have been widely reported, with an incidence of up to 39.5%.[27] Typically, these spikes are transient and are thought to be due in large part to retained viscoelastic. Although healthy eyes can often tolerate brief episodes of high IOP, glaucomatous eyes are more vulnerable to damage from even short periods of high IOP. Additionally, because glaucomatous eyes often have decreased facility of outflow, the risk of IOP spikes is higher than in those with normal outflow function. Therefore, surgeons should be careful to thoroughly remove all viscoelastic from the eye, particularly any dispersive agent that can obstruct the trabecular meshwork for a longer period of time. Moreover, consideration should be given to perioperative prophylaxis with the use of oral carbonic anhydrase inhibitors in high-risk patients.

Besides the potential intraoperative difficulties posed by pseudoexfoliation discussed earlier, there are also postoperative issues to consider. Pseudoexfoliative eyes are at a particularly high risk for IOP spikes, corneal edema, aqueous flare, IOL deposits, cystoid macular edema (CME), anterior capsular phimosis, posterior capsular opacification (PCO), and IOL subluxation.[25] Increased postoperative inflammation may be due to increased blood–aqueous barrier breakdown from relative anterior segment ischemia, leading to CME, anterior capsular contraction, and fibrinoid reaction with posterior synechiae.[28-30] Thus, IOP control and aggressive control of inflammation is critical in these eyes. Anterior capsular phimosis is a risk factor for IOL decentration and tilt, and should be addressed as early as possible **(Fig. 22.6)**. Therapeutic options include neodymium:yttrium-aluminum-garnet (Nd:YAG) laser cruciate incisions or surgical incisions with microforceps and scissors to release centripetal traction on the anterior capsule and zonules. With continued capsular phimosis and zonular compromise, IOL dislocation is possible. The precise incidence of late IOL dislocations is unclear, but it is thought to be uncommon. The treatment of this condition depends on the degree of IOL decentration or dislocation. If decentration is mild, IOL repositioning may be sufficient, but with greater degrees of decentration or dislocation, IOL exchange with placement of an anterior chamber IOL (ACIOL) or an iris- or scleral-sutured IOL may be necessary.

With regard to ongoing long-term IOP control in glaucoma patients, cataract surgery provides a unique opportunity to reevaluate a patient's need for preoperative IOP-lowering therapy. Given the additional medication dependence after cataract

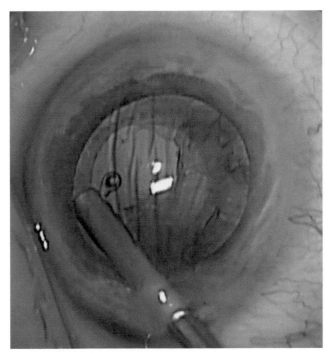

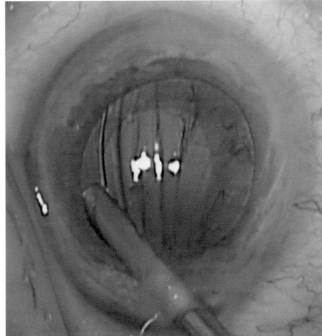

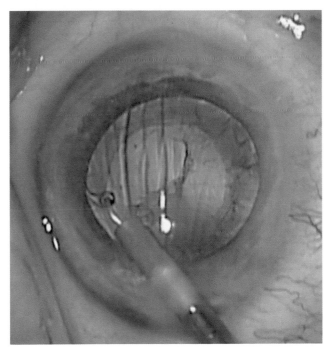

Fig. 22.5 Capsular tension ring being inserted into the capsular fornix via an injector. **(a)** Beginning of the insertion. **(b)** Midway through the insertion as a capsular tension ring (CTR) is advanced. **(c)** Final islet to be released at termination of the CTR insertion.

surgery, it may not be reasonable to simply continue all preoperative glaucoma medications in the postoperative period. Additionally, due to the IOP-lowering effects of cataract surgery, all preoperative glaucoma medications may not be necessary. Careful reassessment of IOP fluctuation along with structural and functional tests is essential after the initial postoperative period.

There is some concern about the use of prostaglandin analogues (PGAs) after cataract surgery due to reports of the development of CME with PGA use.[31–34] The pathophysiology of CME following cataract surgery is thought to involve anterior segment inflammation with release of endogenous inflammatory media-

tors, including PGAs. It is unclear whether exogenous PGA use is directly causative of CME, however, because the majority of case reports linking CME to exogenous PGA use involve patients with other risk factors for CME, such as a ruptured posterior capsule or a prior history of uveitis. Warwar et al,[35] in a large retrospective review of 136 pseudophakic eyes receiving latanoprost reported, only two cases of CME (1.5%). One of these eyes had a ruptured posterior capsule and the other had a history of uveitis prior to the use of latanoprost. In another large multicenter retrospective review of 225 eyes that were started on latanoprost after cataract surgery, only three eyes (1.3%) developed CME, and each had a ruptured posterior capsule necessitating anterior

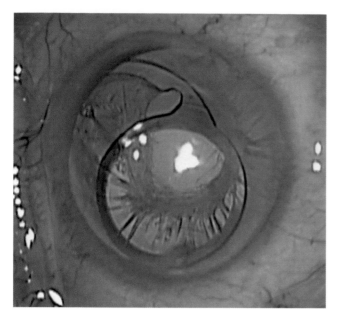

Fig. 22.6 Anterior capsular phimosis leading to a decentered intraocular lens (IOL).

vitrectomy.[36] Thus, it is unclear if PGA use is truly a risk factor for the development of CME after cataract surgery. The ultimate decision to withhold or continue PGA use should be made on a case-by-case basis.

Conclusion

Cataract surgery in glaucoma patients, although sometimes associated with risks relating to postoperative IOP spikes, is commonly beneficial in long-term glaucoma diagnosis and therapy. Improved structural and functional assessment of the optic nerve is one such benefit. A lower average IOP and decreased dependence on glaucoma medications are found in the majority of post–cataract surgery glaucoma patients. The extent of glaucoma damage, the target IOP, and the risk of further vision loss from an IOP spike must be taken into consideration when deciding on surgery. If these issues are of concern, the patient may benefit from a combined glaucoma procedure. With cataract extraction alone, future glaucoma surgical options are preserved and sometimes enhanced following removal of the cataractous lens.

References

1. Trends in Vision and Hearing Among Older Americans, 2001. www.cdc.gov/nchs/data/ahcd/agingtrends/02vision.pdf. Accessed February 19, 2015

2. Leaming DV. Practice styles and preferences of ASCRS members—2003 survey. J Cataract Refract Surg 2004;30:892–900

3. Kim NR, Lee H, Lee ES, et al. Influence of cataract on time domain and spectral domain optical coherence tomography retinal nerve fiber layer measurements. J Glaucoma 2012;21:116–122

4. Rehman Siddiqui MA, Khairy HA, Azuara-Blanco A. Effect of cataract extraction on SITA perimetry in patients with glaucoma. J Glaucoma 2007; 16:205–208

5. Zahid S, Musch DC, Niziol LM, Lichter PR; Collaborative Initial Glaucoma Treatment Study Group. Risk of endophthalmitis and other long-term complications of trabeculectomy in the Collaborative Initial Glaucoma Treatment Study (CIGTS). Am J Ophthalmol 2013;155:674–680, 680.e1

6. Jampel HD, Solus JF, Tracey PA, et al. Outcomes and bleb-related complications of trabeculectomy. Ophthalmology 2012;119:712–722

7. Gedde SJ, Herndon LW, Brandt JD, Budenz DL, Feuer WJ, Schiffman JC; Tube Versus Trabeculectomy Study Group. Postoperative complications in the Tube Versus Trabeculectomy (TVT) study during five years of follow-up. Am J Ophthalmol 2012;153:804–814.e1

8. Husain R, Liang S, Foster PJ, et al. Cataract surgery after trabeculectomy: the effect on trabeculectomy function. Arch Ophthalmol 2012;130:165–170

9. Sałaga-Pylak M, Kowal M, Zarnowski T. Deterioration of filtering bleb morphology and function after phacoemulsification. BMC Ophthalmol 2013;13:17

10. Friedman DS, Jampel HD, Lubomski LH, et al. Surgical strategies for coexisting glaucoma and cataract: an evidence-based update. Ophthalmology 2002;109:1902–1913

11. Matsumura M, Mizoguchi T, Kuroda S, Terauchi H, Nagata M. [Intraocular pressure decrease after phacoemulsification-aspiration+ intraocular lens implantation in primary open angle glaucoma eyes].Nippon Ganka Gakkai Zasshi 1996;100:885–889

12. Mansberger SL, Gordon MO, Jampel H, et al; Ocular Hypertension Treatment Study Group. Reduction in intraocular pressure after cataract extraction: the Ocular Hypertension Treatment Study. Ophthalmology 2012;119:1826–1831

13. Hayashi K, Hayashi H, Nakao F, Hayashi F. Effect of cataract surgery on intraocular pressure control in glaucoma patients. J Cataract Refract Surg 2001;27:1779–1786

14. Liu L. Deconstructing the mechanisms of angle closure with anterior segment optical coherence tomography. Clin Experiment Ophthalmol 2011; 39:614–622

15. Euswas A, Warrasak S. Intraocular pressure control following phacoemulsification in patients with chronic angle closure glaucoma. J Med Assoc Thai 2005;88(Suppl 9):S121–S125

16. Issa SA. A novel index for predicting intraocular pressure after cataract surgery. Br J Ophthalmol 2005;89:543–546

17. Kim DD, Doyle JW, Smith MF. Intraocular pressure reduction following phacoemulsification cataract extraction with posterior chamber lens implantation in glaucoma patients. Ophthalmic Surg Lasers 1999;30:37–40

18. Tong JT, Miller KM. Intraocular pressure change after sutureless phacoemulsification and foldable posterior chamber lens implantation. J Cataract Refract Surg 1998;24:256–262

19. Hansen TE, Naeser K, Nilsen NE. Intraocular pressure 2 1/2 years after extracapsular cataract extraction and sulcus implantation of posterior chamber intraocular lens. Acta Ophthalmol (Copenh) 1991;69:225–228

20. Steuhl KP, Marahrens P, Frohn C, Frohn A. Intraocular pressure and anterior chamber depth before and after extracapsular cataract extraction with posterior chamber lens implantation. Ophthalmic Surg 1992;23:233–237

21. Banov E, Moisseiev J, Blumenthal M. Intraocular pressure following ECCE, ICCE, and IOL implantation. Cataract. 1984;1:21–24

22. Poley BJ. Long term effects of phacoemulsification with intraocular lens implantation in normotensive and ocular hypertension eyes. J Cataract Refract Surg 2008;34:724–742

23. Alió JL, Plaza-Puche AB, Montalban R, Javaloy J. Visual outcomes with a single-optic accommodating intraocular lens and a low-addition-power rotational asymmetric multifocal intraocular lens. J Cataract Refract Surg 2012;38:978–985

24. Visser N, Bauer NJ, Nuijts RM. Toric intraocular lenses: historical overview, patient selection, IOL calculation, surgical techniques, clinical outcomes, and complications. J Cataract Refract Surg 2013;39:624–637

25. Shingleton BJ, Crandall AS, Ahmed II. Pseudoexfoliation and the cataract surgeon: preoperative, intraoperative, and postoperative issues related to intraocular pressure, cataract, and intraocular lenses. J Cataract Refract Surg 2009;35:1101–1120

26. Erie JC, Baratz KH, Mahr MA, Johnson DH. Phacoemulsification in patients with Baerveldt tube shunts. J Cataract Refract Surg 2006;32:1489–1491

27. Pohjalainen T, Vesti E, Uusitalo RJ, Laatikainen L. Phacoemulsification and intraocular lens implantation in eyes with open-angle glaucoma. Acta Ophthalmol Scand 2001;79:313–316

28. Pohjalainen T, Vesti E, Uusitalo RJ, Laatikainen L. Intraocular pressure after phacoemulsification and intraocular lens implantation in nonglaucomatous eyes with and without exfoliation. J Cataract Refract Surg 2001;27:426–431

29. Kato S, Suzuki T, Hayashi Y, et al. Risk factors for contraction of the anterior capsule opening after cataract surgery. J Cataract Refract Surg 2002; 28:109–112

30. Drolsum L, Davanger M, Haaskjold E. Risk factors for an inflammatory response after extracapsular cataract extraction and posterior chamber IOL. Acta Ophthalmol (Copenh) 1994;72:21–26

31. Ayyala RS, Cruz DA, Margo CE, et al. Cystoid macular edema associated with latanoprost in aphakic and pseudophakic eyes. Am J Ophthalmol 1998;126:602–604

32. Moroi SE, Gottfredsdottir MS, Schteingart MT, et al. Cystoid macular edema associated with latanoprost therapy in a case series of patients with glaucoma and ocular hypertension. Ophthalmology 1999;106:1024–1029

33. Rowe JA, Hattenhauer MG, Herman DC. Adverse side effects associated with latanoprost. Am J Ophthalmol 1997;124:683–685

34. Wand M, Gaudio AR. Cystoid macular edema associated with ocular hypotensive lipids. Am J Ophthalmol 2002;133:403–405

35. Warwar RE, Bullock JD, Ballal D. Cystoid macular edema and anterior uveitis associated with latanoprost use. Experience and incidence in a retrospective review of 94 patients. Ophthalmology 1998;105:263–268

36. Lima MC, Paranhos A Jr, Salim S, et al. Visually significant cystoid macular edema in pseudophakic and aphakic patients with glaucoma receiving latanoprost. J Glaucoma 2000;9:317–321

23 Trabeculectomy by Internal Approach: Trabectome

Kevin Kaplowitz, Igor I. Bussel, and Nils A. Loewen

Trabeculectomy performed ab interno with the Trabectome (NeoMedix, Tustin, CA) is an established minimally invasive glaucoma surgery (MIGS) with a decade's worth of published results.[1,2] The surgery is designed to increase conventional outflow via the physiological route. This chapter discusses the indications and technique for, and results and complications of, the using the Trabectome in primary and adjunctive surgery. The Trabectome can be expected to decrease the intraocular pressure (IOP) to an average of 15 mm Hg and the number of medications by one. IOP reduction depends on flow resistance downstream of the trabecular meshwork (TM) and is independent of preoperative IOP. The risk of vision-threatening complications is reported to be less than 1%. Thus, the Trabectome offers an effective and safe option for a wide range of glaucoma patients.

Case Presentation

An 81-year-old woman presents with worsening chronic angle-closure glaucoma having had a Descemet's stripping automated endothelial keratoplasty with cataract surgery several years before. Her visual acuity has decreased to 20/150, with an IOP of 20 mm Hg despite maximal medical treatment including three topical medications and oral acetazolamide. The corneal specialist felt that the number of medications was contributing to anterior corneal edema. There was nearly 180 degrees of peripheral anterior synechiae with iridocorneal touch along the nasal circumference, and the patient was pseudophakic. The visual field showed a superior greater than inferior arcuate defect, and the vertical cup-to-disk ratio was 0.75 with inferior thinning. Surgery was performed with goniosynechialysis using the Trabectome tip to expose the nasal TM, followed by ablation of the TM (**Fig. 23.1**). After 1 year, the IOP had decreased to 12 mm Hg on only timolol drops, which helped allow the cornea to clear and improved the vision to 20/60.

The Procedure

Trabeculectomy was originally described as a mechanism of plasma surgery with a bipolar 550-kHz electrode that could ablate a nasal arc of TM through a gonioscopic view. It was designed to improve the aqueous outflow in cases of open-angle glaucomas while reducing the side-effect profile of external filtration procedures. The Trabectome system consists of four components: the disposable handpiece, the foot pedal, the cautery generator with a peristaltic irrigation-aspiration console, and the stand (**Fig. 23.2**).

Rationale Behind the Procedure

By removing the TM, the aqueous has direct access to Schlemm's canal, which should significantly increase the rate of outflow by decreasing the amount of aqueous outflow resistance. Previous work over several decades has shown that the juxtacanalicular TM and endothelial cells in Schlemm's canal offer the greatest source of aqueous outflow resistance.[3] Because it is believed that only 35% of total resistance to aqueous outflow is found beyond the inner wall of Schlemm's canal, techniques to allow the aqueous to bypass this region should greatly facilitate aqueous egress.[4] There is a nonlinear relationship between the decrease in resistance and the increased area of trabeculotomy, at least partly because Schlemm's canal is septated and is actually wider near the collector channel orifices,[5] so a long ablation arc may expose more collector channel orifices directly to the anterior chamber.

Because the procedure does not rely on external filtering of the aqueous, only a single clear corneal incision is made. By leaving the conjunctiva untouched and without retaining any hardware in the eye, the side-effect profile of the procedure is much closer to that of phacoemulsification than that of traditional glaucoma filtration surgery.

Patient Selection

In the initial clinical report,[1] the Trabectome was described for use in open-angle glaucomas (angles open to at least 20 degrees), because an adequate view of the meshwork is required to engage the instrument. It may be that with a smaller surface area, a narrow angle has a greater propensity for fibrosis or peripheral anterior synechiae (PASs) to close the surgical cleft made after removing the meshwork. This theory has been challenged with clinical data (see Safety, Efficacy, and Results, below). We now routinely operate on cases with a wide range of etiologies, including narrow angles, trauma, scleral buckles, and uveitis, as well as following failed trabeculectomy.[6,7]

To be positioned properly during the surgery, patients must be able to rotate either their neck or their entire axial core so that the surgeon is ensured a view of the angle through the goniolens. If the patient has a secondary glaucoma from increased episcleral pressure, then the IOP would not be expected to be lowered as significantly, because this procedure relies on the episcleral veins for aqueous drainage. Also, the increased episcleral pressure would increase the frequency of blood refluxing through Schlemm's canal, potentially causing recurrent microhyphemas, which pose the risk of episodes of decreased vision and

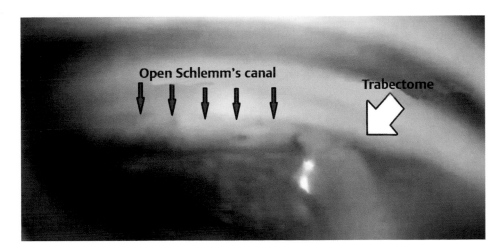

Fig. 23.1 Using the Trabectome for goniosynechialysis in advanced angle-closure glaucoma. Note the poor view through the edematous cornea. The Trabectome is passing from left to right into an area of synechiae, and the opening in Schlemm's canal is seen to the left.

increased IOP.[8] The only contraindication that has been widely reported in the literature is active neovascular glaucoma. This contraindication is not based on any published reports of complications following use of the Trabectome for neovascular glaucoma, but rather it is thought that attempting to ablate a vascularized angle will lead to excessive hyphema with a resultant higher risk of fibrosis closing the surgical cleft. Finally, because the TM is the target tissue, when there is heavier TM

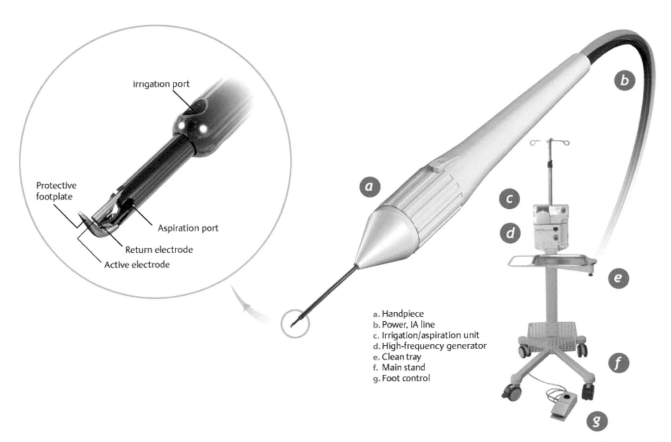

a. Handpiece
b. Power, IA line
c. Irrigation/aspiration unit
d. High-frequency generator
e. Clean tray
f. Main stand
g. Foot control

Fig. 23.2 The Trabectome system. The handpiece *(a) is* connected via tubing and cables *(b)* to an irrigation/aspiration (IA) unit *(c)* and a high-frequency generator *(d)*. The handpiece can be rested on the clean tray *(e)*. The irrigation/aspiration unit, high-frequency generator and clean tray are mounted on a wheeled stand with an adjustable pole *(f)*. The amount of fluid flow is controlled by manual adjustment of the balanced salt solution bottle on the pole above the unit, and the foot pedal *(g)* is used to turn on the irrigation and then the aspiration and ablation.

pigmentation, the surgical target site is highlighted. Patients with pigmentary glaucoma may have better IOP outcomes (see Safety, Efficacy, and Results, below).

Surgical Technique

This section describes the key steps to maximize the potential result of a lower postoperative IOP while minimizing potential complications. It is not absolutely necessary to stop systemic platelet inhibitors or anticoagulants, but this can be considered if it is safe to do so. Stopping blood thinners does not reduce the frequency of postoperative hyphemas because they are the result of flow reversal during early postoperative low pressure. However, if iris vessel bleeding results from traumatic injury with the tip, then the potential for bleeding is increased with these agents.

Stand-Alone Procedure

The tip of the 19.5-gauge handpiece is coated in a proprietary multilayered polymer with a pointed tip necessary to engage the TM while protecting the surrounding tissue from dissipated heat.[9] The electrocautery unit operates at 550 kHz at 0.1 to 10 W.

The aspiration port is only 0.3 mm away from the electrode tip, so that ablated debris is quickly and effectively aspirated to keep the view clear, while the irrigation also helps keep the anterior chamber deep and improves the view.[9] The irrigation and aspiration is controlled with the foot pedal. Position 1 activates continuous, nonlinear aspiration, and position 2 activates ablation. The aspiration has a maximum flow rate of 10 mL/minute.[10] The foot pedal also has a black ball that activates continuous irrigation when it is tapped.

The preoperative preparation is identical to that for topical clear cornea phacoemulsification, with the addition of gonioscopy to confirm that the TM is visible. The surgeon sits temporally. As with phacoemulsification, a paracentesis should be created to inject 1% preservative-free lidocaine. The irrigation bottle should be raised as high as deemed safe for the optic nerve status, because this deepens the angle and improves the view. No viscoelastic is needed and actually could worsen the view by trapping gas bubbles from ablation.

The main incision should be 1.6 to 1.8 mm to enable a tight fit of the handpiece to keep the chamber maintained (**Fig. 23.3**). The incision should be uniplanar and parallel to the iris to improve the facile insertion of the handpiece. To reduce the risk of iris prolapse through the wound, the incision should be created 1 to 2 mm anterior to the limbus. If a beveled incision is made from the limbus, the entry into anterior chamber will also be 1 to 2 mm anterior to the limbus. To ablate more than 90 degrees in total, we recommend enlarging both internal sides of the wound. With a uniplanar wound and flaring the right and left internal corners, there is more room to sweep the handpiece to each side without causing significant corneal striae that will impair the view significantly.

Once the wound is created, a view of the TM must be established. The most commonly used goniolens is the direct modified Swan-Jacobs gonioscopy lens (Ocular Instruments, Bellingham, WA). No coupling gel is required but balanced salt solution should be applied to the cornea before placing the lens. For the clearest and deepest view, there should be almost 60 to 80 degrees between the chamber and the surgeon: 30 to 40 degrees from rotating the microscope downward, and 30 to 40 from rotating the patient's head away from the surgeon. If the patient is unable to rotate the neck, then another option is rotating the entire axial core, although this may make it difficult to stabilize the surgeon's hands. If the view is established but the TM cannot be found, a small amount of fluid egress out of the main wound will enable a temporary hypotony. Hypotony can allow blood to reflux into Schlemm's canal, highlighting the target tissue (**Fig. 23.4**). Ablating the wrong structure likely accounts for many cases where excessive hyphemas are seen in the early postoperative period.

Once the gonioscopic view of the TM has been established, the handpiece is inserted and advanced across the anterior chamber while viewing through the goniolens (**Fig. 23.5**). The TM should be approached with the tip at an angle. The upward angle helps with the engagement of this thin tissue (**Fig. 23.6**). The other technique to improve engagement is to avoid approaching the TM from a perpendicular angle. The angle of approach should instead be greater than 90 degrees from the direction of ablation. Once the TM is engaged, the ablation arc should be swept in a smooth motion, because there is very little resistance once the correct space is entered (**Fig. 23.7**). While the ablation

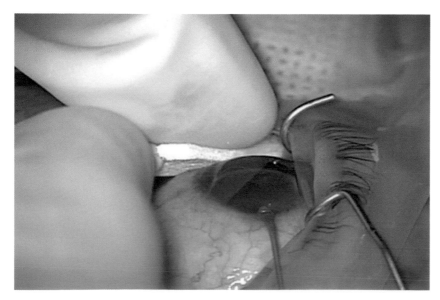

Fig. 23.3 Surgical photograph of the clear corneal incision for Trabectome.

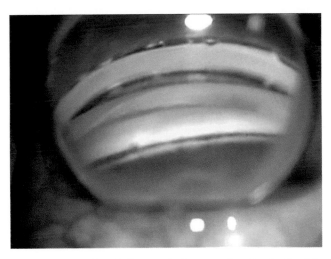

Fig. 23.4 Surgical goniophotograph demonstrating blood reflux into Schlemm's canal prior to ablation of the trabecular meshwork. This was accomplished by inducing temporary hypotony with release of aqueous from the incision and then repressurizing the anterior chamber. The area of blood is the target for the ablation.

is performed, it is vital to exert a very slight inward force to counteract the natural outward pressure that accompanies the sweep, particularly as the tip nears the edge of the gonioscopic image at the superior and inferior poles, where the curvature is not reflected well in the image. The inward pull helps avoid direct damage from the tip to the small collector channels in the outer wall of Schlemm's canal.

The ablation should be started at 0.8 mW, as was described in the original cases.[1] The ideal power has not been investigated since then. If there is insufficient ablation, the power should not need to be increased by more than 1 to 3 mW. If the power is too high, blackened necrotic tissue will be seen at the ablation lip. The first 60 degrees of ablation can usually be accomplished without many adjustments, and we routinely approach 90 degrees of ablation in each direction. Rotating the goniolens in the direction

of ablation can help widen the view at the superior and inferior poles. At the end of the arc, the tip is disengaged from the TM and rotated toward the iris by 180 degrees so that the ablation can be continued in the other direction. By ablating 180 degrees, the aqueous has direct access to at least 240 degrees of outflow because one opening through the TM can provide access to 60 degrees of Schlemm's canal.[11] After the second half of the arc is completed, injecting a viscoelastic crescent near the ablation zone minimizes postoperative hyphema from reflux through Schlemm's canal. Our technique used in a consecutive series of 192 patients led to an IOP ≤ 18 mm Hg in 81%, IOP ≤ 15 in 52%, and an IOP ≤ 12 in 27% after 1 year.[12]

In narrow angles with peripheral anterior synechiae, the smooth tip of the Trabectome handpiece makes an excellent instrument for goniosynechialysis (**Fig. 23.8**). If the PAS is not densely adherent, simply sweeping them downward and posteriorly may remove them from the TM. Forceful movements should not be made, to avoid creating iridodialysis or a cyclodialysis cleft. If the synechiae are more adherent, they can be directly engaged with the tip and very gently peeled off of the TM.

Combined with Phacoemulsification

If the procedure is combined with phacoemulsification, the Trabectome surgery should be completed first. This enables a tighter incision and a watertight chamber during the Trabectome surgery. Following the ablation, the Trabectome is disengaged from the TM and removed from the incision, and viscoelastic can be injected near the ablation arc to minimize hyphema. The main wound can now be enlarged to the necessary size for phacoemulsification, and the wound should now be made triplanar. Capsulotomy and phacoemulsification can proceed as usual. If the angle is quite narrow and does not open with irrigation, the Trabectome surgery is sometimes performed after the removal of the cataract. Indeed, some surgeons prefer this technique to maximize the exposure of the TM. With this technique, the cataract incision should be closed with a suture, and the Trabectome tip can be inserted to one side of the suture. The placement of the suture effectively reduces the incision size to fit the Trabectome tip and helps maintain the anterior chamber. During irrigation and aspiration, some surgeons leave some viscoelastic near the nasal ablation site to minimize postoperative hyphema.

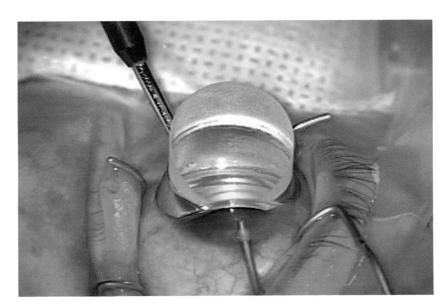

Fig. 23.5 Surgical photograph of the Trabectome tip inserted through the corneal incision and advancing across the anterior chamber with the goniolens.

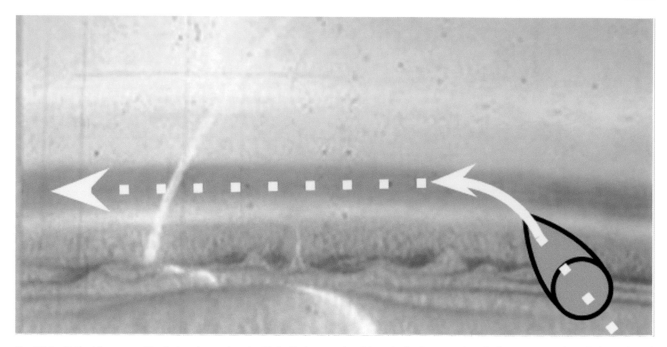

Fig. 23.6 Method for approaching trabecular meshwork with the Trabectome handpiece tip tilted at an angle to facilitate insertion through the meshwork and into Schlemm's canal.

Complications Specific to the Procedure

Trabectome surgery has a safety profile that is similar to phacoemulsification especially when combined with phacoemulsification. An early postoperative hyphema that is the result of temporary flow reversal is common following a Trabectome surgery and should not be viewed as a significant complication. Hyphemas may occur far beyond the immediate postoperative period, but they are extremely rare. A series of 12 patients complained of transient blurring between 2 and 31 months after a Trabectome surgery and were found to have spontaneous reflux that was associated with an increase in IOP that averaged 12 mm

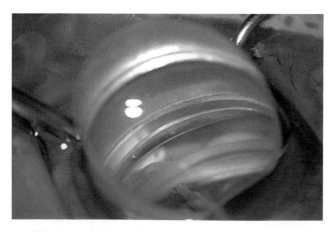

Fig. 23.7 Surgical photograph showing the creation of the ablation arc using the Trabectome. The trabecular meshwork and inner wall of Schlemm's canal has been removed to the right of the handpiece, with exposure of the outer wall of the canal *(white)* and some reflux of blood from collector channels *(red)*.

Hg higher than the previous visit.[8] In our experience of 800 cases, only one patient experienced recurrent hyphema. He had high myopia with an axial length of 27 mm and suffered associated IOP elevations. The hyphema stopped when anticoagulation with aspirin was discontinued and did not recur 6 months later when the aspirin was resumed.

A transient postoperative IOP spike of ≥ 10 mm Hg may be seen in 4 to 10%.[13,14] Another common problem is PAS, which can be found in up to 24% of patients.[1] If PAS leads to an IOP rise, neodymium:yttrium-aluminum-garnet (Nd:YAG) laser-mediated PAS lysis can be performed.[15]

Performing a stand-alone trabeculectomy in phakic eyes does not seem to accelerate cataract progression; after 30 months, only one of 86 cataracts (1.2%) was noted to have significant progression.[16] Cystoid macular edema was reported to occur in only 1.6% of 192 combined phacoemulsification-Trabectome surgeries.[17]

An extensive literature search revealed that the most commonly reported serious complication reported was 10 cases of hypotony (IOP < 5 mm Hg) after 1 month.[2,18] However, there were no details given as to what the target IOP had been, what was the possible etiology, and whether this was clinically significant.

As in all intraocular procedures, endophthalmitis, retinal detachment, and bleeding are possible complications. Only a single case of endophthalmitis with *Enterococcus faecalis* 1 week after phaco–Trabectome surgery was reported when the patient used unsanitary water during a 1-week power outage caused by a hurricane.[19] A single case of a suprachoroidal hemorrhage with no further details given has been reported.[20] No retinal detachment or tears have been described during the initial 3-month postoperative period, even though the Trabectome is often used in surgery performed on patients with high myopia to avoid retinal complications of trabeculectomy and tube shunt implantation. We have observed a shallow retinal detachment in a patient with 28 mm axial length who presented with flashes and floaters 1½ years after phaco-Trabectome surgery that was successfully reattached using gas.

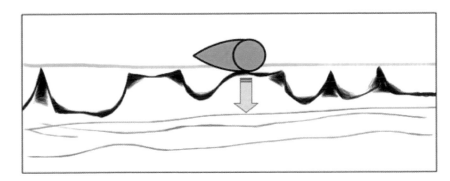

Fig. 23.8 Goniosynechialysis with the Trabectome utilizes the safety of the rounded footplate and takes advantage of irrigation and aspiration for a stable, pressurized anterior chamber in which debris can be quickly removed. The blunt side of the tip is used to exert gentle downward pressure on the synechiae to pull it away from the trabecular meshwork. Schwalbe's line is shown (*gray*).

Four cases of aqueous misdirection have been published, but no details were provided about risk factors such as chronic angle-closure or short axial length, or about whether it was a combined procedure.[17] There are seven reported cases of cyclodialysis cleft and four of them closed spontaneously.[21] One patient referred to us for persistent hypotony at 6 months despite atropine use had a narrow but long cyclodialysis tract that was the result of the patient making a sudden head movement toward the Trabectome tip during surgery. After defining the exact location with ultra-biomicroscopy, we were able to close this tract with a simple, single limbus parallel loop stitch from the outside through the conjunctiva, sclera, and ciliary body, resulting in instant closure without the need for transcameral suturing or cut-down with direct suturing.

Trabectome surgery is effective in traumatic glaucoma with or without angle recession, as we have found in five cases. The angle should be treated in an area that does not have angle recession damage. No cases of sympathetic ophthalmia have been observed.

As of April 2015, no occurrence of vision loss of two or more lines of Snellen visual acuity could be directly attributed to the Trabectome. Although most reports directly specify that no patient lost two or more lines of vision, there is a single paper that notes that 13 patients (5%) lost at least two lines of vision, but it does not specify if the vision loss was related to glaucoma or to a different comorbidity, whether there was a surgical or postoperative complication, or whether those patients had received combined surgery.[22]

How to Recognize and Manage Complications

The majority of postoperative hyphemas are small enough to clear within the first postoperative week and do not require any additional care. Microhyphemas, which can appear similar to postoperative anterior chamber inflammatory cells, still do not require any change in treatment. There are only three published cases requiring a surgical intervention because of a hyphema with an IOP spike.[8,17] Keeping the anterior chamber pressurized and leaving a small amount of viscoelastic near the ablation zone at the end of the procedure may minimize postoperative reflux. If a reoperation is later necessary, intraoperative hyphema has been reported and it is suggested to take measures to avoid hypotony during reoperations, such as ensuring that enough viscoelastic is in the anterior chamber and preplacing sutures for a trabeculectomy.[23]

Gonioscopy should be done routinely after 1 month or sooner if the IOP starts to increase. Even if PASs are seen following Trabectome surgery, it is still not clear what the functional sequelae will be. In a small series of eight patients, one team reported using YAG laser goniopuncture where the laser was applied to

the synechiae at 0.2 to 0.6 mJ for three to 15 shots.[15] The IOP did decrease 21% after 11 months, but there are no further reports of the success of this procedure. If a cyclodialysis cleft is noted, it seems prudent to defer surgical closure as long as possible because at least four of the reported six clefts closed spontaneously.

Additional Considerations and Surgical Tips

- To help limit anterior chamber bleeding, one may use topical apraclonidine or brimonidine preoperatively, or preservative-free epinephrine intracameral injection. Complete irrigation and aspiration will help reduce postoperative hyphema. If blood reflux is significant despite irrigation, consider an air bubble tamponade in the anterior chamber or a small amount of viscoelastic in the nasal angle.

- If the corneal view is poor, reduce corneal striae by not applying compression with the goniolens or torque at the wound edges. If there is peripheral epithelial edema at the incision, removing the epithelium in this area may improve the view.

- If the angle is too narrow, increase the irrigation from the console and make sure the corneal incision is not too large.

- If iris is obstructing the view, advance the tip of the handpiece all the way to the angle so that the irrigation is pushing down onto the anterior surface of the iris and not flowing posterior to the iris to cause billowing anteriorly. Viscoelastic can also be placed in the peripheral angle to push the iris posteriorly.

- Iris prolapse is often caused by improper wound construction, and is best treated with a paracentesis with decompression of the anterior chamber and viscoelastic.

- To aid in finding TM, preoperative gonioscopy is critical to establish angle landmarks. When the anterior chamber is inflated, identify the ciliary body band and scleral spur and work your way anteriorly. As stated, inducing temporary hypotony may cause blood reflux into Schlemm's canal and highlight the area to treat.

- Corneal endothelial or Descemet's membrane damage is usually not clinically significant and does not require treatment, but if it is extensive it should be treated with an air bubble in the anterior chamber to push the tissue back into place.

- Lens damage can be avoided by constricting the pupil in stand-alone cases with pilocarpine or intracameral miotic. One should be prepared with intraocular lens calculations prior to surgery in case the capsule is violated and removal of the lens is necessary.

- Iris damage may be prevented during insertion of the handpiece by starting with a formed anterior chamber and inserting the tip with the irrigation on. If the anterior chamber is still very shallow, place viscoelastic just inside the temporal incision site. To avoid iris damage during tissue ablation, take care not to try to treat more of the angle than is easily visible or accessible. If it occurs, damage is usually at the very limits of the ablation arc.
- A cyclodialysis cleft can be avoided by treating in the proper location (TM instead of ciliary body band) and avoiding sudden movements with the handpiece tip or of the patient's head.

Postoperative Management

In routine cases, for both stand-alone and combined cases, all glaucoma medications can be discontinued on the day of surgery. The postoperative routine should be the same as for phacoemulsification, with the addition of pilocarpine 1 to 2% (i.e., a topical fluoroquinolone), prednisolone acetate 1% or loteprednol 0.5% four times a day, and pilocarpine two to four times on the day of surgery. The antibiotic can be maintained for 1 week and the steroid tapered over 1 month. Pilocarpine can be decreased after 1 month and then discontinued after 1 more month; it is used to flatten the peripheral iris, which may reduce the risk of postoperative fibrosis and peripheral anterior synechiae closing the surgical cleft.[15] Refraction should be delayed until the pilocarpine is stopped.

The two most common reasons for surgical failure are inadequate ablation, such as not entering the correct space and completely ablating the TM,[24] and fibrosis of the surgical cleft. Corneal endothelial cells at Schwalbe's line[25] have been demonstrated to migrate and repair wounded TM and are very likely capable of forming a membrane over the Trabectome cleft.[26] Most failures occur within 6 months; over 5 years with 738 stand-alone Trabectome surgeries, 14% of patients required additional surgery, and 88% of them required their second surgery by postoperative month 6.[27] In another study, the time to reoperation ranged from 3 days to 18 months, and averaged 4.9 months.[28]

Following a failed Trabectome surgery, every type of conventional surgery and laser has been reported as a subsequent procedure, but the most common is trabeculectomy ab externo.[17,22,29] Repeat Trabectome surgery has been reported in some cases without enough data to analyze the efficacy.[29] It has been suggested that testing for an episcleral venous fluid wave (decompressing the anterior chamber and then placing the irrigation/aspiration handpiece directly adjacent to the cleft and triggering irrigation, looking for the surge of balanced salt solution blanching episcleral, conjunctival, or aqueous veins to demonstrate functional patency of the distal collector system) can be used to distinguish between failure due to fibrosis at collector channel orifices versus at more distal structures.[30] The authors suggested that repeat Trabectome surgery will be more successful if a fluid wave cannot be initiated despite a visibly patent surgical cleft, although to test this requires a return to the operating room.

Safety, Efficacy, and Results

All of the published data on the Trabectome uses IOP as the main outcome measure. At this time, there are no papers directly describing stabilization of visual fields or retinal nerve fiber layer thinning as a result of this surgical intervention. Currently, no randomized controlled trial results have been published.

Trabectome and phaco-Trabectome surgery can be expected to decrease the IOP to an average of 15 mm Hg that is relatively independent of preoperative IOP and above the theoretical limit of episcleral venous pressure near 8 mm Hg.[31] This residual outflow resistance is thought to be relatively close to the outer wall of Schlemm's canal.[4] Statistically, IOP is typically reduced by an overall average of 8 mm Hg, or 31%, while concurrently lowering the number of medications by one.[18] The largest study dating back to the original case had 1,878 Trabectome cases (alone or with phacoemulsification) recorded as of 2010.[32] There were data on five patients who had been evaluated a full 6 years after the procedure and they still maintained a 38% mean IOP decrease.

The use of the Trabectome has now been reported in most subtypes of glaucoma, although two thirds of reported cases are still done for primary open-angle glaucoma (POAG). There is some evidence that the Trabectome works even better in secondary open-angle glaucomas. Two prospective studies found greater reductions in IOP in pigmentary or pseudoexfoliation glaucoma than with POAG.[14,17] For pseudoexfoliation, combining the case with phacoemulsification can avoid further accumulation of pseudoexfoliation material. Due to its superior safety profile relative to external filtration procedures, it can be employed earlier in the disease progression, helping to avoid highly complicated surgeries from zonular dehiscence seen later on.

Because different studies use different definitions of success, it is difficult to estimate the average success rate. The longest available success analysis (from the Trabectome Study Group) defined success as IOP ≤ 21 mm Hg while maintaining a 20% IOP decrease from baseline without reoperation, and the success rate was 85% for combined cases after 5 years, and 56% for stand-alone Trabectome cases after 7.5 years, for an overall rate of 66%.[2] Only 7% of those cases had reoperations. These success rates are similar to other studies.[14,33]

The biggest risk factor for failure is a lower baseline IOP, with a hazard ratio of 0.96 per 1 mm Hg.[29] Another study (n = 304) stratified IOP results after combined cases and found that when the baseline IOP was > 25 mm Hg, there was a 45% IOP decrease at 12 months, but if the baseline IOP was < 20 mm Hg, then there was actually a 0.2% IOP increase (although the patients were on 60% fewer medications compared with baseline).[10] This is likely due to a floor effect, where most successful cases will finish with an IOP in the low to mid-teens, regardless of the baseline IOP. Another possible explanation, however, is that with a high baseline IOP, the main goal of the procedure was to lower IOP, whereas in patients with lower baseline IOPs the main goal was reducing medication dependence. The second main risk factor is younger age (hazard ratio 0.98 per year).[29]

The use of the Trabectome has not been compared with any other procedure in a randomized trial. Just to give an overall average to compare with the mean 8 mm Hg (33%) IOP decrease seen with the Trabectome, previous studies suggest that stand-alone phacoemulsification decreases the IOP by 1.5 to 2 mm Hg.[34] The iStent (Glaukos, Laguna Hills, CA) has been shown to reduce the IOP by 8[35] to 27%[36] with an overall mean final IOP of ~ 17 mm Hg. Endoscopic cyclophotocoagulation lowers the IOP by an overall average of 7 mm Hg or 31% in POAG and 18 mm Hg (50% decrease) in advanced secondary glaucomas, mostly neovascular glaucoma.[37] In the multicenter, randomized Tube Versus Trabeculectomy Study, a Baerveldt shunt lowered the IOP by 41% (mean IOP at 5 years was 14.4 mm Hg) and trabeculectomy by 50% (mean IOP at 5 years was 12.6 mm Hg).[38] This compares well with other large studies, including a national survey[39] as well as a meta-analysis, which found that trabeculectomy lowered the IOP 3.8 mm Hg more than aqueous shunts.[40]

Two studies compared the Trabectome to trabeculectomy with mitomycin C but neither was randomized. A prospective study found a 52% IOP decrease following trabeculectomy versus a 30% decrease following Trabectome surgery with a statistically similar success rate in both groups.[13] The second study was retrospective (*n* = 217).[29] After 2 years, the success rate of Trabectome surgery was only 43% versus 76% with trabeculectomy. In exchange for this superior IOP reduction, the complication rate was 35% with trabeculectomy versus only 4% with Trabectome surgery.

Expanding Indications as a Secondary and Adjunctive Procedure

Narrow anterior chamber angles were previously considered a relative contraindication due to the assumed high risk of failure. However, in a prospective study of Trabectome surgery alone and combined with phacoemulsification, the outcomes demonstrated no significant differences between narrow and open angles in the reduction of IOP, medications, and complications, and in the success rates.[7] The Trabectome has also been demonstrated to successfully lower IOP by ~ 30% after failed trabeculectomy and tube shunt surgery.[6,41]

Most recently, Trabectome surgery has also been explored as an adjunctive procedure with tube shunt implantation or as a stepped up procedure after a failed triple ICE (iStent, cataract extraction, and endocyclophotocoagulation) procedure or after

failed canaloplasty. In the latter case, the sutures can be engaged with the tip and drawn into the center of the eye. This leads to a circumferential trabeculotomy, the lips of which can be further ablated in the nasal angle to avoid reapproximation. Similarly, we have removed five iStents in patients referred for postoperative IOP increase. We ablated TM along the nasal circumference, leading to an appropriate IOP reduction. Most of these eyes had persistent inflammation, and one iStent was implanted into the ciliary body, resulting in persistent arterial bleeding associated with high IOP. These trabecular bypass stents were difficult to extract with microforceps due to fibrosis (**Fig. 23.9**) with scar formation on histology.

Cost Considerations

High costs on an individual case basis are attributed to the disposable handpiece, which cannot be reused, as the activation of the power through the outgoing and returning electrode during surgery may result in a change in the coating of the handpiece and improper discharge of energy if used again. The surgical system of the electrosurgical generator and irrigation aspiration console is a one-time, fixed setup cost.

The direct medical cost estimates for 2 million patients with glaucoma in the United States is $2.9 billion annually.[42] This does

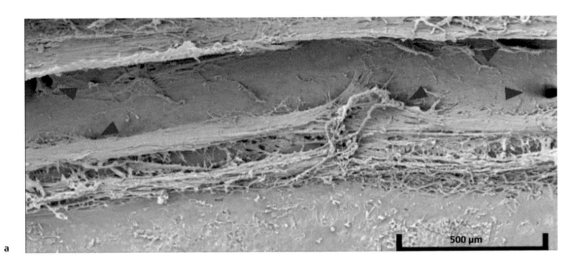

a

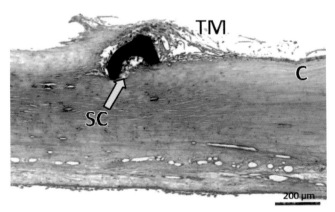

b

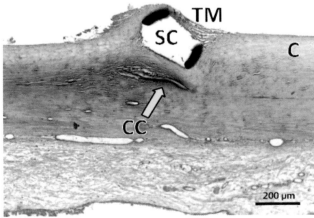

c

Fig. 23.9 Challenges encountered in angle surgery. **(a)** Electron microscopy of Trabectome-ablated Schlemm's canal. *Red arrowheads* indicate collector openings that may occlude by the superior and posterior wound lips in goniotomy or suture trabeculotomy. **(b)** Partial lumen occlusion of a trabecular bypass stent. TM, trabecular meshwork. **(c)** Inadvertent compression of the collector channel (CC) by a scaffold stent. SC, Schlemm's canal.

not account for other direct costs or productivity losses. Given these considerations and the chronic nature of glaucoma, it is worth taking into account the costs savings offered by MIGS procedures compared with glaucoma medications. A cost-analysis study using the Ontario Health Insurance Plan indicated that the cost of treatment with the Trabectome offered modest cost savings compared with medications.[43] Over a projected period of 6 years, successful Trabectome surgeries offered a cumulative cost savings of Canadian $279.23, $1,572.55, and $2,424.71 per patient versus monodrug, bi-drug, and tri-drug therapy, respectively. However, a formal cost-effective study to test these assumptions has yet to be done.

Conclusion

Trabeculectomy ab interno with the Trabectome is a developed surgical technique with an extensive body of experience since 2004. On average, the Trabectome can be expected to lower the IOP by ~ 31% to a final average IOP of around 15 mm Hg. Comparable results may also be achieved with various subtypes of glaucoma, including angle-closure, inactive neovascular, uveitic, traumatic, and postsurgical glaucoma. Vision-threatening complications are limited to case reports at the current time, and total < 1% of reported cases. The Trabectome offers an effective and safe surgical option for a wide range of glaucomas.

References

1. Minckler DS, Baerveldt G, Alfaro MR, Francis BA. Clinical results with the Trabectome for treatment of open-angle glaucoma. Ophthalmology 2005;112:962–967

2. Mosaed S. The first decade of global Trabectome outcomes. Clinical & Surgical Ophthalmology. 2014;32:1

3. Johnson MC, Kamm RD. The role of Schlemm's canal in aqueous outflow from the human eye. Invest Ophthalmol Vis Sci 1983;24:320–325

4. Schuman JS, Chang W, Wang N, de Kater AW, Allingham RR. Excimer laser effects on outflow facility and outflow pathway morphology. Invest Ophthalmol Vis Sci 1999;40:1676–1680

5. Hann CR, Bentley MD, Vercnocke A, Ritman EL, Fautsch MP. Imaging the aqueous humor outflow pathway in human eyes by three-dimensional micro-computed tomography (3D micro-CT). Exp Eye Res 2011;92:104–111

6. Bussel II, Kaplowitz K, Schuman JS, Loewen NA, Trabectome Study Group. Outcomes of ab interno trabeculectomy with the Trabectome after failed trabeculectomy. Br J Ophthalmol 2015;99:258–262

7. Bussel II, Kaplowitz K, Schuman JS, Loewen NA, Trabectome Study Group. Outcomes of ab interno trabeculectomy with the Trabectome by degree of angle opening. Br J Ophthalmol 2015;99:914–919

8. Ahuja Y, Malihi M, Sit AJ. Delayed-onset symptomatic hyphema after ab interno trabeculotomy surgery. Am J Ophthalmol 2012;154:476–480.e2

9. Pantcheva MB, Kahook MY. Ab interno trabeculectomy. Middle East Afr J Ophthalmol 2010;17:287–289

10. Francis BA, Minckler D, Dustin L, et al; Trabectome Study Group. Combined cataract extraction and trabeculotomy by the internal approach for coexisting cataract and open-angle glaucoma: initial results. J Cataract Refract Surg 2008;34:1096–1103

11. Rosenquist R, Epstein D, Melamed S, Johnson M, Grant WM. Outflow resistance of enucleated human eyes at two different perfusion pressures and different extents of trabeculotomy. Curr Eye Res 1989;8:1233–1240

12. Kaplowitz K, Schuman JS, Loewen NA. Techniques and outcomes of minimally invasive trabecular ablation and bypass surgery. Br J Ophthalmol 2014;98:579–585

13. Francis BA, Winarko J. Ab interno Schlemm's canal surgery: Trabectome and i-stent. Dev Ophthalmol 2012;50:125–136

14. Ting JL, Damji KF, Stiles MC; Trabectome Study Group. Ab interno trabeculectomy: outcomes in exfoliation versus primary open-angle glaucoma. J Cataract Refract Surg 2012;38:315–323

15. Wang Q, Harasymowycz P. Goniopuncture in the treatment of short-term post-Trabectome intraocular pressure elevation: a retrospective case series study. J Glaucoma 2012

16. Minckler D, Baerveldt G, Ramirez MA, et al. Clinical results with the Trabectome, a novel surgical device for treatment of open-angle glaucoma. Trans Am Ophthalmol Soc 2006;104:40–50

17. Jordan JF, Wecker T, van Oterendorp C, et al. Trabectome surgery for primary and secondary open angle glaucomas. Graefes Arch Clin Exp Ophthalmol 2013;251:2753–2760

18. Kaplowitz K, Bussel I, Schuman JS, Loewen N. Meta-analysis of ab interno trabeculectomy outcomes. American Glaucoma Society annual meeting, San Diego, 2015

19. Kaplowitz K, Chen X, Loewen N. Two year results for 180 degree Trabectome ablation. American Glaucoma Society annual meeting, San Francisco, 2013

20. Minckler D, Dustin L, Mosaed S. Trabectome UPdate: 2004–2010. Poster, American Glaucoma Society, Naples, FL, 2001

21. Mosaed S, Rhee D, Filippopoulos T. Trabectome outcomes in adult open-angle glaucoma patients: one-year follow-up. Clin Surg Ophthalmol. 2010;28:5–9

22. Ahuja Y, Ma Khin Pyi S, Malihi M, Hodge DO, Sit AJ. Clinical results of ab interno trabeculotomy using the Trabectome for open-angle glaucoma: the Mayo Clinic series in Rochester, Minnesota. Am J Ophthalmol 2013; 156:927–935.e2

23. Knape RM, Smith MF. Anterior chamber blood reflux during trabeculectomy in an eye with previous Trabectome surgery. J Glaucoma 2010;19: 499–500

24. Francis BA, See RF, Rao NA, Minckler DS, Baerveldt G. Ab interno trabeculectomy: development of a novel device (Trabectome) and surgery for open-angle glaucoma. J Glaucoma 2006;15:68–73

25. McGowan SL, Edelhauser HF, Pfister RR, Whikehart DR. Stem cell markers in the human posterior limbus and corneal endothelium of unwounded and wounded corneas. Mol Vis 2007;13:1984–2000

26. Whikehart DR, Parikh CH, Vaughn AV, Mishler K, Edelhauser HF. Evidence suggesting the existence of stem cells for the human corneal endothelium. Mol Vis 2005;11:816–824

27. Minckler D, Mosaed S, Dustin L, Ms BF; Trabectome Study Group. Trabectome (trabeculectomy-internal approach): additional experience and extended follow-up. Trans Am Ophthalmol Soc 2008;106:149–159, discussion 159–160

28. Jea SY, Mosaed S, Vold SD, Rhee DJ. Effect of a failed Trabectome on subsequent trabeculectomy. J Glaucoma 2012;21:71–75

29. Jea SY, Francis BA, Vakili G, Filippopoulos T, Rhee DJ. Ab interno trabeculectomy versus trabeculectomy for open-angle glaucoma. Ophthalmology 2012;119:36–42

30. Fellman RL, Grover DS. Episcleral venous fluid wave: intraoperative evidence for patency of the conventional outflow system. J Glaucoma 2014; 23:347–350

31. Sit AJ, Ekdawi NS, Malihi M, McLaren JW. A novel method for computerized measurement of episcleral venous pressure in humans. Exp Eye Res 2011;92:537–544

32. Vold SD. Ab interno trabeculotomy with the Trabectome system: what does the data tell us? Int Ophthalmol Clin 2011;51:65–81

33. Francis BA. Trabectome combined with phacoemulsification versus phacoemulsification alone: a prospective, non-randomized controlled surgical trial. Clin Surg J Ophthalmol 2010;28:10

34. Shingleton BJ, Pasternack JJ, Hung JW, O'Donoghue MW. Three and five year changes in intraocular pressures after clear corneal phacoemulsification in open angle glaucoma patients, glaucoma suspects, and normal patients. J Glaucoma 2006;15:494–498

35. Craven ER, Katz LJ, Wells JM, Giamporcaro JE; iStent Study Group. Cataract surgery with trabecular micro-bypass stent implantation in patients with mild-to-moderate open-angle glaucoma and cataract: two-year follow-up. J Cataract Refract Surg 2012;38:1339–1345

36. Fernández-Barrientos Y, García-Feijoó J, Martínez-de-la-Casa JM, Pablo LE, Fernández-Pérez C, García Sánchez J. Fluorophotometric study of the effect of the Glaukos trabecular microbypass stent on aqueous humor dynamics. Invest Ophthalmol Vis Sci 2010;51:3327–3332

37. Kaplowitz K, Kuei A, Klenofsky B, Abazari A, Honkanen R. The use of endoscopic cyclophotocoagulation for moderate to advanced glaucoma. Acta Ophthalmol (Copenh) 2015;93:395–401

38. Gedde SJ, Schiffman JC, Feuer WJ, Herndon LW, Brandt JD, Budenz DL; Tube versus Trabeculectomy Study Group. Treatment outcomes in the Tube Versus Trabeculectomy (TVT) study after five years of follow-up. Am J Ophthalmol 2012;153:789–803.e2

39. Edmunds B, Thompson JR, Salmon JF, Wormald RP. The National Survey of Trabeculectomy. II. Variations in operative technique and outcome. Eye (Lond) 2001;15(Pt 4):441–448

40. Minckler DS, Vedula SS, Li TJ, Mathew MC, Ayyala RS. Aqueous shunts for glaucoma (Cochrane review). Cochrane Database Syst Rev 2006;2: CD004918

41. Mosaed S. Effect of Trabectome in Patients with Prior Failed Tube Shunts Surgery. American Glaucoma Society annual meeting, 2014

42. Rein DB, Zhang P, Wirth KE, et al. The economic burden of major adult visual disorders in the United States. Arch Ophthalmol 2006;124:1754–1760

43. Iordanous Y, Kent JS, Hutnik CML, Malvankar-Mehta MS. Projected cost comparison of Trabectome, iStent, and endoscopic cyclophotocoagulation versus glaucoma medication in the Ontario Health Insurance Plan. J Glaucoma 2014;23:e112–e118

24 Trabeculotomy by Internal Approach: Dual Blade

Handan Akil and Brian A. Francis

Intraocular pressure (IOP) is the most important modifiable risk factor for glaucoma.[1] The dysregulation of IOP is thought to be caused by the obstruction of aqueous outflow at the juxtacanalicular trabecular meshwork (TM) and distal outflow structures.[2,3] Performing a goniotomy or trabeculotomy in adults with glaucoma has not been as successful as in cases with congenital glaucoma for lowering IOP.[4] Inferior long-term outcomes in adults might be related to incomplete removal of TM and membrane formation or scarring across the remaining TM leaflets, with subsequent elevation in IOP.[5] More recently, a novel dual-blade ab interno trabeculectomy procedure has been reported to remove TM more completely than traditional trabeculotomy in adult patients.[6,7]

The Kahook Dual Blade (KDB, New World Medical, Inc., Rancho Cucamonga, CA) is a single-use ophthalmic knife designed to make parallel incisions in the trabecular meshwork, creating a free strip of tissue. The device has a micro-engineered profile that enables it to be inserted into the eye through a small clear corneal incision. The stainless steel body is composed of a long thin shaft that facilitates access across the anterior chamber, a pointed tip used to pierce the TM under gonioscopic view, a ramp that lifts and stretches the tissue as the device is advanced, and two blades for tissue cutting (**Figs. 24.1, 24.2, 24.3**). The angle of the distal cutting surface and the size of the device shaft are engineered to facilitate a maximum arc of treatment through a single clear corneal incision.

In a preclinical study of human donor corneoscleral rims, the KDB device was used to perform parallel incisions in the TM, and results were compared with the results of treatment with a microvitreoretinal (MVR) blade and the Trabectome (NeoMedix, Tustin, CA).[6] Specimens were collected and examined histologically under light microscopy. The authors also completed human eye perfusion studies to assess the IOP-lowering efficacy of each approach. Use of the MVR blade resulted in a full-thickness incision through the TM with minimal tissue removal and large residual leaflets. Use of the MVR blade was also associated with damage to the adjacent sclera. The Trabectome produced an opening in the TM with residual tissue and thermal damage to the edges of the residual TM leaflets. Histological analysis of specimens treated with the KDB ophthalmic knife revealed more complete TM tissue removal without damage to adjacent tissues. In this study, all surgeries with the dual-blade, MVR blade, and

Trabectome resulted in a statistically significant reduction of IOP. The dual-blade and Trabectome had a greater percentage decrease in IOP compared with the MVR blade, although this did not reach statistical significance. The size of the arc treated did not correlate with IOP lowering for any of the three devices.

Abdullah et al[7] discussed their initial clinical experience with a novel dual-blade device in a meeting abstract (results not yet published). They designed a multicenter study of 122 eyes that underwent (1) combined cataract and KDB (60%); (2) combined cataract, endoscopic cyclophotocoagulation (ECP), and KDB (14%); (3) combined KDB and ECP (16%); (4) KDB alone (7%); or (5) KDB plus other surgery (4%; percents sum to more than 100% because of rounding). The glaucoma type was mostly primary open-angle glaucoma (70%), with exfoliation, pigmentary dispersion, angle closure, and normal tension glaucoma comprising the rest.

The results for all eyes was a preoperative IOP of 18.9 ± 6.8 mm Hg (mean ± standard deviation), and after 3 months the IOP was reduced to 13.3 ± 4.1 mm Hg. For the 73 eyes that underwent combined cataract and dual-blade surgery, the IOP was reduced from 17.5 ± 5.3 mm Hg to 11.8 ± 2.5 mm Hg. The authors found that 83% of the eyes showed a reduction of at least one IOP lowering medication compared with preoperative values for all surgeries. The percentage of eyes with medication reduction was 69% for the combined cataract and dual-blade surgery cases. The complications noted were hyphema in 10% of patients at 1 day, and one case of additional glaucoma surgery.

Early results of dual-blade ab interno trabeculectomy are encouraging as a combined procedure with cataract extraction and/or ECP, and as a stand-alone surgery. Longer term results are awaited to demonstrate the long-term efficacy.

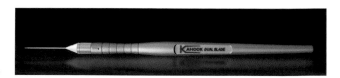

Fig. 24.1 The Kahook Dual Blade (New World Medical, Inc., Rancho Cucamonga, CA) is a single-use disposable ophthalmic knife. (Reprinted with permission from New World Medical, Inc., Rancho Cucamonga, CA.)

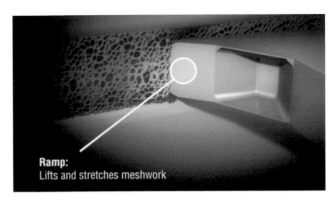

Fig. 24.2 The ramp is designed to lift and elevate the trabecular meshwork prior to the blades creating parallel incisions for tissue removal.

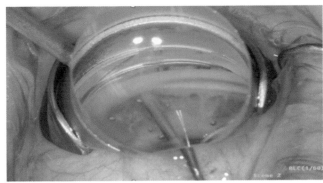

Fig. 24.3 The Kahook Dual Blade is shown cutting through the trabecular meshwork under gonioscopic view.

References

1. Quigley HA, Broman AT. The number of people with glaucoma worldwide in 2010 and 2020. Br J Ophthalmol 2006;90:262–267

2. Grant WM. Experimental aqueous perfusion in enucleated human eyes. Arch Ophthalmol 1963;69:783–801

3. Johnson DH, Tschumper RC. Human trabecular meshwork organ culture. A new method. Invest Ophthalmol Vis Sci 1987;28:945–953

4. Luntz MH, Livingston DG. Trabeculotomy ab externo and trabeculectomy in congenital and adult-onset glaucoma. Am J Ophthalmol 1977;83:174–179

5. Francis BA, See RF, Rao NA, Minckler DS, Baerveldt G. Ab interno trabeculectomy: development of a novel device (Trabectome) and surgery for open-angle glaucoma. J Glaucoma 2006;15:68–73

6. Seibold LK, Soohoo JR, Ammar DA, Kahook MY. Preclinical investigation of ab interno trabeculectomy using a novel dual-blade device. Am J Ophthalmol 2013;155:524–529.e2

7. Abdullah S, Jasek MC, Radcliffe NM, et al. A novel dual-blade device for goniotomy: initial clinical experience. Paper presented at the annual meeting of the Association for Research in Vision and Ophthalmology (ARVO), Seattle, 2016. http://www.arvo.org/webs/am2016/sectionpdf/GL/Session_448.pdf

25 Gonioscopy-Assisted Transluminal Trabeculotomy

Davinder S. Grover and Ronald L. Fellman

Case Presentation

A patient with mild to moderate glaucoma on maximal medical therapy presents with uncontrolled intraocular pressure (IOP) and an open angle with easy-to-define landmarks. The cornea is clear, the anterior chamber is deep, and the patient is not on chronic anticoagulant therapy. The surgeon and patient discuss using a microinvasive technique to improve the flow of aqueous into the patient's natural clogged drainage system. The patient understands that if the flow cannot be improved into its own natural drain, the patient will need further, and more aggressive, surgery to create a new drainage system for the eye. It is explained that the gonioscopy-assisted transluminal trabeculotomy (GATT) procedure, which does not involve scleral or conjunctival incisions, does not negate the option of using more invasive and traditional glaucoma procedures, should they be required in the future. Depending on the patient's lens status, this surgery can be safely performed as a stand-alone procedure or in combination with clear corneal cataract extraction.

The Procedure

Trabeculotomy lowers the IOP by enhancing the aqueous flow through an incised trabecular meshwork (TM)–Schlemm's canal complex consisting of the TM, the juxtacanalicular tissue (JCT), and the inner wall of Schlemm's canal (IWSC); this complex is the area of greatest resistance to aqueous flow. This bleb-less procedure improves aqueous flow through the patient's natural drainage system. Trabeculotomy has evolved from a loupe-assisted ab externo procedure into a modern-day gonioscopy-assisted ab interno circumferential minimally invasive glaucoma surgery (MIGS).

Trabeculotomy was initially designed in 1962 for a young patient with glaucoma secondary to Marfan's syndrome, with the hope that cleaving open a preexisting malformed angle would reduce the IOP.[1] Others extended the surgical concept to adults when they learned of Grant's[2] work, which found that much of the resistance to outflow in adult eyes was in the TM–canal area. Grant believed trabeculotomy reduced outflow resistance by 75%, but subsequent investigations found, at lower perfusion pressures, that trabeculotomy realistically eliminated 40 to 50% of outflow resistance.[3,4] Major advancements in trabeculotomy included the ability to navigate the canal, initially with a suture demonstrated by Redmond Smith,[5] then identifying the canal under a scleral flap,[6] circumnavigating the canal for 360 degrees,[7] and later with a lighted microcatheter.[8,9] Further advancements include the ability to open the canal for 360 degrees from an ab interno approach, without violating the conjunctiva or sclera, namely the GATT procedure.[10]

It is generally recognized that limited trabeculotomy with McPherson's[11] or Harms's trabeculotomes yields suboptimal long-term results in adults. However, over the past decade, progress in technique and technology has improved outcomes in adult glaucomas, especially with circumferential trabeculotomy. For example, Chin et al[12] found that 360-degree suture trabeculotomy ab externo was significantly more effective in lowering the IOP in adult primary and secondary glaucomas than was a limited metal trabeculotomy; the success rate was higher with the circumferential trabeculotomy, 84% versus 31%.

Over the past decade, the indications for circumferential trabeculotomy have widened to encompass more adult glaucomas.[13] This is due to the desire to reduce complications from filtration surgery, particularly bleb-related issues, and instead try to salvage the natural outflow channels of the eye. In addition, over the past decade, there has been a major surge in interest and innovation in angle-based procedures in the treatment of open-angle glaucoma, exemplified by the Trabectome (NeoMedix, Tustin, CA), canaloplasty, and trabecular microbypass with devices such as the iStent (Glaukos, Laguna Hills, CA) or the Hydrus (Ivantis, Irvine, CA).

Canal-based MIGS includes either a trabecular bypass device (iStent) or opening the canal with a Trabectome, suture, or microcather. All of these microinvasive techniques enable the surgeon to tailor the glaucoma procedure to the patient's needs, lifestyle, degree of glaucoma damage, and inherent drainage system functionality. This is a major advancement in glaucoma care.

Rationale Behind the GATT Procedure

The ability to enhance the circumferential flow of aqueous humor into the patient's diseased natural drainage system is a major step forward in glaucoma surgery. Flow into the patient's inherent collector system prevents all of the problems associated with trying to establish an artificial drain, through subconjunctival filtration. This minimally invasive approach avoids the problems related to blebs and tubes, and facilitates a rapid recovery. In addition, MIGS works well in conjunction with modern-day cataract surgery. One problem with MIGS is the inability to assess the condition of the collector channels before surgery. Understanding the status of the patient's inherent drainage system is vital because there may be damage to the intrascleral portion of the collector channels in certain types of open-angle glaucomas. Even if the surgeon successfully implants a trabecular device, or cleaves the trabecular meshwork, the downstream collector channels may not be functional and thus the procedure may be doomed to fail (see Chapter 26).

Patient Selection

Patient selection is critical to the outcome of all ophthalmologic procedures, but especially to the outcome of glaucoma surgeries in which both the health of the collector channels and the unpredictability of wound healing may significantly alter success. Patient selection regarding canal-based surgery is difficult because the success of the canal procedure is tied to the health and integrity of the downstream collector channels, and as of yet, we do not have a reliable preoperative methodology to visualize and assess the collector channels. If the collector channels are badly damaged or occluded, then a canal procedure's effect may be limited. Various studies have reported disparate MIGS outcomes, and we believe that the key factors that correlate with damaged collector channels are more severe disease, long duration of the disease, poorer condition of the ocular surface, and the presence of an intraoperative episcleral venous fluid wave (EVFW).[14] Thus, younger patients are likely to be better candidates for canal-based procedures, as their collector channels have had less time to atrophy. This surgical approach is the opposite of filtration surgery, in which older patients who scar less tend to be better candidates. In addition, trabeculotomy is particularly well suited for patients with primary congenital glaucoma (PCG) and juvenile open-angle glaucomas (JOAG), because their drainage system was malformed and cleavage of the canal restores more normal flow.

Careful preoperative gonioscopy is necessary for all GATT patient candidates, and if aberrant angle vessels or extensive peripheral anterior synechiae (PAS) are seen, we do not recommend the GATT procedure. Also, because one must perform several manipulations within the anterior chamber, a loose or unstable intraocular lens/bag complex is a contraindication to the GATT procedure. Patients with pigmentary and pseudoexfoliation glaucoma are good candidates, as excessive deposition of material typically causes increased resistance in the trabecular meshwork, and GATT is able to target the site of pathology. In addition, we have found the GATT procedure is often a reasonable option for patients with failed glaucoma drainage tubes or trabeculectomies as long as the angle is open. In patients with prior incisional glaucoma surgeries, one must evaluate the location of the tube or sclerostomy to ensure that Schlemm's canal is not involved. We have also had relatively good experience with GATT in patients with steroid-induced glaucoma, glaucoma related to anti–vascular endothelial growth factor (VEGF) treatment, angle recession glaucoma, and certain types of uveitic glaucoma.

Surgical Technique

Following a standard sterile preparation, the eye is draped and a nasal open wire lid speculum holds the eyelids open. A tangential (not radial), 23-gauge needle paracentesis track is placed through either the superonasal or inferonasal cornea. This first paracentesis track serves as the entry site for the microcatheter or thermally blunted suture. A viscoelastic (sodium hyaluronate) is injected into the anterior chamber through the initial tangential paracentesis site. A temporal paracentesis is created. When using a suture, the authors incorporate dye from the tip of the marking pen onto the thermally blunted tip of the 4-0 clear nylon suture (**Fig. 25.1**). This facilitates visualization of the suture tip as it circumnavigates the globe. This is not necessary with an Ellex lighted microcatheter (Ellex Medical Lasers, Adelaide, Australia), for it incorporates a blinking light at the tip of the catheter, facilitating visualization of the probe in the canal. We recommend mastering GATT with the microcatheter first, as we

feel it is easier to learn the key portions of the technique before relying on the suture.

Next, the suture or microcatheter is inserted into the anterior chamber through the entry site with the tip resting in the nasal angle. The microscope and the patient's head are then oriented to allow proper visualization of the nasal angle with a Swan-Jacob goniolens. A 1- to 2-mm goniotomy in the anterior trabecular meshwork is created in the nasal angle with a microsurgical blade through the temporal site. The tip of the blade is used to slightly depress the posterior lip of the cleaved TM tissue to expose the canal. Typically, upon decompression of the eye, blood will reflux into the canal, facilitating identification of angle structures. Microsurgical forceps are then introduced through the temporal site and used to grasp the microcatheter or suture within the anterior chamber. The distal tip of the microcatheter is then inserted into Schlemm's canal at the goniotomy incision. Within the anterior chamber, the microsurgical forceps are used to advance the catheter through the canal circumferentially for 360 degrees.

When using a microcatheter, the surgeon can visco-dilate the canal as the catheter is being passed circumferentially, as this may improve the outcome (this has not been proven). If visco-dilation is performed, one must keep the catheter moving at all times, because if the catheter stops, a Descemet's detachment can occur. The progress of the microcatheter is noted by observing the illuminated tip. When a suture is used, the progress of the suture can be appreciated through the use of a gonioprism or watching for the dye-stained tip externally through the limbus. After the catheter has passed 360 degrees around the canal, the distal catheter tip is grasped in the nasal angle and externalized through the temporal corneal incision, creating the first half of the 360-degree trabeculotomy. Traction is then placed on the proximal aspect of the catheter, thus completing the 360-degree ab interno trabeculotomy (**Figs. 25.2** and **25.3**). The viscoelastic is then removed from the anterior chamber by a two-handed irrigation aspiration system (through the previously created corneal paracenteses) to wash the anterior chamber of blood. Near the end of the procedure, a 25 to 50% anterior chamber filled with viscoelastic can be instilled to help tamponade bleeding from the canal. We vary the amount of viscoelastic fill depending on the degree of blood reflux and the extent and quality of an intraoperative EVFW. Leaving Healon in the anterior chamber protects against immediate postoperative hypotony and may decrease the chance of a significant postoperative hyphema. The wounds are hydrated and checked to ensure a watertight closure. Postoperative steroid (subconjunctival or intracameral) and antibiotic drops are given per the surgeon's discretion. **Figs. 25.2** and **25.3** summarize the key surgical steps with both the suture and catheter.

In certain cases, the suture or microcatheter cannot be passed 360 degrees in one direction and stops at around 180 to 270 degrees. In these cases, the surgeon should create a new paracentesis site 180 degrees from where the catheter stopped, and use a gonioprism to perform an ab interno goniotomy directly over the site where the distal tip stopped. The distal end is retrieved from this new location, opening up part of the canal. A suture/microcatheter can then be passed in the opposite direction through an additional 23-gauge needle incision, thus completing a 360-degree trabeculotomy (**Fig. 25.2**).

If initially the surgeon is unable to insert the microcatheter or suture into the canal, for example starting from an inferonasal approach, then the surgeon should withdraw and create a second superonasal paracentesis track, relocate the microcatheter or suture, and try again navigating the canal in the opposite direction.

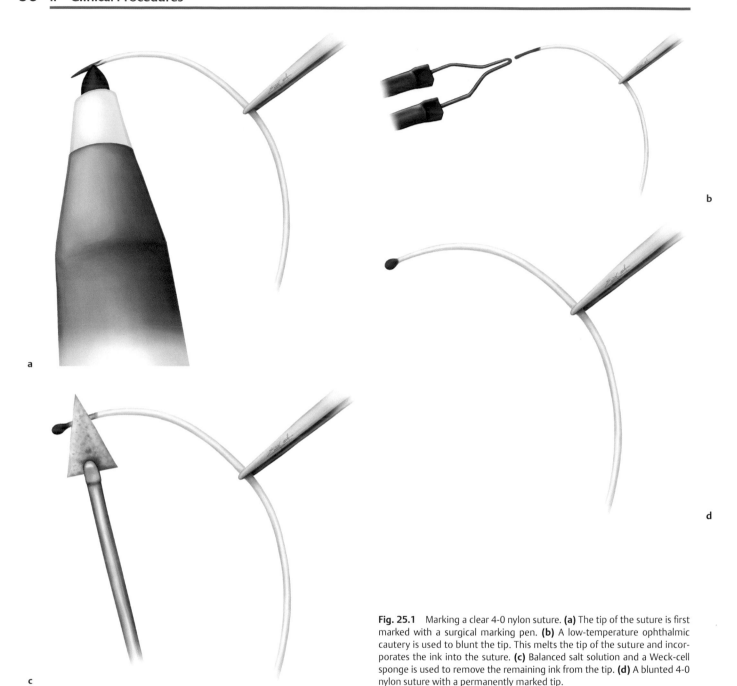

Fig. 25.1 Marking a clear 4-0 nylon suture. **(a)** The tip of the suture is first marked with a surgical marking pen. **(b)** A low-temperature ophthalmic cautery is used to blunt the tip. This melts the tip of the suture and incorporates the ink into the suture. **(c)** Balanced salt solution and a Weck-cell sponge is used to remove the remaining ink from the tip. **(d)** A blunted 4-0 nylon suture with a permanently marked tip.

Stand-Alone Procedure

The GATT procedure can be performed safely in phakic or pseudophakic patients. In phakic eyes, the surgeon may consider constricting the pupil with intracameral acetylcholine chloride to protect the patient's lens. In pseudophakic patients, the surgeon must make sure the intraocular lens (IOL) is stable and that the prior cataract surgery was not complicated, as vitreous in the anterior chamber will likely cause the GATT to fail.

Combined with Cataract Extraction

The GATT procedure can be performed safely in combination with cataract surgery. Although the GATT procedure can be performed before or after standard clear corneal cataract surgery,

the authors prefer to perform GATT first, followed by cataract surgery and IOL implantation. We believe that the flush of balanced salt solution (BSS) in the anterior chamber throughout the procedure may serve as a lavage of the distal collector system and also serve to minimize the risk of postoperative hypotony.

Complications Specific to the Procedure

Circumferential trabeculotomy with either a microcatheter or suture universally causes a hyphema. Usually the postoperative hyphema is small, but in rare cases it may be significant, necessitating a return to the operating room to perform an anterior chamber washout. Most routine hyphemas resolve within 7 to

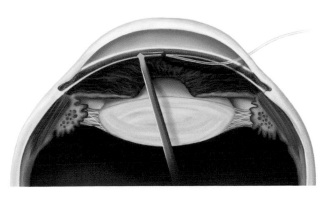

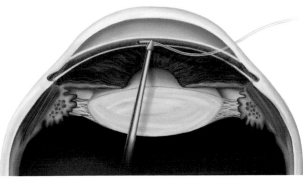

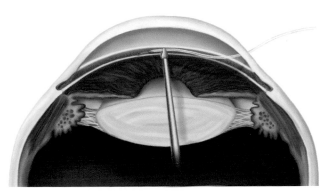

Fig. 25.2 A gonioscopy-assisted transluminal trabeculotomy (GATT) procedure with a 4-0 nylon suture. **(a)** A goniotomy is created with a microsurgical blade. **(b)** Microsurgical forceps are used to cannulate Schlemm's canal through the goniotomy site. **(c)** The marked 4-0 nylon suture is being passed through the canal. **(d)** The suture has stopped, having been passed 270 degrees around the canal. The *white arrow* points to the tip of the marked suture. Given the marking, the tip can be seen externally, without the aid of a gonioprism. **(e)** One can appreciate the marked suture tip with the aid of a gonioprism. **(f)** A goniotomy is performed through the trabecular meshwork overlying the marked suture tip. (*continued on page 104*)

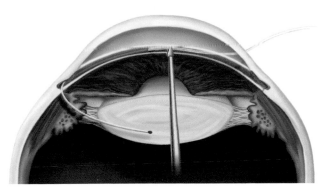

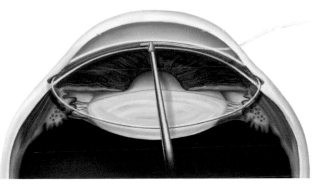

a

b

c

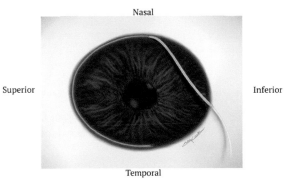

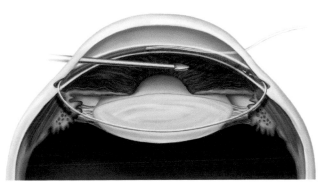

Nasal

Superior

Inferior

Temporal

d

e

f

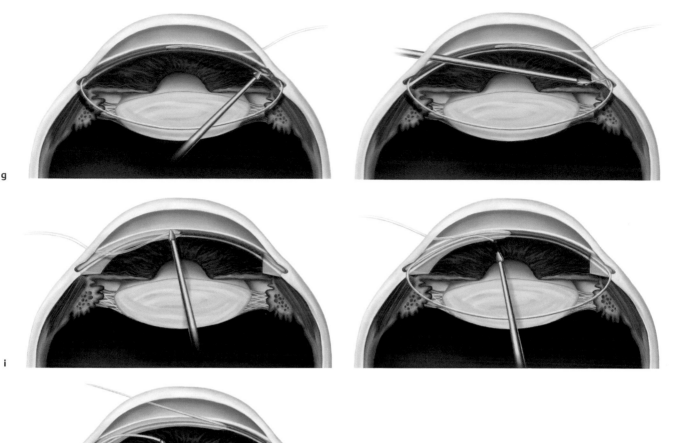

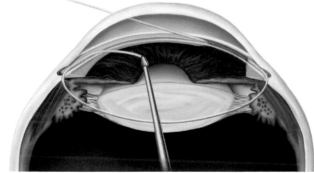

Fig. 25.2 (*continued*)   **(g)** The suture is retrieved through the goniotomy site. **(h)** Traction is placed on the distal and proximal portion of the suture. **(i)** The suture is then passed in the clockwise direction in an effort to treat the remaining 90-degrees. **(j)** The suture has been passed 360 degrees around the canal, and the distal end has been retrieved. **(k)** Traction is placed on the proximal and distal end of the suture, thus treating the remaining 90 degrees and completing the entire 360-degree trabeculotomy.

10 days. A rare complication of trabeculotomy surgery is an iridodialysis or cyclodialysis. This may occur due to excessive manipulation during angle surgery. A Descemet's detachment has been reported with various types of angle surgery; we have seen this occur rarely with the GATT procedure. We have seen an unstable IOL complex worsen following the GATT procedure.

Recognizing and Managing Complications

The physician should always be alert for complications related to postoperative hyphema. This may necessitate topical or oral antiglaucoma medications, and if unsuccessful, a return to the operating room to wash out the anterior chamber. Blood in the anterior chamber may induce scarring in the angle, and we prefer to perform an anterior chamber washout if a substantial hyphema is noted at postoperative week 1. Careful gonioscopy is required at every visit to observe for angle closure related to PAS. If this appears to be a problem, the patient is prescribed pilocarpine 1% at bedtime or twice daily to try to pull the peripheral iris out of the operative site. Approximately 10 to 30% of patients, depending on their diagnosis, will fail the GATT procedure and

require filtration or tube shunt surgery. This is likely a feature of poor downstream collector channels or aberrant canal-based wound healing.

Postoperative Management

After surgery, all patients should be given topical broad-spectrum antibiotics and topical steroids. Pilocarpine can be used in the immediate postoperative period if the IOP is > 15 mm Hg; this may help keep the trabecular shelf open. The trabecular shelf is the remaining layer of tissue that is cleaved open during trabeculotomy. This tissue is hinged at the scleral spur and usually falls over the iris and becomes tethered to it. This affords an easy view into the canal with its glistening back white wall. The topical antibiotics are discontinued at postoperative week 1. The topical steroids (prednisolone acetate 1%) are tapered over 1 to 2 months, depending on the inflammation. Topical drops of a nonsteroidal anti-inflammatory drug (NSAID) can be used in addition to steroids to help control inflammation. A steroid response can still occur in patients even though their trabecular meshwork has been cleaved open for 360 degrees. The mechanism for this is poorly understood,[15] but may be related to the transformation of outer wall scleral fibrocytes into glycoprotein

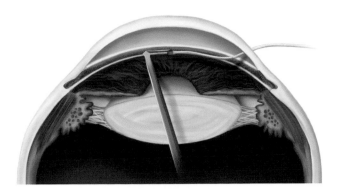

Fig. 25.3 **(a–f)** Intraoperative picture series of a GATT surgery performed with a microcatheter. (*continued on page 106*)

a

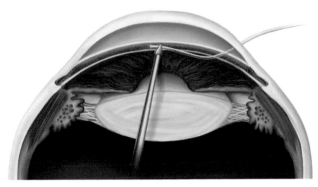

b

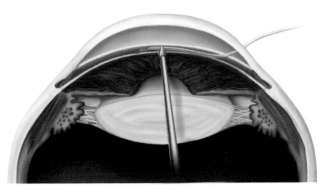

c

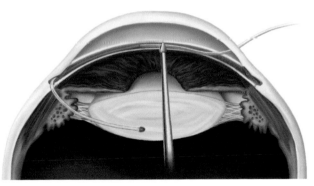

d

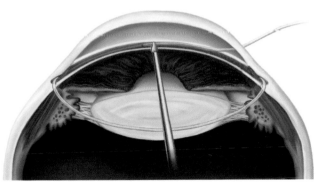

Nasal

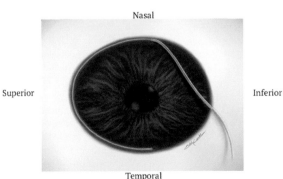

Superior

Inferior

Temporal

e

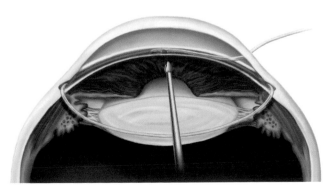

f

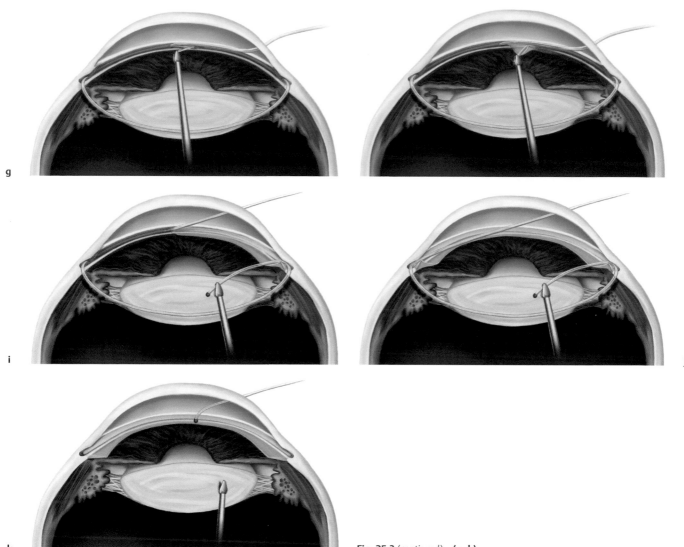

Fig. 25.3 (*continued*) **(g–k).**

secreting myofibroblasts, thereby obstructing the downstream collector channels. In these situations, we have prescribed topical NSAIDs to control inflammation while rapidly tapering topical steroid drops. The patient's IOP should be treated during the postoperative period as per the surgeon's discretion, but once the topical steroid drops are eliminated, the IOP will fall. Typically, patients are seen on postoperative day 1, at the end of week 1, and then at the end of month 1. Patients are then followed a month or two after that, and then every 3 months, and eventually every 6 months. Gonioscopy should be performed at the 1-month visit and then regularly to ensure that the trabecular shelf remains open and free of PAS.

Safety, Efficacy, and Clinical Results

The GATT technique has been shown to be highly safe and effective with results similar to (if not better than) the previously published results on ab externo circumferential trabeculotomy. We reported on the initial results of GATT.[10] This first study described in detail the technique as well as its safety and efficacy. In this short-term follow-up cohort, there were 85 eyes of 85 patients with at least 6 months of follow-up. At 12 months, there were 57 eyes in the primary open-angle glaucoma (POAG) group.

This group had an average decrease in IOP of 11.1 mm Hg and required 1.1 fewer medications. At 12 months in the secondary open-angle glaucoma group, there were 28 eyes. This group had an average decrease in IOP of 19.9 mm Hg and required 1.9 fewer medications. The cumulative proportion of failure at 1 year ranged from 0.1 to 0.32, depending on the specific subgroup.

We reported on a different subgroup separately, which evaluated the efficacy and safety of GATT in treating primary congenital glaucoma and JOAG. This study evaluated 14 eyes of 10 patients who underwent a GATT with longer than 1 year of follow-up.[16] The age in this study population ranged from 17 months to 30 years. The mean IOP decreased from 27.3 to 14.8 mm Hg. There was a mean decrease in the number of glaucoma medications from 2.6 to 0.86.

We subsequently followed a larger cohort for a longer period of time and found relatively similar midterm results as compared with our initial report in adults. This midterm cohort consisted of 198 eyes of 198 patients with a preoperative IOP of ≥ 18 mm Hg and no history of a prior incisional glaucoma surgery. This cohort was divided into six groups, as follows: group 1, POAG patients who underwent an isolated GATT surgery; group 2, POAG patients who underwent both a GATT surgery and a cataract surgery; group 3, pseudophakic POAG patients who underwent an isolated cataract surgery; group 4, secondary open-angle glaucoma (SOAG) patients who underwent an isolated GATT; group 5, SOAG patients who underwent a combined phaco-GATT; group 6, pseudophakic SOAG patients who underwent an isolated GATT surgery. Briefly, at 18 months, there was a substantial, statistically significant, and sustained reduction in IOP as well as glaucoma medications across all six groups. Depending on the group, at 18 months, the cumulative proportion of failure ranged from 0.1 to 0.3 and the cumulative proportion of eyes that required reoperation for IOP control ranged from 0.07 to 0.25.

Regarding safety, one third of the patients had a hyphema at 1 week, but the bleeding was transient and resolved in 95% of cases at 1 month and in 100% of cases at 3 months. Other clinically significant complications in this study group include two eyes with an iridodialysis, and one hemorrhagic Descemet's detachment. The case of iridodialysis did not lead to long-term hypotony and resolved within a few months.

Conclusion

The GATT procedure is a novel, safe, minimally invasive, conjunctiva-sparing glaucoma surgery that can be performed as a stand-alone procedure or in combination with cataract surgery. The midterm results are similar to previously published results for ab externo circumferential trabeculotomy as well as GATT. Equally exciting is the fact that this procedure does not involve the conjunctiva, and therefore does not affect the potential success of subsequent, more invasive, traditional glaucoma surgeries such as a trabeculectomy or a glaucoma drainage implant.

References

1. Allen L, Burian HM. Trabeculotomy ab externo. A new glaucoma operation: technique and results of experimental surgery. Am J Ophthalmol 1962;53:19–26
2. Grant WM. Further studies on facility of flow through the trabecular meshwork. AMA Arch Opthalmol 1958;60(4 Part 1):523–533
3. Ellingsen BA, Grant WM. The relationship of pressure and aqueous outflow in enucleated human eyes. Invest Ophthalmol 1971;10:430–437
4. Johnstone MA, Grant WG. Pressure-dependent changes in structures of the aqueous outflow system of human and monkey eyes. Am J Ophthalmol 1973;75:365–383
5. Smith R. A new technique for opening the canal of Schlemm. Preliminary report. Br J Ophthalmol 1960;44:370–373
6. Lynn JR, Berry PB. A new trabeculotome. Am J Ophthalmol 1969;68:430–435
7. Beck AD, Lynch MG. 360 degrees trabeculotomy for primary congenital glaucoma. Arch Ophthalmol 1995;113:1200–1202
8. Sarkisian SR Jr. An illuminated microcatheter for 360-degree trabeculotomy [corrected] in congenital glaucoma: a retrospective case series. J AAPOS 2010;14:412–416
9. Girkin CA, Marchase N, Cogen MS. Circumferential trabeculotomy with an illuminated microcatheter in congenital glaucomas. J Glaucoma 2012; 21:160–163
10. Grover DS, Godfrey DG, Smith O, Feuer WJ, Montes de Oca I, Fellman RL. Gonioscopy-assisted transluminal trabeculotomy, ab interno trabeculotomy: technique report and preliminary results. Ophthalmology 2014; 121:855–861
11. McPherson SD Jr. Results of external trabeculotomy. Am J Ophthalmol 1973;76:918–920
12. Chin S, Nitta T, Shinmei Y, et al. Reduction of intraocular pressure using a modified 360-degree suture trabeculotomy technique in primary and secondary open-angle glaucoma: a pilot study. J Glaucoma 2012;21:401–407
13. Godfrey DG, Fellman RL, Neelakantan A. Canal surgery in adult glaucomas. Curr Opin Ophthalmol 2009;20:116–121
14. Fellman RL, Grover DS. Episcleral venous fluid wave: intraoperative evidence for patency of the conventional outflow system. J Glaucoma 2014;23:347–350
15. Overby DR, Bertrand J, Tektas OY, et al. Ultrastructural changes associated with dexamethasone-induced ocular hypertension in mice. Invest Ophthalmol Vis Sci 2014;55:4922–4933
16. Grover DS, Smith O, Fellman RL, et al. Gonioscopy assisted transluminal trabeculotomy: an ab interno circumferential trabeculotomy for the treatment of primary congenital glaucoma and juvenile open angle glaucoma. Br J Ophthalmol 2015;99:1092–1096

26 Episcleral Venous Fluid Wave: A Snapshot of Patency of the Trabecular Outflow Pathway

Ronald L. Fellman and Davinder S. Grover

The success of canal-based minimally invasive glaucoma surgery (MIGS) is dependent on the patency and function of the trabecular outflow pathway. Specifically, the collector channels downstream of nearby canal-based surgery sites must be intact and functional to enhance the flow of aqueous humor. Studies have shown that these collectors may be damaged in glaucoma,[1] but currently we do not have a clinically available method to visualize these small collectors or determine their capacity.

The flow through the trabecular pathway is quite complex and still poorly understood, both from an anatomic and physiological viewpoint **Fig. 26.1** illustrates the attempt to map the flow of aqueous humor through the tortuous trabecular path-

way, demonstrating that there are at least 11 sites of resistance along this path.

We found an easy intraoperative method to visualize the patency of the nearby downstream collectors after a Trabectome procedure; we call it the episcleral venous fluid wave (EVFW).[2] The characteristics of the wave of balanced salt solution that courses through the opened canal and veins represent the overall health of the nearby collector channels and tend to correlate with outcomes (**Fig. 26.2**). The EVFW is an intraoperative visible outcome marker, much like a bleb after a filter, that predicts the outcome of the canal-based procedure.

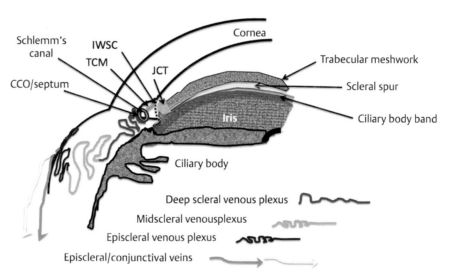

Fig. 26.1 The path of trabecular aqueous outflow. Aqueous humor has a long journey from the anterior chamber to the episcleral and conjunctival outlet veins. There are multiple sites of resistance along this pathway, and most are poorly understood. Trabeculotomy eliminates 50% of the outflow resistance. Even though the trabecular meshwork–Schlemm's canal complex is cleaved open with trabeculotomy, downstream resistance in the intrascleral collector channels (ISCCs) is considerable. The flow of aqueous through these ISCCs is hidden by the sclera, but intraoperative flow to the downstream visible episcleral veins (episcleral venous fluid wave, EVFW) may reveal the overall condition of these hidden channels. The septum comprises part of the CCO and simultaneously serves as a wall for the deep angulated ISCCs that parallel Schlemm's canal (Murray Johnstone, personal communication). Note the first part of the deep ISCCs *(red)* are nearly parallel, not radial, to the canal. JCT, juxtacanalicular tissue; IWSC, inner wall of Schlemm's canal; TCM, transcanalicular microtubules; CCO, collector channel opening.

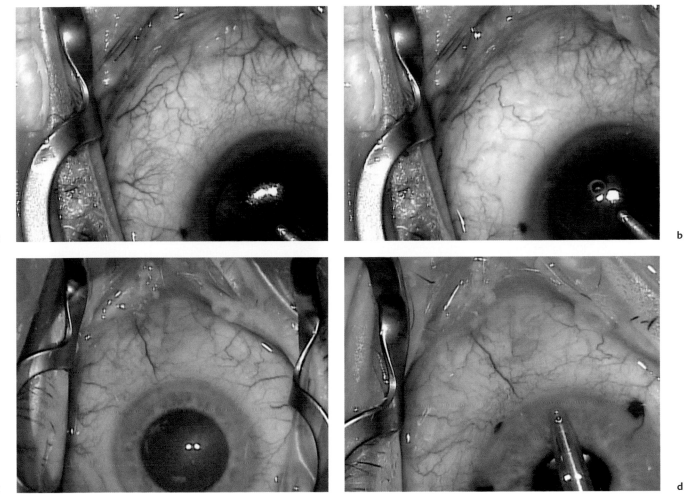

Fig. 26.2 The episcleral venous fluid wave (EVFW) that is elicited during irrigation and aspiration (I/A) of phaco-Trabectome surgery, and correlation with trabecular outflow. **(a)** Appearance of episcleral veins with low intraocular pressure (IOP) and no flow of balanced salt solution (BSS) to the episcleral veins. The episcleral vasculature is easy to see because the pressure is greater in these veins compared with the anterior chamber. **(b)** Marked blanching and washout of blood with diffuse wave (EVFW). The episcleral vasculature is washed out by a surge of BSS due to a reversal of the pressure gradient during I/A at maximal bottle height. There is a diffuse blanching with the wave spreading out over a wide arc. Patients with a diffuse wave have an intact and functional collector channel system. These patients tend to have a lower postoperative IOP and require fewer antiglaucoma medications than patients with a poorly defined wave. **(c)** Near absence of EVFW. Appearance of episcleral veins with low IOP, no flow of BSS to the episcleral vasculature. The episcleral vessels are easy to see before the EVFW. **(d)** There is minimal flow to the downstream collectors, near complete absence of the EVFW. Even with maximal bottle height, there is minimal flow of BSS into the downstream collectors. This is most likely due to obstruction in the ISCCs, a sign of significant glaucomatous damage to the trabecular outflow pathway. These patients are more likely to need further glaucoma surgery to create a new drainage system, because their inherent collector system is not salvageable or sufficiently functional.

References

1. Nesterov AP. Pathological physiology of primary open angle glaucoma: the aqueous circulation. In: Cairns JE, ed. Glaucoma, vol 1. Orlando, FL: Grune and Stratton; 1986:335–336

2. Fellman RL, Grover DS. Episcleral venous fluid wave: intraoperative evidence for patency of the conventional outflow system. J Glaucoma 2014; 23:347–350

27 360-Degree Ab Interno Trabeculotomy

Steven R. Sarkisian, Jr. and Evan Allan

Case Presentation

An 80-year-old man presents to clinic with controlled intraocular pressure (IOP) in the mid-teens on two medications. He is phakic, and has mild-to-moderate open-angle glaucoma (OAG) by Humphrey visual field. Given his mild level of disease and relatively controlled IOP, treatment is cataract motivated. He likely does not need a filtration surgery and the associated risks. Surgery with the TRAB360™ surgical instrument (Sight Sciences, Menlo Park, CA) is a potential option that can be done in conjunction with phacoemulsification to minimize IOP spikes after cataract surgery and to decrease the medication burden.

The Procedure

The gold standard for the surgical treatment of glaucoma has historically been trabeculectomy with the use of antifibrotics. However, despite effectively lowering the IOP, the trabeculectomy procedure is not without the risk of postsurgical complications. Postsurgical hypotony and a lifetime risk of blebitis are two of the most serious postoperative complications after a trabeculectomy procedure.

More recently, increasing interest in rejuvenating the natural trabeculocanalicular outflow pathway has led to advancement in the surgical approach to treating OAG that avoids shunting aqueous humor to a nonphysiological drainage site and is less likely to result in postoperative hypotony.

Trabeculotomy lowers the IOP by improving the flow of aqueous through Schlemm's canal and adjacent collector channels without bleb formation.[1-5] Currently, the most common approach to trabeculotomy is ab externo, which requires an extensive conjunctival and scleral flap dissection that may diminish the success rate of a subsequent trabeculectomy. A few ab interno methods have been described, including using the Trabectome (NeoMedix, Tustin, CA) and gonioscopy-assisted transluminal trabeculotomy using either suture or novel dual-blade devices.[6] A drawback to the Trabectome is its inability to perform 360-degree trabeculotomy.

A novel device that can perform 360-degree ab interno trabeculotomy is the TRAB360. This procedure is a minimally invasive way to surgically treat OAG. Further, this procedure results in lower the IOP without the formation of a conjunctival bleb.

The TRAB360 surgical Instrument is a "trabeculotome," a nonpowered instrument intended for the manual cutting of the trabecular meshwork, or trabeculotomy (**Fig. 27.1**). It can be used to mechanically cut up to 360 degrees of trabecular meshwork.

Rationale Behind the Procedure

The TRAB360 offers several advantages over traditional, incisional glaucoma surgery and even other currently performed minimally invasive glaucoma surgery (MIGS).

First and foremost, traditional filtration or shunting surgery is fraught with both early and late complications, such as bleb leak, hypotony, suprachoroidal hemorrhage, blebitis, and endophthalmitis. The consequences can be severe. Patients with earlier disease burdens, may be amenable to more conservative surgery. Because the TRAB360 is bleb-less and conjunctiva-sparing, if the patient loses control of the IOP over time, further filtration or shunting options can still be used.

Research already has demonstrated the safety and efficacy of trabeculotomy in the adult population. Data for trabeculotomy in adults shows a sustained effect with good IOP lowering. This has been traditionally done externally and can be done either for 180 degrees or 360 degrees.[7-11] The TRAB360 enables 360 degrees of trabecular meshwork unroofing.

Other MIGS procedures have downsides, which include difficult dissection or intraocular maneuvers, the high cost of equipment, and the need for a power source. Moreover, one does not need to worry about identifying Schlemm's canal externally, which can be difficult in external trabeculotomy or canaloplasty. Lastly, there is no need for capital investment in equipment or a power source.

Patient Selection

During a surgeon's learning curve with the device, suitable patients would include those with mild-to-moderate glaucoma that is generally controlled on medications. Once a surgeon is familiar with the use of the device, the procedure may be considered for more advanced OAG patients or those with higher IOP. Patients can be either phakic or pseudophakic, but they must have an open angle with a good view of the angle. The patient also should be able to tolerate some postoperative blurring secondary to transient hyphema. Other candidates for the procedure are patients for whom the surgeon does not want to subject to the risks of a filtration or shunting procedure, and patients with extremely poor conjunctiva (thin or scarred) or ocular surface disease.

Surgical Technique

The surgeon begins by using a keratome (1.5 to 2.8 mm) to make a temporal incision. Care must be taken to avoid any blood vessels at the limbus, as any bleeding can obscure the view by interfering with the interface. If the surgery is being performed topically, topical anesthetic will be instilled into the anterior chamber followed by a cohesive viscoelastic. It is important not to underinflate, as the view will be distorted more easily, but overinflation will collapse Schlemm's canal, causing distortion of angle anatomy or difficulty entering the canal. Viscoelastic is then placed on the cornea.

The most important step surgically is obtaining a view of the angle anatomy and recognizing the structures. The patient's

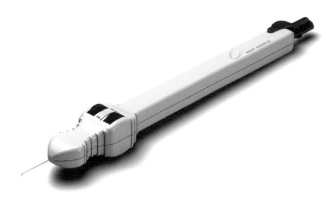

Fig. 27.1 The TRAB360 device. Note the blue "roller" on the surface and the metallic tip through which the blue nylon probe is guided. (Courtesy of Sight Sciences, Inc.)

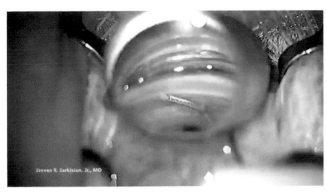

Fig. 27.2 The nylon probe of the TRAB360 device is seen entering Schlemm's through a small piercing in the trabecular meshwork created by the tip of the metallic guide.

head should be rotated away from the surgeon ~ 30 degrees and the microscope tilted toward the surgeon ~ 30 degrees. This is similar to other angle-based surgeries. A gonioprism or double mirror such as the Swann Jacobs, Hill, Vold, or Ritch lenses are used to assess the view of the angle. Often it is beneficial to increase magnification. It is essential to know the angle anatomy, because intraoperative gonioscopy with viscoelastic in the eye can be different from gonioscopy in the clinic as the viscoelastic may change the iris approach. It is not unheard of in patients with lightly pigmented trabecular meshwork and an overinflated anterior chamber for the surgeon to mistakenly identify the anterior ciliary body as the trabecular meshwork.

Next, the trabecular meshwork is incised with the tip of the device and the probe is advanced into Schlemm's canal (**Fig. 27.2**). The device should be parallel to the iris, lest the surgeon distort the view by pushing on the posterior lip or the side of the incision. Sometimes the surgeon may have to back up the tip of the device from the insertion site and guide the probe into Schlemm's canal. At this juncture, it is important not to guide the probe posterior to trabecular meshwork or to allow the probe to deflect off of the trabecular meshwork. If this should occur and not be recognized, the result can be trauma to the iris, iris root, or ciliary body. A cyclodialysis cleft can also occur.

Once the probe has been advanced 180 degrees, the surgeon uses a push-pull motion to unroof the trabecular meshwork to achieve 180 degrees of trabeculotomy (**Fig. 27.3**). Care must be taken not to allow the probe to back itself out during the trabeculotomy. Healon is placed to tamponade bleeding, and the

device is reversed to perform the same procedure on the other 180 degrees of the angle.

Healon is then rinsed from the eye with either irrigation and aspiration or a balanced salt solution on a canula.

Complications Specific to the Procedure

As with any angle-based surgery, hyphema is almost universal, but it typically resolves by the end of week 1. In previously pseudophakic patients with a broken anterior hyaloid face, significant hyphema can result in vitreous hemorrhage. This is more common in patients with a history of vitreous loss.

As mentioned above, iris, iris root, or ciliary body damage can occur or even cyclodialysis cleft if the surgery is not done correctly and the probe goes behind the iris root unnoticed. If it is in the canal from the beginning, it will remain there for its entire course.

Lastly, as with all angle surgery, one must be aware of the risk of steroid response glaucoma.

How to Recognize and Manage Complications

Most complications with the TRAB360 are transient and to be expected. We tell patients they will experience a "snow-globe" effect as the blood settles with gravity and then recirculates with eye movement; thus, intermittent blurring is expected.

Patients with late scarring of the outflow system invariably present with high IOP. They should be managed acutely with medical therapy and may require filtration surgery. Usually, it is wise for the surgeon to inform patients for any of the ab interno procedures involving removal of the trabecular meshwork of the possibility of performing a "two-stage" procedure in cases in which the less invasive surgery intended to restore the natural outflow fails, requiring a more invasive surgery to bypass the natural system and create a new system consisting of a reservoir under the conjunctiva, namely glaucoma filtration surgery, which entails a higher risk of complications.

Postoperative Management

Our patients all receive a topical antibiotic to be taken q.i.d. for a week, a nonsteroidal anti-inflammatory drug (NSAID) if combined with phacoemulsification, pilocarpine 2% b.i.d. for 1 month,

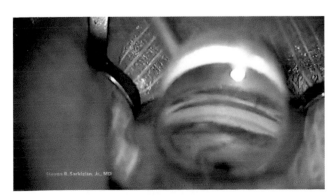

Fig. 27.3 The ab interno trabeculotomy is performed with a "push-pull" motion with the TRAB360 device to complete the first half of the complete trabeculotomy.

Table 27.1 Diagnosis Prior to Surgery, by Eye

Diagnosis	No. of Eyes	Percent
OAG, K-Scar	1	3.85%
POAG	24	92.3%
PXG	1	3.85%
Total	26	100.0%

Abbreviations: OAG, angle-closure glaucoma; POAG, primary angle-closure glaucoma; PXG, pseudoexfoliative glaucoma.

Table 27.2 Patient Race, by Eye

Race	No. of Eyes	Percent
Asian	1	3.85%
African American	5	19.23%
White	20	76.92%
Total	26	100.0%

and a low-dose steroid (Lotemax/fluorometholone [FML]/Vexol) to be tapered over 1 month. These patients can be exquisitely sensitive to steroid response. As long as no hyphema is present, and anterior chamber reaction is resolving, we aggressively taper steroids in steroid responders.

Safety, Efficacy, and Clinical Results

We have investigated the TRAB360 and reported our results at the American Society of Cataract and Refractive Surgery (ASCRS) in 2015. We reviewed charts for patients from February 2014 through January 2015 ($n = 21$ patients, 26 eyes). Mean ($\pm$ standard deviation) age at surgery, by eye, was 80.7 $\pm$ 11.8 years. Mean follow-up posttrabeculotomy was 131.5 $\pm$ 101.6 days. Five patients had bilateral trabeculotomies, two had the right eye only, and 14 had the left eye only. Diagnoses prior to surgery are listed in **Table 27.1**. Only one diagnosis was recorded per eye. Demographics are reported by eye in **Table 27.2**.

Table 27.3 Mean Intraocular Pressure (IOP) ($\pm$ Standard Deviation [SD]) in mm Hg by Time Period

Time	No. of Eyes	IOP (mmHg)	Range	p-Value*
Preoperative	26	19.8 $\pm$ 6.4	9.0–35.0	NA
Day 1	25	13.6 $\pm$ 8.7	5.0–50.0	0.0094
Week 1	26	12.7 $\pm$ 5.3	5.0–24.0	< 0.0001
Month 1	22	14.4 $\pm$ 5.1	6.0–27.0	0.0021
Month 2	12	12.8 $\pm$ 4.7	7.0–22.0	0.0083
Month 3	14	13.2 $\pm$ 3.4	8.0–20.0	0.0065
Month 6	7	12.0 $\pm$ 2.4	10.0–17.0	0.0029**
Month 9	7	11.9 $\pm$ 2.3	10.0–16.0	0.0014**
Month 12	0	–	–	–
Final visit	26	13.5 $\pm$ 4.6	5.0–22.0	< 0.0001

*Paired *t*-test, postoperative versus preoperative IOP.
**Inferential results should be interpreted with caution due to the small number of eyes.

Mean preoperative IOP was 19.8 $\pm$ 6.4 mm Hg. Mean postoperative IOP values, along with significance levels for paired pre/post comparisons, are listed in **Table 27.3**.

Mean preoperative visual acuity (VA) was 0.69 $\pm$ 0.51 Log-Mar corresponding to ~ 20/45 on the Snellen chart. Postoperative visual acuities are listed in **Table 27.4**, with red highlighting indicating significantly worse VA (vs preoperative) and green highlighting indicating improved VA (vs preoperative). Roughly speaking, VA worsened significantly immediately postoperative, then returned to preoperative levels by the end of month 1.

Mean number of medications preoperative was 1.1 $\pm$ 1.2. Postoperative numbers of medications are presented in **Table 27.5**, indicating a significantly higher number of medications (vs preoperative) and green highlighting indicating a lower number of medications (vs preoperative). Because of the small range of values for this variable (0, 1, 2, 3, or 4), Wilcoxon signed-rank test results are also reported.

Surgical success was defined as those eyes not meeting criteria for surgical failure. This was broken down between complete (no medications) or qualified (with medications). Failure was deemed to have occurred if any of the following conditions were met: (1) IOP above or below threshold (consecutive IOPs of $\geq$ 21 mm Hg or < 6 mm Hg at the last two postoperative visits); (2) additional procedures performed including cyclodestruction; or (3) serious complications, such as VA of no light perception vision, suprachoroidal hemorrhage, malignant glaucoma, endophthalmitis, retinal detachment, or serous choroidal effusions that either necessitated surgical drainage or had a kissing appearance.

No patients required further glaucoma procedures at final follow-up. No patients failed both IOP criteria and surgical complication criteria.

For IOP thresholds of 21 and 18 mm Hg, one patient failed with a severe complication 3 months after surgery (retinal detachment). No patients failed for hypotony. The total success rate was 96.2%. Complete and qualified success were noted to be 73.1% and 19.2%, respectively. When the threshold was decreased to 16 mm Hg, total success was 76.9%, with complete and qualified success rates of 65.4% and 11.5%, respectively (**Table 27.6**).

Complications were observed as follows. Universal transient hyphema was noted. Transient corneal edema was observed in seven cases. No cases of persistent edema were observed. Three patients had minimal iris root trauma or cyclodialysis, neither of which was clinically significant. No cases of hypotony or IOP spikes were noted. After initially looking well at the end of week 1 postoperatively, one patient was noted to have a vitreous hemorrhage at the 1-month postoperative visit. No retinal tears or detachments were noted by the retina service. He was followed by the retina service and diagnosed with a macula-off retinal detachment at 3 months after surgery. Otherwise, no other complications were observed.

Table 27.4   Mean Visual Acuity (VA) by Time Period

Time	No. of Eyes	VA (LogMar)	VA (Snellen)	Range	p-Value*
Preoperative	26	0.69 ± 0.51	45	20–100	NA
Day 1	24	1.50 ± 1.26	263	15–2000	0.0045
Week 1	25	1.08 ± 1.18	207	20–2000	0.1215
Month 1	22	0.66 ± 1.11	102	5–800	0.7841
Month 2	12	0.54 ± 0.62	43	20–150	0.3220
Month 3	13	0.43 ± 1.20	101	4–2000	0.1846
Month 6	7	0.18 ± 0.18	24	20–30	0.0018**
Month 9	7	0.31 ± 0.22	28	20–40	0.0003**
Month 12	0	–	–	–	–
Most recent	26	0.72 ± 1.40	174	4–2000	0.8945

*Paired t-test, postoperative versus preoperative VA in LogMAR.
**Inferential results should be interpreted with caution due to the small number of eyes.

Table 27.5   Mean Number of Medications (± SD) by Time Period

Time	No. of Eyes	No. of Medications	Range	p-Value*	p-Value†
Preoperative	26	1.1 ± 1.2	0.0–4.0	NA	NA
Day 1	25	0.3 ± 0.7	0.0–2.0	0.0020	0.0002
Week 1	26	0.2 ± 0.5	0.0–2.0	0.0010	0.0009
Month 1	22	0.1 ± 0.5	0.0–2.0	0.0004	0.0001
Month 2	12	0.1 ± 0.3	0.0–1.0	0.0021	0.0020
Month 3	14	0.4 ± 0.6	0.0–2.0	0.0009	0.0020
Month 6	7	0.3 ± 0.8	0.0–2.0	0.0038**	0.0313**
Month 9	7	0.0 ± 0.0	0.0–0.0	0.0082**	0.0625**
Month 12	0	–	–	–	–
Final visit	26	0.2 ± 0.5	0.0–2.0	0.0003	0.0001

*Paired t-test, postoperative versus preoperative number of medications.
†Wilcoxon signed-rank test versus preoperative number of medications.
**Inferential results should be interpreted with caution due to the small number of eyes.

Table 27.6   Surgical Outcomes by IOP Threshold

Outcome	21 mm Hg	18 mm Hg	16 mm Hg
Success			
Complete	19 (73.1%)	19 (73.1%)	17 (65.4%)
Qualified	5 (19.2%)	5 (19.2%)	3 (11.5%)
Total	26 (96.2%)	26 (96.2%)	20 (76.9%)
Failure			
Surgical complications	1 (3.8%)	1 (3.8%)	1 (3.8%)
IOP at or over threshold	1 (3.8%)	1 (3.8%)	5 (19.2%)

Conclusion

The TRAB360 is a novel device that can be utilized to perform circumferential 360-degree trabeculotomy. It has several advantages over the current methods used to perform this procedure and seems to be safe and efficacious. Long-term follow-up of more patients will help us to confirm our initial findings; however, the data from Chin et al,[8] Grover et al,[10] and the other reports mentioned above from authors doing the same procedure with a suture or a catheter demonstrate that ab interno trabeculotomy is an important and less invasive method for lowering IOP. Moreover, these data show that doing a complete 360-degree trabeculotomy will yield a lower IOP than doing a partial trabeculotomy. We contend that the use of the TRAB360 device is much easier and less invasive, with fewer incisions than the other methods currently available due to its unique design and the fact that it was designed from the beginning as a MIGS procedure for ab interno use.[8,10]

References

1. Gregersen E, Kessing SV. Congenital glaucoma before and after the introduction of microsurgery. Results of "macrosurgery" 1943-1963 and of microsurgery (trabeculotomy/ectomy) 1970-1974. Acta Ophthalmol (Copenh) 1977;55:422–430

2. Haas J. Principles and problems of therapy in congenital glaucoma. Invest Ophthalmol 1968;7:140–146

3. Harms H, Dannheim R. Epicritical consideration of 300 cases of trabeculotomy "ab externo." Trans Ophthalmol Soc U K 1970;89:491–499

4. McPherson SD Jr, McFarland D. External trabeculotomy for developmental glaucoma. Ophthalmology 1980;87:302–305

5. Smith R. A new technique for opening the canal of Schlemm. Preliminary report. Br J Ophthalmol 1960;44:370–373

6. Seibold LK, Soohoo JR, Ammar DA, Kahook MY. Preclinical investigation of ab interno trabeculectomy using a novel dual-blade device. Am J Ophthalmol 2013;155:524–529.e2

7. Vold SD. Ab interno trabeculotomy with the Trabectome system: what does the data tell us? Int Ophthalmol Clin 2011;51:65–81

8. Chin S, Nitta T, Shinmei Y, et al. Reduction of intraocular pressure using a modified 360-degree suture trabeculotomy technique in primary and secondary open-angle glaucoma: a pilot study. J Glaucoma 2012;21:401–407

9. Ahuja Y, Ma Khin Pyi S, Malihi M, Hodge DO, Sit AJ. Clinical results of ab interno trabeculotomy using the Trabectome for open-angle glaucoma: the Mayo Clinic series in Rochester, Minnesota. Am J Ophthalmol 2013; 156:927–935.e2

10. Grover DS, Godfrey DG, Smith O, Feuer WJ, Montes de Oca I, Fellman RL. Gonioscopy-assisted transluminal trabeculotomy, ab interno trabeculotomy: technique report and preliminary results. Ophthalmology 2014; 121:855–861

11. Nakasato H, Uemoto R, Isozaki M, Meguro A, Kawagoe T, Mizuki N. Trabeculotomy ab interno with internal limiting membrane forceps for open-angle glaucoma. Graefes Arch Clin Exp Ophthalmol 2014;252: 977–982

28 Trabecular Bypass: iStent

John P. Berdahl, Christine L. Larsen, and Thomas W. Samuelson

Case Presentation

A 69-year-old man presented for a second opinion regarding surgical intervention for relatively well-controlled primary open-angle glaucoma (POAG) in the setting of visually significant cataracts. He had borderline elevated intraocular pressure (IOP) despite maximally tolerated medical therapy. His referring physician was recommending a trabeculectomy, but the patient had researched various options and wanted to explore iStent implantation.

The patient was a high myope with a moderate superior arcuate field defect in the right eye and nonspecific visual field changes in the left eye (**Fig. 28.1**). Nuclear sclerosis reduced his best corrected vision to a level of 20/40 in both eyes. Angles were open on gonioscopy, with a moderate amount of trabecular meshwork pigment. Applanation tonometry assessed the IOP as 23 OD and 22 OS on three topical medications (Lumigan and Cosopt) and in the setting of average pachymetry.

In preoperative discussion with the patient, he expressed his expectations for visual improvement after the cataracts were removed. The surgeon informed him of the typical risks involved with the surgery. In addition, the patient was aware that the goal of stent implantation was to reduce the medication burden required to maintain adequate IOP. He understood that he would likely still require some topical therapy to keep his glaucoma under control.

The patient underwent a successful cataract surgery with iStent placement in the right eye, and, 1 month later, in the left eye. Postoperatively, the patient's Cosopt medication was discontinued, but he continued to use Lumigan in both eyes. His topical steroid was tapered relatively rapidly over 2 weeks, as inflammation was under good control. Approximately 6 weeks after the second eye surgery, he had uncorrected distance vision of 20/20 in both eyes and an IOP of 19 OD and 18 OS on Lumigan alone.

The Procedure

The iStent (or trabecular micro-bypass stent) has become a key procedure in minimally invasive glaucoma surgery (MIGS). The MIGS procedures have a higher safety profile and a more rapid recovery time in comparison with more invasive filtering surgery. They also have demonstrated the ability to reduce both the IOP as well as the patient's need for medications, a significant benefit considering concerns regarding compliance rates among glaucoma patients.[1] Moreover, unlike most other glaucoma surgical interventions, iStent implantation does not diminish the superb visual and refractive outcomes inherent to modern phacoemulsification. The iStent was developed by Glaukos Corp. (Laguna Hills, CA), with the first implantation in the United States performed in 2005.[2] The stent is designed to fit into and remain within Schlemm's canal. Made from nonferromagnetic titanium, it consists of an inlet (or "snorkel") connected at a 40-degree angle to the implanted portion. The stent itself is then attached to the tip of a 26-gauge disposable insertion instrument, which has been sterilized by gamma radiation (**Fig. 28.2**). The pointed end facilitates entry into the canal and the direction of this point corresponds to the designation of a right- or left-handed model. Both right and left iStents have been developed to ease implantation, depending on the preference of the surgeon. The implanted portion includes a half-cylinder opening, which combined with heparin coating, helps to prevent blockage or fibrosis. Three retention arches help to ensure that the device will be held in place within the canal. The iStent is the smallest known medical device to be implanted into the human body. It is 1.0 mm in length, 0.33 mm in height, and with a weight of 60 µg. The snorkel has a length of 0.25 mm and bore diameter of 120 μm^3 (**Fig. 28.3**).

Rationale Behind the Procedure

As with many other MIGS procedures, the iStent works at the level of the trabecular meshwork (TM). Research on the physiology of POAG has demonstrated that the diseased TM is the primary site of reduced outflow facility resulting from increased outflow resistance.[4] Approximately 75% of the resistance occurs at the juxtacanalicular meshwork. As the alternative designation for the iStent (the trabecular micro-bypass stent) implies, implantation of the device enables aqueous to bypass the increased TM resistance to outflow and provides a direct channel into Schlemm's canal and the subsequent collector channels (**Fig. 28.4**).

The U.S. iStent Study Group performed a large comparative study in POAG patients already undergoing planned cataract surgery to compare the effect of cataract removal alone with cataract removal in combination with iStent placement.[5] Prior to this study, several pilot studies had been performed demonstrating the effectiveness of iStent implantation at lowering IOP. Zhou and Smedley[6] investigated the effectiveness of a trabecular bypass on outflow facility and IOP. A series of equations explored this relationship and demonstrated that in normal healthy eyes, the facility of outflow increases by 13% and 26% in the presence of a unidirectional and bidirectional bypass, respectively. Via enhanced outflow facility, the IOP could be reduced to physiological levels. Bahler et al[7] took this a step further, investigating the effect of a TM bypass on IOP in cultured human anterior segments. A single stent placed into Schlemm's canal provided the greatest change in pressure (21.4 ± 3.8 mm Hg to 12.4 ± 4.2, $p <$ 0.001) with the addition of more stents providing further lowering of pressure, but to a lesser degree.

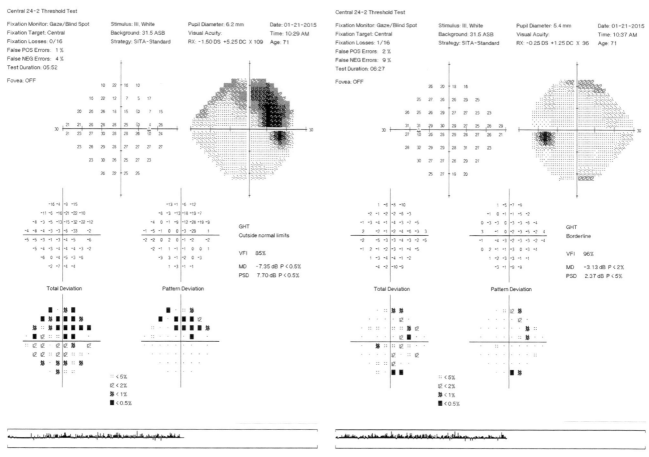

Fig. 28.1 (a,b) The patient's visual fields as described. Both eyes meet criteria for mild-to-moderate glaucoma as defined by the International Classification of Diseases (ICD-9) glaucoma staging codes. The iStent is approved for use in both mild and moderate glaucoma.

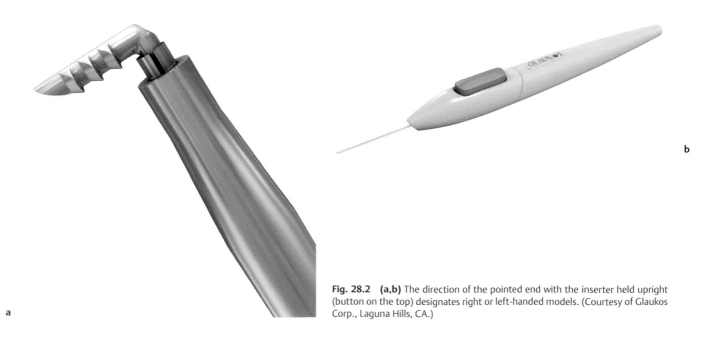

Fig. 28.2 (a,b) The direction of the pointed end with the inserter held upright (button on the top) designates right or left-handed models. (Courtesy of Glaukos Corp., Laguna Hills, CA.)

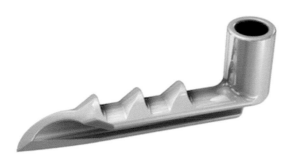

Fig. 28.3 The iStent is the smallest known medical device to date to be implanted in humans. (Courtesy of Glaukos Corp., Laguna Hills, CA.)

Patient Selection

In 2012, the Food and Drug Administration (FDA) approved the iStent for use in combination with cataract extraction for patients with mild to moderate open-angle glaucoma who were using one to three ocular hypotensive medications.

Ideal candidates are those with stable and well-controlled disease. Those who are demonstrating progression on their current medication regimen may require more aggressive surgical intervention, such as filtration surgery. The aforementioned ideal candidate also typically requires pressure lowering, but not to an extreme level (i.e., target IOP around the mid-teens or higher). The general goal is to reduce the dependency on topical medication and not necessarily increase the aggressiveness of treatment.

As can be extrapolated from the characteristics of an ideal candidate, poor candidates would be those with a very low target IOP. Patients with a very shallow anterior chamber should also be avoided, as implantation can be more difficult, with an increased risk of iris or endothelial damage, although the angle in such patients will likely be much deeper once the native lens has been removed. Similarly, iStent placement has been reported in primary angle-closure glaucoma patients in combination with goniosynechialysis. The aforementioned difficulties with implantation may be encountered in these patients, and there may also be a predisposition to recurrent scarring over the angle.

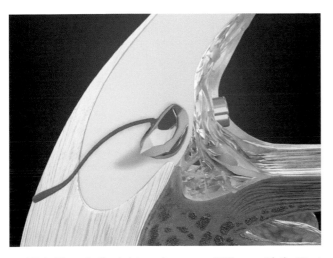

Fig. 28.4 The reduction in intraocular pressure (IOP) seen with the iStent is related to the creation of a direct-access pathway of aqueous to collector channels via bypass of the diseased trabecular meshwork. (Courtesy of Glaukos Corp., Laguna Hills, CA.)

As the functionality of the iStent relies on bypassing the diseased TM to allow aqueous to access an otherwise functional outflow system, secondary glaucomas related to elevated episcleral venous pressure (e.g., Sturge-Weber) would not be amenable to stent implantation. Patients with neovascular glaucoma are contraindicated because of both the increased bleeding risk and the reduced function of the outflow system.[8]

While surgeons are first developing their implantation skills and becoming more comfortable with the procedure, it may be of benefit to select patients who would do well with cataract surgery alone. These patients will still likely do well postoperatively should implantation be unsuccessful. Other favorable traits for initial cases might include highly cooperative individuals with at least moderate pigmentation of the TM and well discernible angle structures. Also, if surgeons favor right or left eyes for phacoemulsification, they are likely to favor those eyes for initial iStent cases as well.

Surgical Technique

Mastering intraoperative gonioscopy is a key to success with iStent implantation. For surgeons who do not perform gonioscopy often, it is useful to examine patients in the clinic to better familiarize oneself with the angle anatomy. In addition, practicing intraoperative gonioscopy during routine cataract cases proves to be beneficial prior to implanting the first stent. Gently touching the anterior meshwork with a viscoclastic cannula can also help one become more comfortable with the hand position.

Once the cataract surgery is completed and the intraocular lens (IOL) has been implanted, injection of a miotic helps to pull the iris away from the angle, and the insertion of viscoelastic material will aid in anterior chamber maintenance (**Fig. 28.5a**). For initial cases, it is desirable to remove all of the ophthalmic viscosurgical device (OVD) from within the retropupillary space and capsular bag before the pupil is constricted. Later, once more experience is achieved, many surgeons will choose to wait until the iStent has been successfully implanted before the OVD is removed and the miotic instilled. The patient's head and the operating microscope are rotated 30 to 40 degrees in opposite directions to facilitate a gonioscopic view of the angle. The surgical goniolens is placed on the cornea with a coupling solution (Goniosol, OVD), and the angle is viewed under high magnification. Care is taken not to place pressure on the eye with the goniolens, as resultant corneal striae will impede the view (**Fig. 28.5b**) Likewise, the surgeon should avoid putting pressure on the wound with the insertion trochar to avoid expressing the OVD from the eye with the subsequent loss of visualization. Once a clear view of the TM is achieved, the applicator is inserted into the anterior chamber through the clear cornea temporal incision and advanced across the anterior chamber toward the nasal angle. As mentioned previously, there are two different designs designating the direction of the pointed end. The intent of the unique iStent design is that after implantation, the body of the stent points toward the inferior angle such that right stents are used in right eyes and left stents are used in left eyes. Evidence that right or left orientation makes any clinical difference, however, is lacking. As such, most surgeons believe that right- and left-hand models are interchangeable (i.e., right and left iStents can be used in both right and left eyes) depending on what feels more comfortable (forehand or backhand) in the dominant hand of the surgeon.

The anterior one third of the TM is approached at a 15-degree angle and is perforated by the tip. The implanted portion is advanced into the canal. By slightly adjusting the angle after perforation (lowering the heel and raising the toe), the stent will slide into the canal more easily (**Fig. 28.5c**). Once securely positioned

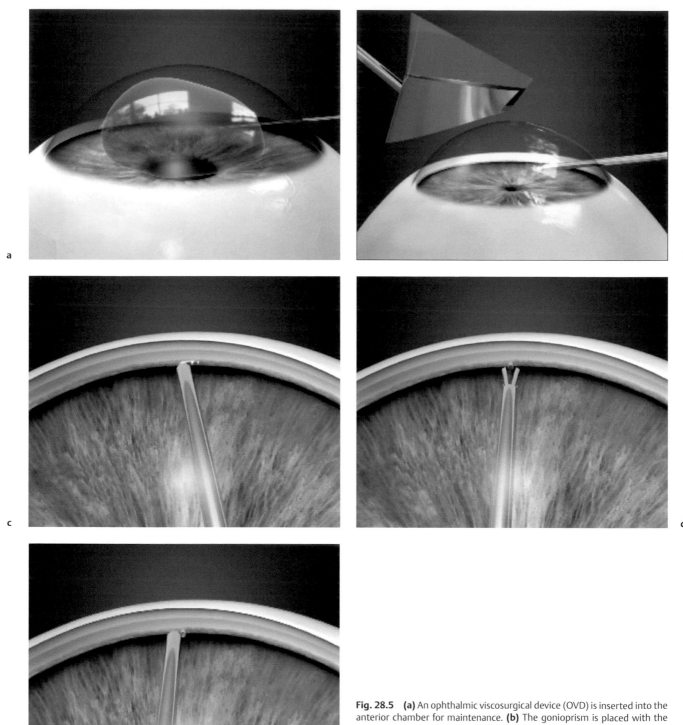

Fig. 28.5 **(a)** An ophthalmic viscosurgical device (OVD) is inserted into the anterior chamber for maintenance. **(b)** The gonioprism is placed with the nondominant hand with a coupling solution, and care is taken not to place pressure on the cornea. **(c)** The iStent is advanced to the nasal angle and inserted into the trabecular meshwork. **(d)** Blood seen exiting the snorkel after insertion is a clue that accurate placement has been achieved. **(e)** The inserter is used to gently push the inlet and to verify that it has memory. (Courtesy of Glaukos Corp., Laguna Hills, CA.)

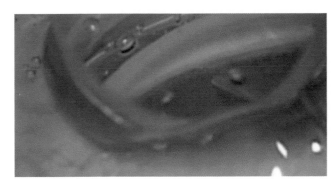

Fig. 28.6 Subsequent to successful insertion, the stent is seen running parallel to the iris plane with a patent snorkel and retention arches well covered with trabecular meshwork pigment. (Courtesy of Thomas Samuelson, MD.)

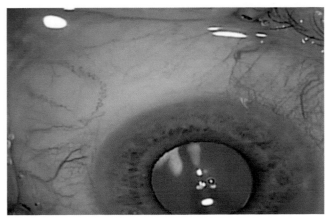

Fig. 28.7 A corresponding area of conjunctival blanching is seen in the area of iStent implantation, indicative of increased aqueous flow into the collector and episcleral venous system. (Courtesy of Thomas Samuelson, MD.)

with the ridges of stent covered by meshwork tissue, the device is released by pushing the button on the applicator (**Fig. 28.5d**). Subtle posterior pressure and relaxing of the hand will ensure a stable release.

After release, the iStent should appear in a stable position, with the heel well seated within the canal. The device will be viewed running parallel to the iris plane. The applicator tip is then used to gently push the inlet to verify that it has memory (i.e., with minimal displacement, it will return to the original position) (**Fig. 28.5e**). Subsequent to successful placement, it is mandatory that the viscoelastic material be thoroughly removed at the conclusion of the procedure (**Figs. 28.6 and 28.7**).

Stand-Alone Procedure

Currently, the iStent is approved for use in combination with cataract extraction. In addition, placement of more than one stent is considered an off-label use. As described previously, Bahler et al[7] found that the implantation of more than one stent into the canal of cultured human anterior segments provided additional pressure lowering to that achieved with a single stent, but to a lesser degree. Several studies and case reports have since been published demonstrating the efficacy of implanting multiple stents.[9–11] In general, an additive effect on IOP reduction has been seen with the placement of additional implants. In studies thus far, the further reduction of both the IOP as well as topical ocular hypotensive use that is seen with multiple stent implantation shows promise for iStent use in patients with more advanced disease (**Fig. 28.8**). Further prospective study is warranted.

Among these multi-stent studies, the potential for iStent implantation in phakic patients and after previous filtering surgery has also been demonstrated.[10,11] A prospective study by Ahmed et al[11] involved 39 phakic patients with unmedicated baseline IOP between 22 and 38 mm Hg. Patients received two stents placed through a clear corneal incision. The mean unmedicated IOP decreased from 25.3 ± 1.8 mm Hg preoperatively to 17.1 ± 2.2 mm Hg at 13 months postoperatively.

Complications

The advantages of the iStent procedure include sparing of the conjunctiva and avoidance of the long-term complications and short-term risks associated with trabeculectomy and tube shunt surgery. More specifically, issues of hypotony are avoided because episcleral backpressure remains.

With any surgical procedure, however, adverse events can occur. Studies involving the iStent thus far have not demonstrated

any significant added risk in comparison with cataract surgery alone. Publications from the iStent Study User Group at both 12 and 24 months showed the overall incidence of adverse events and long-term safety profile was similar between cataract surgery alone and cataract surgery with iStent implantation. There were no unanticipated adverse device effects[5,12] (**Table 28.1**).

How to Recognize and Manage Complications

Although the overall risks and adverse events seen postoperatively with iStent placement are similar to those with cataract surgery alone, there are some intraoperative issues that may be encountered, and steps that can be taken to ensure a successful implantation.

When viewing the angle gonioscopically at the time of stent placement, Schlemm's canal is often highlighted by heme within. This is beneficial for canal identification, but it can also impede the view as heme is released after perforation of the TM. If the angle anatomy becomes obscured, irrigation and aspiration may be utilized to clear the blood, or additional viscoelastic may push it out of the way. Blood visualized flowing out of the snorkel after insertion is a good sign, indicating correct positioning

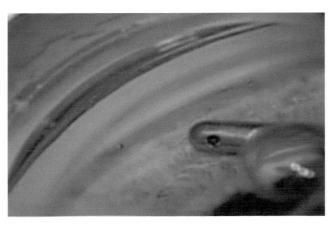

Fig. 28.8 Two stents in good position within Schlemm's canal. (Courtesy of Thomas Samuelson, MD.)

Table 28.1 Intraoperative Findings and Complications as Seen in the iStent User Group Through 24 Months

Finding/Complication	iStent Group (*n* = 116)	Control Group (*n* = 117)
Vitreous removal	5 (4.3%)	3 (2.6%)
Intraocular lens exchange (torn haptic)	0	1 (0.9%)
Intraoperative stent exchange	1 (0.9%)	–
Stent malposition	1 (0.9%)	–
Iris touch	7 (6%)	–
Endothelial touch	1 (0.9%)	–

Source: Data from Craven ER, Katz LJ, Wells JM, Giamporcaro JE; iStent Study Group. Cataract surgery with trabecular micro-bypass stent implantation in patients with mild-to-moderate open-angle glaucoma and cataract: two-year follow-up. J Cataract Refract Surg 2012;38:1339–1345.

within the canal. Blood reflux through the snorkel is a better indicator than blood flowing around the device or from other disrupted tissue.

Excessive anterior chamber fill with viscoelastic can result in pressure on the meshwork and collapse of Schlemm's canal. After IOL placement, viscoelastic should be completely removed from both the anterior chamber and posterior to the iris. Going behind the lens with the irrigation and aspiration tip can help to ensure that all viscoelastic has been removed. Successful evacuation of all OVDs is the most important step in preventing early postoperative IOP spikes. After the instillation of a miotic, the amount of viscoelastic reintroduced into the anterior chamber is enough to provide stability and adequate visualization of the canal without resulting in pressure on the meshwork. After stent placement, the viscoelastic is again thoroughly removed in attempts to avoid a 1-day postoperative pressure spike.

As mentioned previously, avoidance of patients with shallow anterior chambers can help prevent issues with endothelial damage or iris root tears. Should these occur, the stent can still be safely inserted, but the patient may require more frequent postoperative care with the presence of corneal edema or a hyphema that may result.

Another important precaution relates to the re-grasping maneuver should the iStent need repositioning. Although the stent can be readily re-grasped by the inserter, care must be exercised to be certain that the re-grasping prongs do not accidently grasp the iris along with the stent. Should this occur, an iridodialysis or iris trauma could result.

Postoperative Management

Open-angle glaucoma patients are more susceptible to IOP elevation after surgery regardless of whether cataract surgery is performed alone or in combination with iStent placement. Again, aggressive viscoelastic removal is important and can help to reduce the possibility of a pressure spike. In addition to an early postoperative pressure increase, these patients are also at increased risk of experiencing a steroid response. It may be beneficial to taper steroids more rapidly. For example, if IOP is elevated at the 1-week follow-up appointment on prednisolone q.i.d., the steroid can be decreased to b.i.d. and discontinued

at week 2 or 3 as long as inflammation is under control. The supplemental benefit of a nonsteroidal anti-inflammatory drug often enables earlier discontinuation of steroidal agents, thus averting or minimizing an IOP spike.

It typically takes 6 to 8 weeks after surgery to reach a new steady state for IOP. Glaucoma medications may be discontinued on a case-by-case basis. Lower risk eyes and those with a lower medication burden (i.e., one or two topical medications) may be able to have all glaucoma treatment withdrawn. For patients requiring two or more medications or for higher risk patients, medications should be discontinued more cautiously and one at a time.

Other potentially encountered issues in the postoperative period include the presence of a hyphema, with possible occlusion of the stent with blood, or occlusion by iris tissue. Treatment of a hyphema in this case is no different from the normal standard of care. Should the stent become blocked with iris tissue, the neodymium:yttrium-aluminum-garnet (Nd:YAG) laser or argon laser can be utilized to successfully clear the blockage if the IOP becomes uncontrolled.[5,9]

Safety, Efficacy, and Clinical Results

The initial results of the iStent Study Group, the largest study to date, were published in 2011. The study involved 239 patients, with 116 patients receiving the stent. Patients involved in the study were those with mild-to-moderate glaucoma who had an unmedicated IOP between 22 and 36 mm Hg. The primary efficacy measure was defined as unmedicated IOP ≤ 21 mm Hg at 1 year and was seen in 72% of treatment eyes versus 50% of controls. A secondary outcome was unmedicated IOP reduction ≥ 20% at 1 year and was seen in 66% of treatment eyes versus 48% of controls. Approximately half as many patients in the iStent group were using topical drops compared with the cataract-only group at 1 year, suggesting that the iStent may delay or eliminate the need for medications after cataract surgery (a mean reduction in medications of 1.4 for the iStent group and 1.0 for the cataract-only group).

As referenced previously, the incidence of adverse events seen with cataract surgery plus iStent placement versus cataract

Table 28.2   Reported Postoperative Ocular Complications as Seen in the iStent User Group Through 24 Months

Finding/Complication	iStent Group (*n* = 116)	Control Group (*n* = 117)
Anticipated early postoperative event*	20 (17.2%)	22 (18.8%)
Posterior capsule opacification	7 (6%)	12 (10.3%)
Elevated intraocular pressure	4 (3.4%)	5 (4.3%)
Elevated intraocular pressure requiring oral or IV medications or surgery	1 (0.9%)	3 (2.6%)
Stent obstruction	5 (4.3%)	–
Blur or visual disturbance	4 (3.4%)	8 (6.8%)
Stent malposition	3 (2.6%)	–
Iritis	1 (0.9%)	6 (5.1%)
Conjunctival irritation from hypotensive medication	1 (0.9%)	3 (2.6%)
Disk hemorrhage	1 (0.9%)	3 (2.6%)

*Corneal edema, anterior chamber cell, corneal abrasion, discomfort, subconjunctival hemorrhage, blurred vision, or floaters.
Source: Data from Craven ER, Katz LJ, Wells JM, Giamporcaro JE; iStent Study Group. Cataract surgery with trabecular micro-bypass stent implantation in patients with mild-to-moderate open-angle glaucoma and cataract: two-year follow-up. J Cataract Refract Surg 2012;38: 1339–1345.

surgery alone was similar in the iStent Study Group. No unanticipated adverse device effects were seen. The goal of improved vision was achieved in ≥ 95% of subjects for both groups.

A subsequent paper published by the iStent Study Group looked at the same end points at 24 months.[12] It found that the proportion of patients with an IOP of < 21 mm Hg without medication was significantly higher in the stent group. The mean IOP was stable between the 1- and 2-year end points in the stent group, but was slightly increased in the control group (17.0 ± 3.1 versus 17.8 ± 3.3). The total number of hypotensive medications was shown to be significantly less in the stent group at 12 months. This finding was additionally maintained at 24 months, but was no longer statistically significant. It should be noted that the original study was powered to detect a difference only out to 1 year. Again, postoperative complications and adverse events were similar between groups at 24 months **(Table 28.2).** Several publications have since demonstrated similar findings in terms of iStent efficacy and safety profile.[13,14]

Research continues on advancements in iStent technology. A second-generation model is being developed. The iStent inject system consists of a head connected to a narrow thorax that is attached to a wider flange. The head is inserted directly into the canal without the necessity of adjusting the angle for implantation. It resides within the canal and contains four evenly spaced ports for fluid passage. The injector can contain two stents for implantation **(Fig. 28.9).** Similarly, Bahler et al[15] studied the influences of the new model on the outflow facility of cultured human anterior segments. Outflow facility was found to increase and IOP to decrease with a single stent placement. An additional increase in outflow facility was demonstrated with the placement of a second stent. Thus, this second-generation bypass stent may prove to have similar potential compared with first-generation models in the treatment of mild-to-moderate

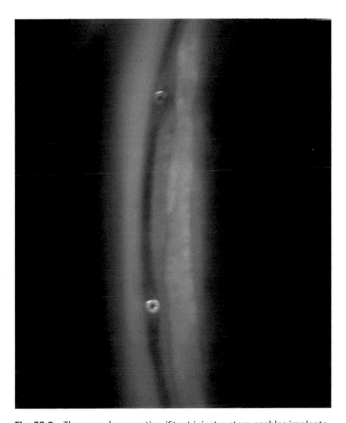

Fig. 28.9   The second-generation iStent inject system enables implantation of two stents within a single injector system. (Courtesy of Thomas Samuelson, MD.)

open-angle glaucoma and carries the additional benefit of greater ease of implantation.

Treating glaucoma patients to reach target IOP levels has been traditionally achieved via medications, laser, or filtering surgery. The significant increase in risk that comes with trabeculectomy or tube shunt placement has led to the development of new therapeutic approaches, such as the iStent, to fill the gap. In both research and clinical experience to date, implantation of the stent in combination with cataract surgery has provided statistically significant improvement in IOP as opposed to cataract surgery alone. A potential added benefit is seen in the reduction of ocular hypotensive medication dependency. Among MIGS procedures, the iStent provides a promising benefit to mild-to-moderate open-angle glaucoma patients with a favorable safety profile and sparing of conjunctival tissue should a more aggressive intervention be necessary in the future.

References

1. Okeke CO, Quigley HA, Jampel HD, et al. Adherence with topical glaucoma medication monitored electronically the Travatan Dosing Aid study. Ophthalmology 2009;116:191–199

2. Karmel M. Glaucoma treatment paradigm driven by new interventions. EyeNet Magazine 2011;November:41–45

3. Francis BA, Singh K, Lin SC, et al. Novel glaucoma procedures: a report by the American Academy of Ophthalmology. Ophthalmology 2011;118:1466–1480

4. Rosenquist R, Epstein D, Melamed S, Johnson M, Grant WM. Outflow resistance of enucleated human eyes at two different perfusion pressures and different extents of trabeculotomy. Curr Eye Res 1989;8:1233–1240

5. Samuelson TW, Katz LJ, Wells JM, Duh YJ, Giamporcaro JE; US iStent Study Group. Randomized evaluation of the trabecular micro-bypass stent with phacoemulsification in patients with glaucoma and cataract. Ophthalmology 2011;118:459–467

6. Zhou J, Smedley GT. A trabecular bypass flow hypothesis. J Glaucoma 2005;14:74–83

7. Bahler CK, Smedley GT, Zhou J, Johnson DH. Trabecular bypass stents decrease intraocular pressure in cultured human anterior segments. Am J Ophthalmol 2004;138:988–994

8. Karmel M. Two approaches to MIGS: iStent and Trabectome. EyeNet Magazine 2014;November:36–41

9. Belovay GW, Naqi A, Chan BJ, Rateb M, Ahmed IIK. Using multiple trabecular micro-bypass stents in cataract patients to treat open-angle glaucoma. J Cataract Refract Surg 2012;38:1911–1917

10. Roelofs K, Arora S, Dorey MW. Implantation of 2 trabecular microbypass stents in a patient with primary open-angle glaucoma refractory to previous glaucoma-filtering surgeries. J Cataract Refract Surg 2014;40:1322–1324

11. Ahmed IIK, Katz LJ, Chang DF, et al. Prospective evaluation of microinvasive glaucoma surgery with trabecular microbypass stents and prostaglandin in open-angle glaucoma. J Cataract Refract Surg 2014;40:1295–1300

12. Craven ER, Katz LJ, Wells JM, Giamporcaro JE; iStent Study Group. Cataract surgery with trabecular micro-bypass stent implantation in patients with mild-to-moderate open-angle glaucoma and cataract: two-year follow-up. J Cataract Refract Surg 2012;38:1339–1345

13. Arriola-Villalobos P, Martínez-de-la-Casa JM, Díaz-Valle D, Fernández-Pérez C, García-Sánchez J, García-Feijoó J. Combined iStent trabecular micro-bypass stent implantation and phacoemulsification for coexistent open-angle glaucoma and cataract: a long-term study. Br J Ophthalmol 2012;96:645–649

14. Augustinus CJ, Zeyen T. The effect of phacoemulsification and combined phaco/glaucoma procedures on the intraocular pressure in open-angle glaucoma. A review of the literature. Bull Soc Belge Ophtalmol 2012;320:51–66

15. Bahler CK, Hann CR, Fjield T, Haffner D, Heitzmann H, Fautsch MP. Second-generation trabecular meshwork bypass stent (iStent inject) increases outflow facility in cultured human anterior segments. Am J Ophthalmol 2012;153:1206–1213

29 Premium Intraocular Lenses in Minimally Invasive Glaucoma Surgery

Joel M. Solano and John P. Berdahl

Subspecialty ophthalmologists share a common focus on a small organ, but their goals of patient management can vary. For example, if a glaucoma specialist and a cataract refractive specialist are caring for the same patient, one might be aiming for an extra point of intraocular pressure (IOP) reduction while the other may favor an extra quarter diopter of cylinder reduction. Although it is natural for physicians to give greater emphasis to factors they encounter on a daily basis, it is becoming increasingly important to broaden the subspecialist's scope of concern.

As the population ages, so does its collective desire for improved outcomes. The physician has to adapt to meet these growing patient needs. Today's ophthalmologist must incorporate a wider view of patients' concerns and identify patients' goals to confirm their alignment with the goals of the referring physician.

Historically, glaucoma surgery has been highly invasive and frequently associated with postoperative complications.[1] The notion of making a complex situation worse by introducing refractive goals was a step too far. Fortunately, the introduction of minimally invasive glaucoma surgery (MIGS) has allowed us to align pressure goals and physician expectations with the desired refractive goals of the patient.

Minimally invasive glaucoma surgery, a term coined by Iqbal "Ike" Ahmed, is defined by the following principle features: ab interno procedure, biocompatibility with minimal disruption of normal anatomy/physiology, high safety profile, efficacy of IOP lowering, and quick recovery time. The iStent (Glaukos Corp., Laguna Hills, CA) is currently the only approved MIGS device for use in the United States, and it has a high safety profile when combined with cataract surgery.[2] The iStent is refractively neutral and enables us to make a pressure intervention without introducing additional optical aberrations.

This chapter illustrates our approach to patients undergoing phaco-MIGS. We shall discuss issues regarding ocular surface disease, excimer support, IOP spikes, and the monocular patient. The chapter ends with a patient case to illustrate some of these concepts.

Phaco-MIGS: Determining Expectations and Goals

Paramount to establishing a surgical plan combining MIGS and refractive cataract surgery is determining the patient's objectives. When identifying a patient with glaucoma and cataracts in need of surgical intervention, the next step is to determine if the patient wants to be less dependent on spectacles.

Many patients state that they do not mind wearing glasses, whereas others have a strong desire to be more glasses independent. Patients having phaco-MIGS have three refractive options:

remain in spectacles postoperatively, opt for distance spectacle independence, or aim for spectacle independence/reduction at distance and near.

Remain in Spectacles Postoperatively

For patients who do not mind wearing glasses after surgery, the surgeon can offer a standard monofocal lens with a refractive error goal matching the patient's desires. Typically the refractive error goal is a spherical equivalent of plano, but on occasion patients desire reading myopia; the choice is theirs, but the patient should be counseled to expect spectacle usage for most, if not all, tasks. The surgeon can allow any residual spherical or cylindrical error of their prescription to be addressed in the final spectacles. These patients will need biometry to help assess the needed intraocular lens (IOL) power to best meet their goals. **Table 29.1** illustrates the supporting testing needed when addressing the cylinder at the time of surgery versus use of spectacles to correct any remaining postoperative astigmatism.

Spectacle Independence

For patients who desire greater independence from glasses, there are two options: glasses independence at distance or glasses independence at distance and near. Carefully addressing astigmatism can help these patients achieve their goals.

Some patients do not mind wearing reading glasses or computer glasses and thus choose the option that is most likely to get them independent from glasses at distance. Other patients wish to be as independent as possible from glasses for both distance and near. For this latter group of patients, the surgeon can discuss their preference for monovision versus presbyopia-correcting IOLs including multifocal and accommodating lenses. The patient's anatomy, physiology and particularly visual field findings can be used to guide options given to patients wishing presbyopia-correcting IOLs.

Distance Spectacle Independence

The options for glasses independence at distance are no different for the glaucoma patient than they are for patients without glaucoma. When a patient desires glasses independence for distance vision, they can be offered a combination of tests to help them achieve their goals.

Achieving emmetropia for spectacle free-distance vision requires accurate targeting of both spherical and cylindrical components of the refractive error. The ideal preoperative evaluation

Table 29.1   Testing for Addressing Astigmatism

	Keratometry	Topography	Biometry	Refraction	Intraoperative Aberrometry
Cylinder addressed in spectacles			X		
Cylinder addressed at the time of surgery	X	X	X	X	X

includes assessing the patient's keratometry, topography, refraction, and biometry. These tests help to closely predict the postoperative residual cylinder.

To better target the postoperative refractive error, intraoperative wavefront aberrometry can be used at the time of surgery for confirmation of IOL calculations and residual astigmatism. The ocular response analyzer (ORA) can be valuable when targeting the cylinder and can guide tools like on-axis surgery, astigmatic keratotomy (AK) with the femtosecond laser or manual AK, toric IOLs, or a combination of these depending on the amount of preoperative astigmatism **(Table 29.1)**.

Spectacle Independence at Distance and Near

In glaucoma patients, options for spectacle independence at both distance and near include multifocal IOLs, monovision, and accommodating IOLs. The patients' visual field evaluation helps guide them in their choices.

A visual field free from defects is needed prior to offering multifocal IOLs to glaucoma patients. Contrast sensitivity is reduced in both glaucoma and in multifocal IOLs,[3,4] and the benefit of spectacle independence is unlikely to outweigh the reduced image quality seen when placing a multifocal IOL in a patient with glaucoma and visual field changes, especially considering that glaucoma can progress.

For the group of patients exhibiting visual field defects, the physician can consider monovision and accommodating IOLs for improved spectacle independence.

Monovision in glaucoma is similar to monovision in the unaffected population. Ideal monovision patients are those who have tried the method through contact lenses or happen to have natural monovision and enjoy the vision they experience. For patients who have not experienced monovision, but are interested in its possibility, the clinician should require a contact lens trial; however, this can be challenging in an older population and will not be perfect if there is a visually significant cataract. Typically the dominant eye is reserved for distance correction, and the nondominant eye for near. A thorough discussion with the patient regarding the risks of disease progression and subsequent difficulty with monovision is essential. With monovision it is important to understand the visual fields and ensure that defects are mild and not interfering with tracking.

Alternatively, an accommodating IOL could be considered in glaucoma patients with visual field defects. The Crystalens accommodating IOL does not have the multifocality that causes a reduction in contrast sensitivity seen with multifocals. Thus, the Crystalens is a reasonable option for patients with glaucoma wishing to have some near vision with their distance correcting IOL. When considering a Crystalens, a thorough preoperative exam is important. Avoid using the Crystalens in patients with pseudoexfoliation due to the risk of an unstable zonule-bag complex and to the risk of capsular contraction leading to a Z-syndrome.

Finally, have a frank discussion with patients suffering from moderate to severe glaucoma who wish to use the Crystalens. When presented with all options, including each option's limitations, it is not infrequent to hear a patient wanting anything that will give them some visual advantage over the standard monofocal lens. Therefore, great importance should be placed on presenting patients with all of their options while respecting their purchasing value. The decision ultimately belongs to the patient, not the doctor.

Special Considerations
Surface Disease

Patients who are receiving treatment for glaucoma suffer from the same surface diseases that impede ideal visual outcomes in a refractive clinic. In fact, many of the IOP-lowering medication regimens can further worsen surface disease, making spectacle independence challenging. Glaucoma and cataract surgeons alike must do a thorough examination and treat the ocular surface to ensure the best refractive outcomes. A healthy surface is critical to realizing any potential gains that the surgeon has primed for reaching emmetropia.

Specifically the surgeon should focus on dryness, meibomian gland dysfunction (MGD), and anterior basement membrane dystrophy (ABMD). Dryness and MGD should be treated preoperatively and the same holds true for ABMD when the surface is irregular and causing difficulty with biometry measurements. On occasion subtle ABMD is not treated preoperatively and may need to be addressed in the symptomatic postoperative refractive IOL patient with phototherapeutic keratectomy (PTK).

Excimer Support

Glaucoma specialists often do not have an excimer at their disposal, which makes offering options for spectacle independence difficult but not impossible. Just like a comprehensive ophthalmologist who offers premium IOL services might have a local refractive surgeon to team with, a glaucoma specialist should form a similar relationship.

The cost of fully committing to performing refractive cataract surgery is significant, but for the financially restricted physician, the cost can be as minimal as acquiring a method of measuring keratometry and a marking pen for axis alignment.

Premium lenses can be offered without excimer support, but many patients would benefit from an enhancement to enjoy their full visual potential. One such technology that currently exists in United States Food and Drug Administration (FDA) trials is the light-adjustable IOL,[5] which enables post–phaco-IOL patients to have their postoperative refractive error adjusted in the immediate period following surgery.

Surgical Intraocular Pressure Spikes in the Glaucoma Patient

It is worth giving thought to the maximal rise in IOP that can be experienced with various surgical interventions (**Table 29.2**).

With phacoemulsification alone, pressures of 60 mm Hg can be experienced during sculpting and irrigation/aspiration. The rise in pressures observed with femtosecond surgery depend on the type, due to differences in retention pressure from suction. With femtosecond cataract surgery, the IOP rise is lower than with femtosecond laser-assisted in-situ keratomileusis (LASIK) at 14 mm Hg and 130 mm Hg, respectively.

To avoid the IOP rise to levels over 100 mm Hg observed with femtosecond LASIK, patients can be offered photorefractive keratectomy (PRK) as an alternative. In either case the surgeon should be mindful when thinning the cornea due to subsequent artificial effects on the measured IOP. Patients should be instructed on the relation between thin corneas and IOP so that they can inform their future eye care providers, and pressures can be appropriately adjusted.

The Monocular Patient

The monocular patient requires special consideration, and it is recommended that they wear a safety lens after cataract surgery. Options for spectacle independence should still be considered. Monocular patients who are a good steward of their health and who will wear the safety lens can be offered premium lenses. There are low-risk situations when these patients would benefit from having the best possible vision. One might argue that by targeting good uncorrected vision, surgeons are giving these patients a means of going without their safety lens. Nonetheless, aiming for the optimal visual potential remains in the patient's best interest.

Case Presentation

A 59-year-old woman presents with complaints of difficulty with night driving because of glare. She had undergone myopic LASIK surgery 10 years ago. Her family history was significant

Table 29.2 Intraocular Pressure (IOP) Rise for Given Surgical Technique

Surgical Technique	IOP Rise	Duration of IOP Rise
Phacoemulsification	> 60 mm Hg	5 to 30 minutes
Femtosecond cataract	14 mm Hg	30 to 120 seconds
Femtosecond LASIK	130 mm Hg	30 to 90 seconds

for glaucoma, and she was using latanoprost nightly to both eyes.

Her best corrected visual acuities were 20/40 OU, but with brightness acuity testing dropped to 20/150 OD and 20/200 OS. Her IOP was 15 OU, with a previously established goal of upper teens OU (a goal established after LASIK surgery).

Pertinent exam findings included open angles with trace pigmentation OU, 1+ nuclear cataracts with 2+ posterior subcapsular cataracts on axis OU, and cup-to-disk ratios of 0.9 OU. Visual fields and topography are shown in **Fig. 29.1** and **Fig. 29.2**. Optical coherence tomography (OCT) of the nerves and maculas was normal OU.

With her history of LASIK surgery, it was important to carefully review her visual objectives. Her hobbies included playing tennis and computer games. She reported enjoying books but did not describe herself as an avid reader. She reported that she highly desired to be less dependent on spectacles and wished to review options for spectacle independence.

Given this background we discussed the Crystalens. Although multifocal IOLs could be considered, there was concern about reducing her contrast sensitivity. Further, the Crystalens comes in a toric lens, which would allow treatment of her corneal cylinder at the time of her cataract and iStent surgery.

The ocular response analyzer was used intraoperatively to confirm and guide the choice of toric Crystalens and to direct the placement of its axis. Plano was targeted for her dominant right eye and –0.5D spherical power was targeted for her nondominant eye.

One month postoperatively, her visual acuity was 20/25 J5 OD and 20/60 J3 OS. Her refraction was plano –0.50 × 160 OD and –0.75 sphere OS. Her pressures were 16 OU despite self-discontinuation of latanoprost therapy. It was recommended that she remain off latanoprost given that she was at her predetermined IOP goal.

Three months postoperatively, the patient reported that her distance vision was not optimal. The right eye measured 20/30 but refracted to 20/20 with –0.25 –0.50 × 175.

Photorefractive keratectomy (PRK) to her right eye was discussed, and she elected to proceed with the treatment. Post-PRK she was 20/20 in the right eye uncorrected and quite happy with her vision.

Pressures have been at her IOP goal and she continues to be followed for her glaucoma. Her visual fields remain stable, and she is pleased with her vision.

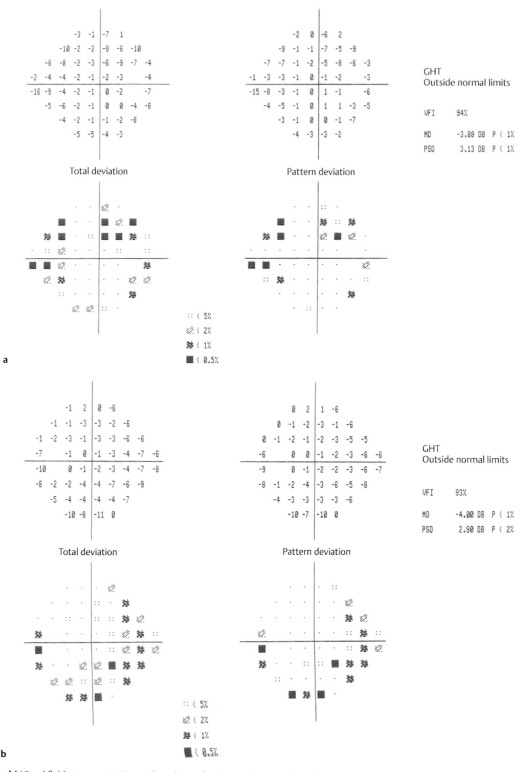

GHT
Outside normal limits

VFI   94%

MD   -3.88 DB   P < 1%
PSD   3.13 DB   P < 1%

Total deviation   Pattern deviation

:: < 5%
⌺ < 2%
✻ < 1%
■ < 0.5%

a

GHT
Outside normal limits

VFI   93%

MD   -4.00 DB   P < 1%
PSD   2.90 DB   P < 2%

Total deviation   Pattern deviation

:: < 5%
⌺ < 2%
✻ < 1%
■ < 0.5%

b

Fig. 29.1 (a,b) Visual fields at presentation, with each eye showing early arcs and nasal steps.

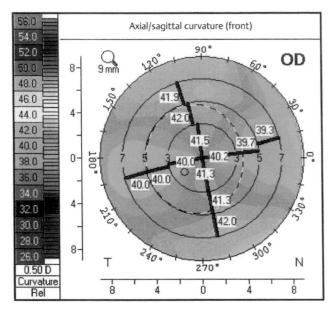

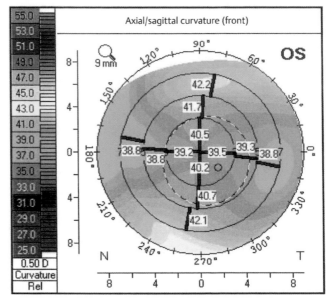

Fig. 29.2 **(a,b)** Topography at presentation, illustrating fairly regular astigmatism in corneas with flatter than normal curvatures (in a patient with a known history of myopic LASIK).

Conclusion

Patient expectations continue to evolve over time. As patients age, they are faced with multiple coexisting diseases. As glaucoma specialists, it is important to remember that when treating glaucoma there is also the potential and opportunity to treat refractive errors.

Thinking of refractive error and glaucoma as comorbidities helps us to fully realize the visual gains of each patient encounter. Many surgeons hesitate to offer options for spectacle independence in the setting of glaucoma with vision loss, but patients truly value these options for reaching their maximum visual potential.

References

1. Gedde SJ, Herndon LW, Brandt JD, Budenz DL, Feuer WJ, Schiffman JC, Tube Versus Trabeculectomy Study Group. Postoperative complications in the Tube Versus Trabeculectomy (TVT) study during five years of follow-up. Am J Ophthalmol 2012;153:804–814.e1

2. Samuelson TW, Katz LJ, Wells JM, Duh Y-J, Giamporcaro JE; US iStent Study Group. Randomized evaluation of the trabecular micro-bypass stent with phacoemulsification in patients with glaucoma and cataract. Ophthalmology 2011;118:459–467

3. McKendrick AM, Sampson GP, Walland MJ, Badcock DR. Contrast sensitivity changes due to glaucoma and normal aging: low-spatial-frequency losses in both magnocellular and parvocellular pathways. Invest Ophthalmol Vis Sci 2007;48:2115–2122

4. Souza CE, Muccioli C, Soriano ES, et al. Visual performance of AcrySof ReSTOR apodized diffractive IOL: a prospective comparative trial. Am J Ophthalmol 2006;141:827–832

5. Ford J, Werner L, Mamalis N. Adjustable intraocular lens power technology. J Cataract Refract Surg 2014;40:1205–1223

30 Trabecular Bypass: Hydrus

Husam Ansari and Reay H. Brown

The Hydrus microstent (Ivantis, Inc., Irvine, CA) is a minimally invasive glaucoma surgery (MIGS) device designed to lower the intraocular pressure (IOP) while avoiding the complications of traditional glaucoma filtration surgeries. The Hydrus microstent is unique among the MIGS devices in that it provides both trabecular bypass and scaffolding of a three-clock-position arc of Schlemm's canal, placing the trabecular meshwork on stretch and providing enhanced access of aqueous humor to downstream collector channels. This chapter reviews the Hydrus surgical technique, patient selection, and initial clinical results.

Case Presentation

A 79-year-old woman with primary open-angle glaucoma (POAG) presented complaining of decreased vision in her left eye. She had difficulty with reading and driving at night due to glare from oncoming headlights. Her glaucoma was controlled with the use of a topical β-blocker and prostaglandin analogue. She desired cataract surgery to improve her visual function, and despite maintaining adherence to medical therapy, she was very interested in reducing her need for topical medications for glaucoma control. Preoperatively, her best-corrected visual acuity (BCVA) with mild myopic, astigmatic correction was 20/60, and IOP was 15 mm Hg. She had moderate nuclear sclerosis and her angle was open to grade 4, with moderate pigmentation of the trabecular meshwork (TM). There was inferior notching of the optic nerve rim and superior nasal step on visual field testing. With a visually significant cataract and moderate POAG controlled on two medications, it was determined that the patient was a good candidate for cataract extraction combined with implantation of a Hydrus microstent.

The patient underwent uncomplicated cataract extraction, intraocular lens implantation, and Hydrus microstent implantation in the left eye. The Hydrus microstent was deployed into the nasal angle. Her postoperative course was uncomplicated, with steady improvement in her BCVA and immediate cessation of topical glaucoma medications. Two years after surgery, her visual acuity was 20/20 without correction, her IOP was 15 mm Hg without any glaucoma medications, and the Hydrus microstent was in its original position.

The Hydrus Microstent

The Hydrus microstent is an 8-mm nitinol implant that enhances aqueous humor outflow via three mechanisms (**Fig. 30.1**). First, the distal end of the device pierces through the TM and rests in Schlemm's canal (SC) while the proximal end of the device (the inlet) remains in the anterior chamber (AC), providing unobstructed flow of aqueous humor from the AC to SC. Second, the three windows on the anterior face of the device stretch the TM, providing an alternate pathway for aqueous through the TM

along the three-clock-position length of the device. Third, the device scaffolds SC, facilitating access of aqueous humor in the canal to downstream collector channels along the length of the device. The extended scaffolding concept distinguishes the Hydrus from the iStent (Glaukos Corp., Laguna Hills, CA), a previously approved MIGS device that also targets the trabecular bypass. The iStent also has a nonluminal section placed into the SC but with a shorter span of scaffolding.

In preclinical studies, the microstent has been shown to have excellent long-term biocompatibility in nonhuman primates and rabbits, and has been shown to increase outflow facility, decrease outflow resistance, and maintain patency of collector channel ostia in human cadaver eyes.[1-5] The device is implanted through a clear corneal incision under gonioscopic visualization using a preloaded handheld inserter and is readily combined with phacoemulsification cataract extraction (**Fig. 30.2**).

Patient Selection

The ideal initial patient for the Hydrus microstent has mild-to-moderate open-angle glaucoma controlled on one or two topical medications, requires IOP in the mid-teens, has moderate to dense pigmentation of the TM, and needs cataract surgery. These patients already have decided to have surgery to improve their vision and can be counseled that the Hydrus procedure adds minimal risk to the cataract surgery with the goal of decreasing their IOP and reducing or eliminating their need for glaucoma medications. The TM pigmentation will enhance the surgeon's view of the AC angle target tissue, making it easier to place the Hydrus within the SC.

Surgical Technique

Patients undergoing Hydrus implantation combined with cataract surgery may receive the surgeon's usual preoperative eyedrop regimen for cataract surgery. Topical or retrobulbar anesthesia may be utilized. After cataract extraction and intraocular lens implantation, intracameral miotics are helpful to improve the view of the angle. The AC is subsequently filled with viscoelastic.

Next, correct positioning of the patient and the operating microscope must be attained. The surgeon usually is seated temporally, although working superiorly is also possible. The microscope should be tilted 30 to 40 degrees toward the surgeon while the patient's head is tilted 30 to 40 degrees away from the surgeon (**Fig. 30.3**). With the patient and microscope positioned this way, a handheld direct gonioprism coupled to the cornea with viscoelastic provides an excellent view of the nasal AC angle.

Prior to entering the eye with the inserter, the surgeon must take several steps to ensure a smooth deployment of the device. The surgeon's index finger is placed on the advancement wheel on the inserter. The surgeon may pronate or supinate his or her

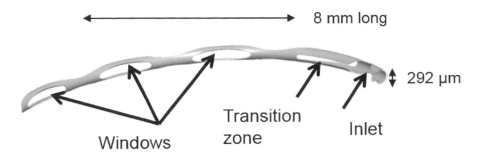

8 mm long

292 μm

Windows

Transition zone

Inlet

Fig. 30.1 The Hydrus microstent. Once the device is inserted, the distal windows reside in Schlemm's canal and stretch the trabecular meshwork, whereas the inlet and proximal portion of the transition zone remain in the anterior chamber to provide trabecular bypass. (Courtesy of Ivantis, Inc.)

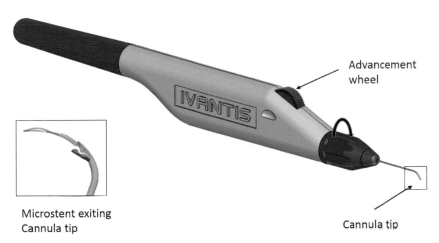

Advancement wheel

Microstent exiting Cannula tip

Cannula tip

Fig. 30.2 The Hydrus microstent inserter. The blue dial allows for rotation of the tip on the long axis of the cannula. The device is deployed by rotation of the advancement wheel with the surgeon's index finger. (Courtesy of Ivantis, Inc.)

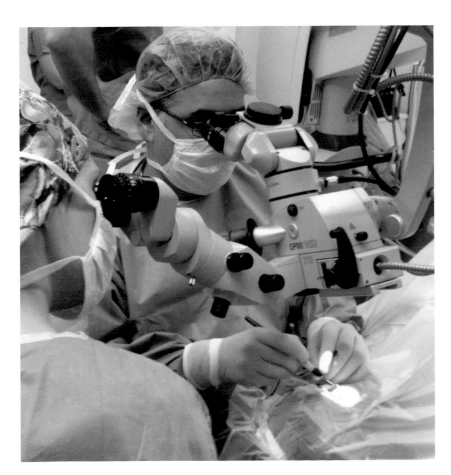

Fig. 30.3 Surgical positioning immediately prior to placement of the gonioprism on the cornea. The operating microscope is tilted 30 to 40 degrees toward the surgeon while the patient's head is tilted 30 to 40 degrees away from the surgeon.

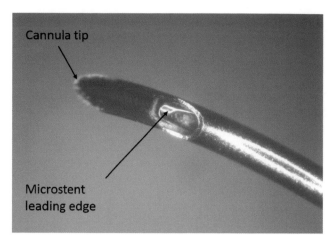

Fig. 30.4 The "ready" position. The distal end of the Hydrus is advanced forward enough to be visible in the tip of the cannula. (Courtesy of Ivantis, Inc.)

wrist to whatever position is most comfortable and then rotate the cannula tip of the inserter on its long axis to achieve the optimal angle of deployment. The microstent should be lubricated by dipping the cannula tip in viscoelastic and then partially advancing and then retracting the microstent by rotating the advancement wheel. Immediately prior to entering the eye, the surgeon should ensure that the distal end of the microstent is visible in the cannula tip but is not protruding from the cannula (**Fig. 30.4**). Placement of the distal end of the device in this "ready" position minimizes the amount of wheel rotation needed to initiate deployment once the cannula incises the TM.

For the right-handed surgeon seated temporally, the optimal location of the corneal incision is at the 45-degree meridian. This can be the incision used for cataract surgery or an alternate

1.5-mm incision if the cataract surgery incision is not optimally located. The cannula should be passed across the AC tangential to the pupillary margin (not across the center of the pupil) toward the 135-degree meridian in the nasal angle (**Fig. 30.5**). By initiating deployment at the 135-degree meridian, the entire three-clock-position section of the angle that will host the device can be visualized without the need to reposition the gonioprism during deployment.

At the TM, the tip of the cannula is angled anteriorly toward Schwalbe's line and depressed into the TM (**Fig. 30.6**). Rotation of the advancement wheel with the index finger deploys the device. It is critical to rotate the wheel without moving the inserter within the eye. It can be helpful to count the windows as they come out of the tip. Once the third window is visualized, the surgeon can prepare for disengagement of the inserter. The wheel is advanced until a hard stop is noted. The wheel is then dialed slightly backward, disengaging the inserter from the device. With a slight backward pivot of the entire inserter within the corneal incision, the inserter is completely freed from the device and removed from the eye. If necessary, an intraocular hook can be used to engage the inlet to slightly advance or retract the device within SC. The ideal final position is for the TM incision to be within the transition zone of the device, all three windows in the SC, and the inlet in the AC (**Fig. 30.7**). Finally, the viscoelastic is removed and the corneal incisions are closed with hydration or sutures as needed for wound stability.

Complications

The Hydrus procedure can be complicated by the same issues that challenge all ab interno angle procedures: establishing and maintaining a view of the angle, identifying the TM, corneal striae, blood reflux, surgeon learning curve, and excessive patient movement. After filling the AC with viscoelastic prior to implanting the device, the use of a Barraquer 15- to 21-mm Hg tonometer (Ocular Instruments, Inc., Bellevue, WA) can be helpful to

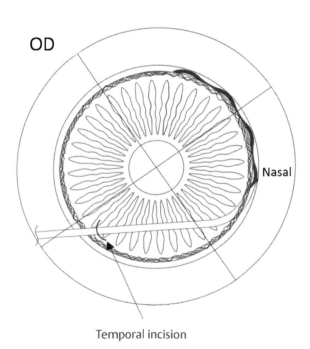
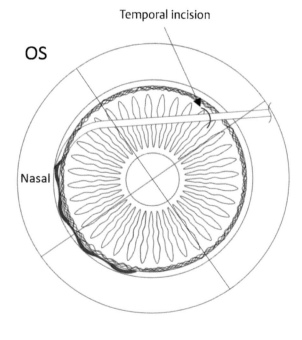

Fig. 30.5 The cannula should be passed across the anterior chamber (AC) tangential to the pupil margin to ensure that the entire arc of the angle that will host the device can be visualized without the need to reposition the gonioprism during deployment. (Courtesy of Ivantis, Inc.)

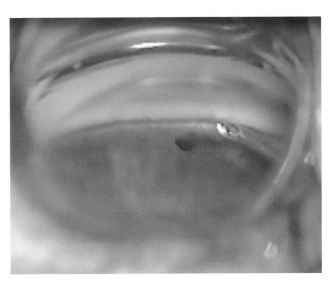
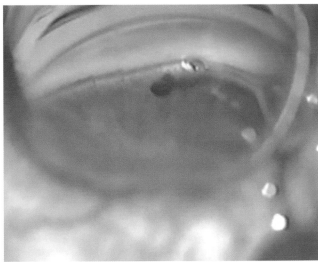

a   b

Fig. 30.6 **(a)** Intraoperative photograph showing the angle of approach of the cannula tip to the trabecular meshwork. **(b)** Depression of the cannula tip into the trabecular meshwork immediately prior to initiating deployment.

ensure that the IOP is sufficiently high to avoid corneal striae during the procedure but also not so high as to collapse the SC, making delivery of the device more difficult. If the TM is less deeply pigmented, blood reflux can be used to identify it, or trypan blue can be used to stain the meshwork. With trypan blue staining, even a nonpigmented meshwork can be identified easily.

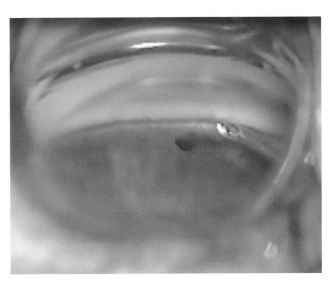

Fig. 30.7 The Hydrus microstent in the anterior chamber angle. (Courtesy of Jason Jones, MD, Sioux City, IA.)

The length of the Hydrus device and the need to thread its full extent into the tight space of the SC creates some unique challenges. The surgeon needs to maintain visualization of a three-clock-position section of the angle throughout the surgery. Because of the duration of deployment, any sudden or excessive movement by the patient or the surgeon may lead to incorrect insertion. Placing the distal tip of the device in the "ready" position within the cannula prior to entering the eye is critical for minimizing the duration of the deployment. If excessive patient movement is precluding safe insertion, topical procedures can be converted to retrobulbar anesthesia and insertion can be reattempted. If the device is entering somewhere other than the SC, a hard stop may be encountered earlier than expected, indicating that the distal tip of the device is encountering tissue that it cannot penetrate. Alternatively, the cannula tip may get pushed off from the TM incision point, allowing the middle and proximal window to deploy in the AC instead of in the SC. Whenever possible, this situation must be recognized prior to disengaging the device from the inserter so that the device may be retracted and redeployed at another location (either via the same corneal incision or a new one at a different meridian). Once disengaged, the device is not easily reloaded onto the inserter.

Postoperative Management

Postoperative management is performed according to the surgeon's usual protocol for cataract surgery, with topical steroid, nonsteroidal, and antibiotic medication and follow-up visits typically at 1 day, 1 week, and 1 month after surgery. Glaucoma medications are discontinued in the operative eye immediately after surgery and can be added back either temporarily or permanently as needed based on the IOP.

Clinical Results

Initial clinical experience with the Hydrus microstent demonstrates a low rate and low severity of adverse events while lowering IOP and reducing glaucoma medications. Pfeiffer and colleagues[6] randomized patients with mild-to-moderate POAG (defined as a mean deviation no worse than –12 dB on preoperative Humphrey visual field testing) to receive Hydrus microstent implantation combined with cataract surgery (treatment group) or cataract surgery alone (control group). One hundred eyes from 100 patients were randomized to the two arms at a 1:1 ratio and followed for 2 years with washed-out diurnal IOP measurements at baseline, 12 months, and 24 months. Washed-out mean diurnal IOP in the treatment group was significantly lower at 24 months compared with control (16.9 ± 3.3 vs 19.2 ± 4.7 mm Hg), as was the mean number of medications used (0.5 ± 1.0 vs 1.0 ± 1.0). Furthermore, the proportion of patients with a 20% decrease in washed out IOP was higher in the treatment group compared with control (80% vs 46%) as was the proportion of patients using no glaucoma medications at 24 months in the treatment group compared with control (73% vs 38%). In this study, the microstent was found to be safe. There were no cases of stent migration, repositioning, or removal. Two of 50 patients in the Hydrus arm of the study experienced a transient IOP spike of greater than 10 mm Hg above baseline. The most common adverse event associated with the stent was focal (less than one clock position) peripheral anterior synechiae (PAS) near the inlet of the stent (nine of 50 patients). However, no effect of these PAS on IOP or medication usage was observed.

Another study by Tetz and colleagues[7] evaluated the use of the Hydrus in combination with cataract surgery and as a stand-alone procedure in patients with mild, moderate, and advanced POAG, pseudoexfoliation glaucoma, and pigmentary glaucoma. In this study, 40 patients received the Hydrus microstent as a stand-alone procedure. In this arm, the mean IOP was lowered from 21.6 mm Hg at baseline to 18.3 mm Hg at 24 months. Furthermore, the mean number of medications used lowered from 1.7 at baseline to 0.4 at 24 months. The combined surgery arm yielded results similar to those in the study by Pfeiffer and colleagues.

The pivotal study for United States Food and Drug Administration (FDA) approval, which recently completed enrollment, is similar to the study of Pfeiffer and colleagues in its design.[8] This suggests that the initial FDA label for the Hydrus microstent in the United States will require it to be implanted at the time of cataract surgery in patients with mild-to-moderate POAG, not as a stand-alone procedure and not in advanced POAG patients. As experience with the procedure increases and more data become available, the use of the Hydrus microstent as a stand-alone procedure in either phakic or pseudophakic individuals may be considered.

Conclusion

The Hydrus microstent will be an excellent addition to our glaucoma surgical armamentarium. The learning curve for the surgical technique is on a par with other ab interno procedures targeting the AC angle, and the device-specific complications are rare. There is an impressive body of laboratory evidence and a growing body of clinical evidence that the Hydrus is safe and effectively lowers IOP. The Hydrus microstent, whether implanted alone or in combination with cataract surgery, has the potential to reduce the treatment burden of glaucoma by lowering the IOP or by reducing the number of glaucoma mediations.

Financial Disclosure

Husam Ansari has received research support from Ivantis, Inc. and Allergan, Inc.

Reay H. Brown has received consulting fees from Ivantis, Inc., Transcend, Inc., and Allergan, Inc. He receives royalties from Rhein, Inc., and has sold patents to Glaukos, Inc.

References

1. Grierson I, Saheb H, Kahook MY, et al. A novel Schlemm's canal scaffold: histological observations. J Glaucoma 2015;24:460–468

2. Camras LJ, Yuan F, Fan S, et al. A novel Schlemm's Canal scaffold increases outflow facility in a human anterior segment perfusion model. Invest Ophthalmol Vis Sci 2012;53:6115–6121

3. Gulati V, Fan S, Hays CL, Samuelson TW, Ahmed II, Toris CB. A novel 8-mm Schlemm's canal scaffold reduces outflow resistance in a human anterior segment perfusion model. Invest Ophthalmol Vis Sci 2013;54:1698–1704

4. Hays CL, Gulati V, Fan S, Samuelson TW, Ahmed II, Toris CB. Improvement in outflow facility by two novel microinvasive glaucoma surgery implants. Invest Ophthalmol Vis Sci 2014;55:1893–1900

5. Johnstone MA, Saheb H, Ahmed IIK, Samuelson TW, Schieber AT, Toris CB. Effects of a Schlemm canal scaffold on collector channel ostia in human anterior segments. Exp Eye Res 2014;119:70–76

6. Pfeiffer N, Garcia-Feijoo J, Martinez-de-la-Casa JM, et al. A randomized trial of a Schlemm's canal microstent with phacoemulsification for reducing intraocular pressure in open-angle glaucoma. Ophthalmology 2015; 122:1283–1293

7. Tetz M, Pfeiffer N, Scharioth G, et al. Two-year results from a prospective multicenter study of a Schlemm's canal scaffold for intraocular pressure reduction in patients with open-angle glaucoma undergoing cataract surgery. J Cataract Refract Surg 2015; in press

8. Samuelson TW. Twenty-four month results from a multi-center study of Hydrus as a stand-alone therapy. The HYDRUS I trial. Presented at the American Society of Cataract and Refractive Surgeons annual meeting, San Francisco, 2013

31 Excimer Laser Trabeculostomy

Michael S. Berlin

Case Presentations

Case 1: Gonioscopic Procedure for Excimer Laser Trabeculostomy Alone

A 71-year-old woman presented with open-angle glaucoma (OAG) and cataract in both eyes (OU). Her right eye was uncontrolled with maximally tolerated topical medications: latanoprost at bedtime and dorzolamide and timolol fixed-combination b.i.d. with an intraocular pressure (IOP) of 28 mm Hg. Her corrected visual acuity (VA) was 20/40 OU. Her visual field and optic disk cupping at 0.7 were consistent with moderate glaucomatous loss, with both showing progression. Surgical options were discussed, including lensectomy, trabeculectomy, lensectomy combined with trabeculectomy, and excimer laser trabeculostomy (ELT) with the expectation that eventual lensectomy might be forthcoming.

Excimer laser trabeculostomy under gonioscopic observation was performed on the patient's right eye. Ten channels were created through the trabecular meshwork (TM) into Schlemm's canal (SC) following the current 10-channel protocol.

The postoperative IOP was 21 mm Hg on day 1, whereas postoperative therapy included dexamethasone and Garamycin. Glaucoma medications were discontinued. Postoperative gonioscopy revealed laser-induced effects within the trabecular meshwork. Initially, the holes appeared round but over time appeared ovular with slight pigmentation around the edges. At 1 month post-ELT, the patient's IOP was 16 mm Hg with no medications. At 3 months, her IOP was 14 mm Hg without medications. At 1 year, her IOP was 12 mm Hg, which was a 57% reduction from her preoperative IOP. Two years later, with visible crater openings into the SC and an unmedicated IOP of 16 mm Hg, the patient underwent lensectomy with intraocular lens (IOL) implantation. Five years later, her post-lensectomy IOP has remained within the range of 15 to 17 mm Hg, a 39% decrease in IOP that has been sustained without medications, even after a second intraocular surgery (**Fig. 31.1**).

Case 2: Combined Phacoemulsification and Gonioscopic ELT Procedure

A 73-year-old man presented for lensectomy with a dense cataract and OAG in his left eye with marked visual field (VF) defects and significant disk cupping, with a cup-to-disk ratio of 0.8. When first examined, his IOP was 25 mm Hg on the α-agonist Brimonidine. He was stable on a medication treatment regimen for nearly a decade with no further progression. At the time of cataract surgery, he was offered the option of adding ELT to potentially eliminate his need for postoperative glaucoma medications.

Phacoemulsification was performed through a 2.4-mm clear corneal incision without complication followed by ELT. The post-operative therapy included dexamethasone phosphate 0.1 mg/mL plus tobramycin 0.3 mg/mL fixed-combination eyedrops administered q.i.d. over a period of 4 weeks. His preoperative washout IOP was 27 mm Hg. His postoperative IOP was 12 mm Hg on day 1, 11 mm Hg at 1 month, 12 mm Hg at 1 year, 14 mm Hg at 2 years, and 13 mm Hg at 3 years, a 53.0% decrease in IOP. The patient's VA improved from the preoperative 20/100 to 20/20 at 1 month, 20/25 at 1 year, and remained stable for the entire 3 years of follow-up. In addition to stable VA, the patient's IOP has also remained stable over the past 3 years, and the patient has not required the use of any topical hypotensive medication during this period. Although the primary diagnosis and treatment was for a mature cataract, the addition of an ELT procedure was anticipated to lower the IOP more than cataract surgery alone to reduce the patient's topical medication requirement. This goal was successfully achieved (**Fig. 31.2**).

Case 3: Combined Phacoemulsification and Endoscopic ELT Procedure

An 83-year-old man presented with moderate cataract and early to moderate OAG in his left eye on maximum tolerated medications including prostaglandin analogue, β-blocker, and carbonic anhydrase inhibitor, with progressive glaucomatous VF defects. His IOP was 15 mm Hg in his left eye on presentation. He had been treated with medications for over a decade, increasing from monotherapy to his current regimen. However, even on maximal medications, his VF defects continued to progress. He elected to proceed with phacoemulsification combined with endoscopic ELT. Preoperative washout IOP in his left eye was 29 mm Hg.

After combined phacoemulsification plus ELT, the patient's vision improved from 20/40 to 20/25 and his IOP was 14 mm Hg without glaucoma medication at 1 week after the procedure and remained stable for over 2 years with no further progression of VF defects. His immediate postoperative therapy included dexamethasone phosphate 0.1 mg/mL and tobramycin 0.3 mg/mL fixed-combination eyedrops q.i.d. tapered over a period of 4 weeks. The ELT procedure in this patient was performed endoscopically, which often enables better visualization of the TM than a gonioscopic approach. In combined cases in which ELT follows rather than precedes lensectomy, endoscopic ELT is considered a better alternative than gonioscopic ELT due to the possibility of corneal edema or Descemet's folds at the end of the cataract surgery, as is often seen following the removal of a dense cataract with a hard nucleus. In addition, the 2.4-mm clear corneal tunnel for the phacoemulsification readily enables an endoscopic approach without further enlargement of the incision.

Even though this patient's cataract was considered only moderate, a combined procedure was preferred due to his progressive glaucomatous field loss while on maximum tolerated medical

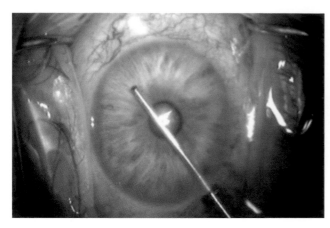

Fig. 31.1 Phakic excimer laser trabeculostomy (ELT). The ELT probe traverses the anterior chamber (AC) in this phakic ELT procedure under gonioscopic visualization. Following paracentesis and AC deepening with an ophthalmic viscosurgical device (OVD), the probe is placed into the eye then under gonioscopic control, and 10 channels are created into the lumen of Schlemm's canal (SC). (Courtesy of U. Giers, Germany.)

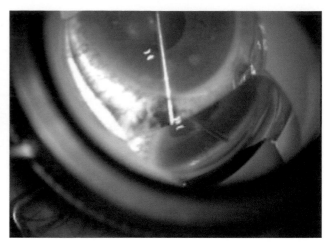

Fig. 31.2 Combined lensectomy and ELT. Following phacoemulsification and implantation of an intraocular lens (IOL), through the phaco incision or the paracentesis incision, the ELT probe is positioned across the AC to contact the trabecular meshwork (TM) under gonioscopic control to create 10 channels into the lumen of the SC. (Courtesy of U. Giers, Germany.)

therapy. It was anticipated that cataract removal with an ELT procedure would reduce both the IOP and the medication requirements. An endoscopic approach for ELT is also preferred when visualization of the anterior chamber angle through a goniolens is inadequate, such as in patients with advanced corneal scarring, band keratopathy, or a failed corneal graft **(Figs. 31.3 and 31.4).**

The Procedure

Excimer laser trabeculostomy is a minimally invasive glaucoma surgery (MIGS) procedure. A 308-nm xenon chloride excimer laser is utilized to remove the tissue obstructing aqueous outflow due to its precision and its effectively nonthermal laser/tissue interaction properties. Additionally, ELT reestablishes physiological aqueous outflow through the TM in a manner that does not provoke a healing response, and consequently enables a sustained reduction in IOP. The ELT procedure is performed via a clear corneal incision in which direct visualization of the target tissue, using a goniolens or an endoscope, provides immediate feedback to the surgeon. ELT, when compared with more invasive glaucoma surgical procedures such as trabeculectomy, is almost as efficacious in both lowering the IOP and decreasing the need for pressure-lowering medication, while being far less traumatic. The sparing of conjunctiva is a major advantage of this technique, because the option of performing a subsequent trabeculectomy, if necessary, would not be precluded. This MIGS procedure, another option in the armamentarium of the glaucoma and cataract surgeon, offers a robust safety profile, rapid stabilization of IOP, and clinically verified long-term efficacy with minimal negative impact on the patient's quality of life. As such, it may become a replacement option for topical glaucoma therapies, which are associated with high costs, compliance issues, and topical and systemic side effects with long-term use.

The ELT concept is similar to that utilized by 193-nm ultraviolet (UV) excimer lasers for corneal surface ablation. The 193-nm wavelength enables precise removal of corneal tissue, facilitating successful refractive surgery without thermal degradation of the corneal collagen to ensure clarity. However, this 193-nm wavelength is not useful for intracameral procedures because it is absorbed by the cornea and is not readily transmissible by fiber optics. In contrast, the 308-nm UV excimer-laser–generated light is fiber-optic transmissible, and after extensive preclinical

experimentation it became the wavelength of choice for nonthermal, precisely targeted, ab interno fistulizing procedures and subsequently for ELT procedures. The initial ocular application of 308-nm excimer lasers was for nonhealing full-thickness ab interno sclerostomy. ELT was developed after careful measurements of the distance between the anterior chamber (AC) and the SC were taken and laser/tissue interaction details were quantified, enabling calculations for the creation of nonhealing ELT channels.[1]

Prior procedures aimed at eliminating the outflow obstruction localized to the juxtacanalicular trabecular meshwork (JCTM) and the inner wall of the SC region attempted to use mechanical devices and thermal lasers to perforate the TM. These have been shown to adequately bypass the outflow obstruction for the short term. However, they have been unsuccessful in the long term due to the amount of adjacent tissue damage related to the nature of the technique or device. Adjacent tissue damage evokes a healing response that eventually closes the openings. As laser

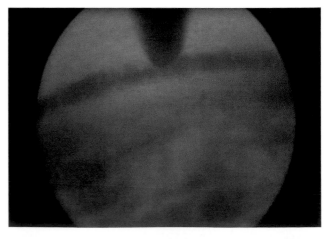

Fig. 31.3 Combined Lensectomy and ELT. Following phacoemulsification and implantation of an IOL, through the phaco incision or the paracentesis incision or both, a coaxial ELT probe (or an endoscope and a separate ELT probe) is positioned across the AC to contact the TM under endoscopic control to create 10 channels into the lumen of the SC.

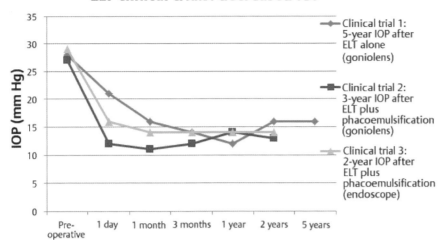

ELT clinical trials: decreased IOP

Legend:
- Clinical trial 1: 5-year IOP after ELT alone (goniolens)
- Clinical trial 2: 3-year IOP after ELT plus phacoemulsification (goniolens)
- Clinical trial 3: 2-year IOP after ELT plus phacoemulsification (endoscope)

Fig. 31.4 Comparison of ELT case study procedures. IOP, intraocular pressure.

technology evolved, several novel lasers were similarly used, but none enabled long-term patent openings. Krasnov[2] reported moderate success using a 943-nm ruby laser to perform "trabeculopuncture." Other laser trabeculopuncture attempts have included Hager's[3] use of an argon laser (488 + 514 nm) and Fankhauser's group's[4] use of a neodymium:yttrium-aluminum-garnet (Nd:YAG) laser (continuous wave of 1,064 nm). All have been unsuccessful due to early and late postoperative scarring. These and other laser trabeculopuncture attempts also limit prospective options for subsequent procedures,[5,6] as they induce destruction of local tissue and scar formation. In addition, with large openings and markedly increasing aqueous outflow, the compositional alterations of the aqueous humor augment the tissue-destructive healing responses.

Unlike ELT, current clinical laser treatments for glaucoma are based on procedures to modify the TM's function without physically bypassing TM flow obstruction. Following initial attempts using lasers ab interno to perforate the TM or to create full-thickness sclerostomies, Wise[7] found that a continuous-wave, long-pulsed, argon laser (488 + 514 nm) could successfully modify the TM to increase outflow without perforation. Their argon laser trabeculoplasty (ALT) procedure effectively lowered the IOP, but it functioned by creating thermal damage to the target tissue, causing coagulative necrosis of the TM.[7] In contrast to ALT procedures, laser trabeculoplasty (LTP) is now more commonly performed with solid-state (532 nm, frequency-doubled Nd:YAG) and diode (810 nm) lasers.

Studies comparing the efficacy of these lasers demonstrate minimal differences in efficacy, longevity, or repeatability. The efficacy of LTP in lowering the IOP has been well documented in the literature.[8–10] However, long-term studies have shown that the IOP-lowering efficacy of LTP decreases over time from a 77% success rate at 1 year, to 49% at 5 years, and finally to 32% at 10 years.[11]

Alternatively, selective laser trabeculoplasty (SLT) relies on selective absorption of short laser pulses to generate and spatially confine heat to pigmented targets within TM cells.[12,13] Based on the principle of selective photothermolysis, SLT uses a Q-switched, frequency-doubled 532-nm Nd:YAG laser. Laser Q-switching enables an extremely brief and high-powered light pulse to be delivered to the target tissue, which is intracellular pigment. Intracellular energy absorption and the short duration of the pulse are critical in preventing collateral damage to the surrounding tissues.[14]

The ELT procedure was developed with the goal of creating a long-term, nonhealing, anatomic modification of the TM to bypass outflow obstructions. It was finalized once the parameters of the target tissue anatomy,[15,16] localization of SC, and ablation rates for the 308-nm wavelength used on target tissue were determined. Target tissue anatomic considerations must specifically address decreasing trauma to the outer wall of the SC, so as to minimize healing responses. The outer wall endothelium contains fibroblasts, whereas the inner wall endothelium does not. Avoiding trauma to the outer wall is paramount to the successful long-term maintenance of outflow. Another anatomic consideration is the space between the inner and outer walls of SC, which can be less than 20 μm. The accuracy of a tool used to perforate the inner wall, such that it does not disturb the outer wall, must be of this same scale. The laser penetration depth is fixed by the number of pulses, similar to the penetration depth control in laser-assisted in-situ keratomileusis (LASIK). Perforation of the inner wall of the SC depends on the canal's distance from the fiber tip, which may vary due to the angle of placement and the amount of pressure on the fiber. This distance was determined by numerous preclinical experiments.[17,18] The ablation precision of the 308-nm excimer laser on this tissue, with 1.2 μm of tissue removal per pulse, enables the ELT procedure's efficacy.

In a study of the effects of 308-nm excimer laser energy applied ab interno to the limbal sclera of rabbit eyes, long-term decreases in IOP were achievable.[19] The use of this 308-nm wavelength, unlike that of earlier procedures with thermal lasers, enables laser tissue interactions that are less likely to evoke a cicatricial response in the TM or sclera. In addition, direct tissue contact of the fiber-optic delivery system ensures minimal exposure of adjacent tissue to radiation and maximizes ablation efficacy. The development of current ELT technologies and techniques are based on evidence that the TM and scleral tissue could be successfully removed without adjacent tissue damage, scar formation, or channel closure. High ablation accuracy enables the precise targeting of the TM through the inner wall of the SC without perforating the outer wall of the SC.

Conjunctiva sparing is another advantage of ELT because subsequent trabeculectomy would not be compromised. ELT, when compared with more invasive glaucoma surgical procedures (i.e., trabeculectomy), is almost as efficacious in lowering the IOP and reducing the use of glaucoma medication.[19]

The ELT procedure potentially enables a pneumatic canaloplasty. Both endoscopic and gonioscopic views of ELT have

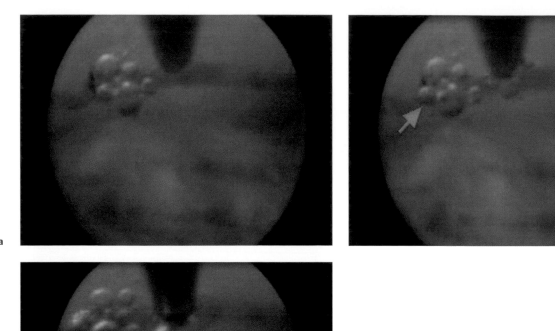

a

b

c

Fig. 31.5 Photos of the ELT procedure demonstrating pneumatic canaloplasty. **(a)** Coaxial endoscopic view of target ELT TM region overlying the SC for the second channel after the first channel has been created. Note bubbles at the first channel site. **(b)** The second channel is created into the lumen of the SC. **(c)** Bubble expansion is observed at the first ELT site, confirming channel patency into the SC at both sites. (Courtesy of J. Funk, Zurich, Switzerland.)

revealed gas bubble formation in the channel tissue and around the probe tip in the anterior chamber as a result of photoablation of the TM tissue. It is theorized that this process dilates the SC. When the ablation penetrates the outflow obstruction, gas is able to enter the SC through the newly formed channels in the TM. The pressure of this gas dilates the SC, displaces the SC's outer wall from the probe, and dilates adjacent collector channels to improve aqueous outflow, lowering the IOP. Observing gas bubbles exiting the adjacent openings confirms the continuity of flow from the SC. This hypothesis has yet to be confirmed via real-time imaging or histological studies. Such studies will improve our understanding of these pneumatic effects on the procedure and enable modifications to potentially further improve outcomes **(Fig. 31.5)**.

Rationale Behind the Procedure

The MIGS procedures use a microincision of 1 to 2 mm and can easily be combined with cataract surgery. The microincision facilitates the intraoperative maintenance of the anterior chamber, retains normal ocular anatomy, minimizes changes in refractive outcome (neutral to induce astigmatism), and adds to procedural safety. The invasive character of trabeculectomy and the incidence of serious complications after the procedure limit its use to later-stage and recalcitrant glaucoma patients. Issues regarding medication costs, patient compliance, and toxicity of preservatives suggest that medicinal therapeutic options also have limitations. Thus, there remains an unmet patient need for

treatments that could effectively treat mild-to-moderate glaucoma. In recent years, several MIGS procedures have been developed to fill the gap left by traditional treatment options. All have advantages and disadvantages, but no current technique fulfills all of the following requirements: (1) ab interno microincision; (2) minimal trauma; (3) efficacy (i.e., both lowering the IOP and reducing medication use); (4) rapid recovery; and (5) high safety profile.

The ELT was first used in a clinical setting by Vogel and Lauritzen[20] in 1997 following preclinical development by Berlin et al.[18] The ELT treats the primary pathology responsible for most OAG by decreasing the outflow resistance at the JCTM and the inner wall of the SC.[20,21] The TM itself is responsible for 60 to 80% of aqueous outflow resistance.[22] Using specified laser parameters, ELT evaporates human tissue by means of essentially non-thermal photoablation, thus denaturing the organic structures without producing undesirable marginal necrosis.[23] ELT excises the uveoscleral, corneoscleral, and juxtacanalicular meshwork, as well as the inner wall of the SC without damaging the outer wall of the SC or the collector channels.[24] No filtering fistula or bleb is created.[17,25,26]

The ELT surgical procedure is performed on an outpatient basis under local anesthesia (e.g., topical, peribulbar, or retrobulbar). Following paracentesis and stabilization of the anterior chamber with a viscoelastic agent, a fiber-optic probe is introduced and advanced across the AC and brought in direct contact with the TM **(Fig. 31.6)**. Probe placement is controlled by direct observation using either a goniolens or an endoscope. In the

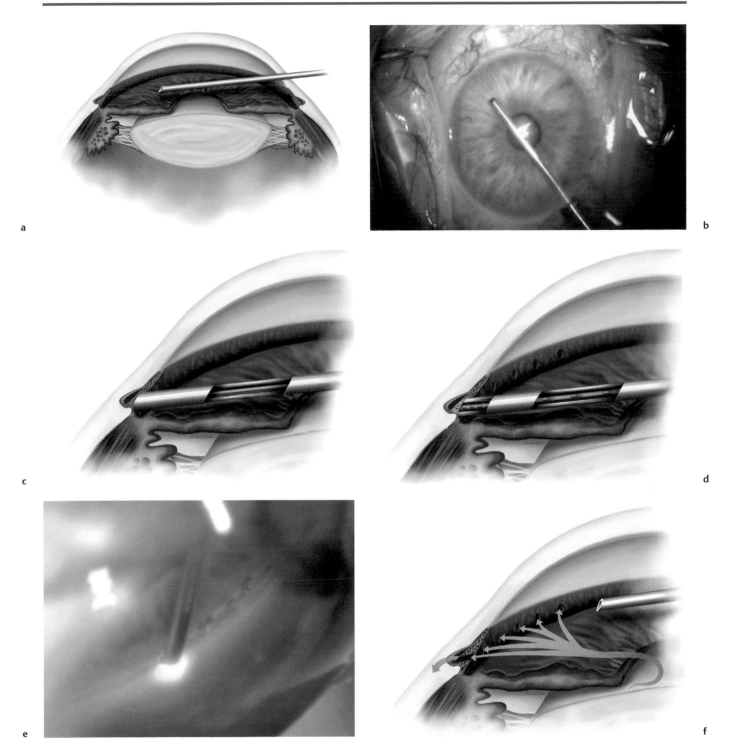

Fig. 31.6 Diagrams and photos of the excimer laser trabeculostomy procedure. The laser fiber is introduced into the AC through **(a)** a clear cornea paracentesis incision and **(b)** advanced across the AC to the **(c)** TM of the opposite quadrant. **(d)** When the fiber tip is in contact with and slightly compressing the TM, laser pulses are initiated. **(e)** Tissue fluorescence produced by the ultraviolet (UV) laser pulses may be visualized gonioscopically. **(f)** A series of laser channels of ~ 180 µm diameter each enables flow from the anterior chamber into Schlemm's canal. (**b,e**: courtesy of U. Giers, Germany.)

current protocols, six to 10 channels are created into the SC (**Fig. 31.7**).

Multichannel protocols ensure that at least several channels enter into the SC and can be readily created once the ELT fiber is in the AC, simply by treating additional sites along the TM. Failure to access the SC may occur if the SC is not adequately targeted. There are several reasons for inadequate targeting of the SC, such as lack of visualization beyond the TM, for example when the SC is compressed and thereby no longer filled with a visible blood column, or if probe positioning precludes the creation of a fistulizing channel not only due to inadequate targeting of the SC but also because the fixed number of pulses that

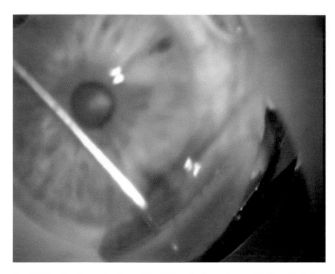

Fig. 31.7 Gonioscopic view of the ELT probe in contact with the TM during creation of channels. The SC may not be visible when the IOP is elevated greater than episcleral venous pressure following viscoelastic injection into the AC. (Courtesy of U. Giers, Germany.)

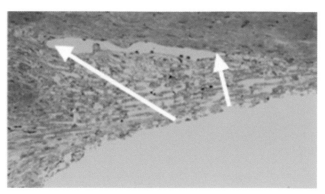

Fig. 31.8 Not all ELT sites enter the SC. Critical factors for ensuring adequacy of each ELT channel connecting from the AC into the lumen of the SC, due to the fixed number of pulses removing a fixed depth of tissue, include adequate localization of SC and probe angulation. Arrows point to the anterior and posterior extent of Schlemm's canal, with overlying trabecular meshwork intact.

ablate a defined depth in current protocols does not enable adequate tissue removal to perforate the TM tissue, due to physiological variations in thickness, SC location, and angulation of the probe (**Fig. 31.8**).

The probe is then removed and the viscoelastic agent is removed by irrigation/aspiration. Most commonly, the probe insertion is superior or superotemporal and the laser channels are located inferiorly or inferonasally. Blood reflux confirms entry into the SC and is a common but inconsequential occurrence (**Fig. 31.9**).

Patient Selection

The ELT procedure significantly reduces the IOP in patients with mild-to-moderate primary open-angle glaucoma (POAG), pigmentary glaucoma, or pseudoexfoliative glaucoma in which an IOP in the low to mid-teens is sufficient. ELT may be conveniently combined with cataract surgery and is also a good option for patients who find it difficult to adhere to a prescription medication regimen. Patients with advanced glaucoma or normal-tension glaucoma, which require very low target pressures in the low teens or even single digits, do not qualify for ELT.

Other patient criteria for ELT include those who would be candidates for medical therapy, laser treatment, and glaucoma filtering surgery. A history of prior eye surgery is not an exclusion criterion for ELT (e.g., history of uncomplicated cataract surgery, retinal laser surgery, SLT, vitrectomy, or extraocular muscle surgery).

Surgical Techniques

The ELT procedure is performed using a 308-nm xenon monochloride (XeCl) laser. The laser is automated to internally calibrate and control the output fluence in accordance with the manufacturer's specifications. Unlike solid-state lasers, this XeCl gas laser requires a short warm-up time during which the output energy is stabilized. The sterile, nonreusable fiber-optic delivery

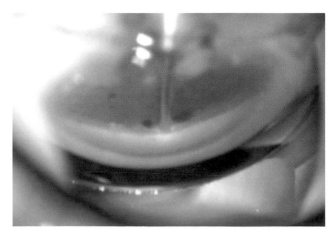

a

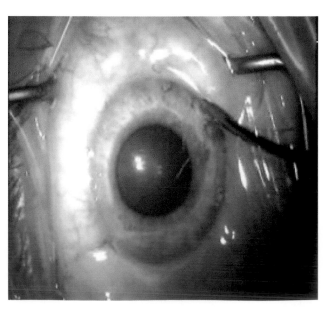

b

Fig. 31.9 **(a)** Blood from the SC verifies appropriate targeting and depth, gonioscopic view. In this series of created channels, occasional tissue fluorescence is visible during a UV laser pulse. **(b)** Induced blood reflux around the tip of the probe verifies patency and enables documentation of the number of successful channels into the SC. (Courtesy of U. Giers, Germany.)

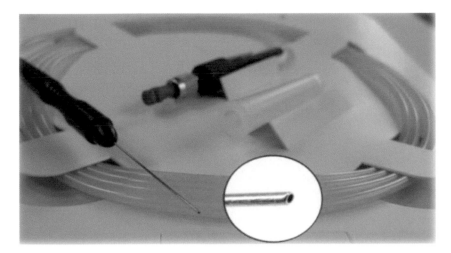

system is coupled to the laser (**Fig. 31.10**). The output beam is then adjusted at the fiber tip to ensure suprathreshold fluence for tissue ablation at the fiber tip. The console includes a power meter to enable this calibration, which is automatically performed prior to each procedure, similar to the tuning of a phacoemulsification handpiece before use.

Topical, peribulbar, or retrobulbar local anesthesia is administered. Alternatively, the procedure can be performed under general anesthesia in special cases. In ELT alone, topical pilocarpine 2% is used preoperatively to constrict the pupil. In phakic patients, this may also assist in protecting the lens. Alternatively, intracameral Miochol (acetylcholine 10 mg/mL) may be used. ELT is performed in the following manner:

1. A 1- to 1.5-mm paracentesis is created in the superotemporal perilimbal cornea at the 2 o'clock position for left eyes and at the 10 o'clock position for right eyes (**Fig. 31.11**); in combined cataract and ELT procedures, the previously created phaco-tunnel (2.0 to 2.4 mm) may be used in a similar fashion.

2. A viscoelastic device (ophthalmic viscosurgical device [OVD], e.g., Healon) fills the AC through the paracentesis (**Fig. 31.12**). The viscoelastic also deepens the

chamber angle and enables the procedure to be done even in an angle of Shaffer grade 2. Depending on the surgeon's preference, the IOP may be unchanged or increased by this injection, enabling or precluding visualization of the SC by blood reflux.

3. The laser probe is inserted into the AC through the paracentesis (**Fig. 31.13**) and is advanced to the opposite chamber angle via gonioscopic (using the surgeon's preferred goniolens) or endoscopic visualization (**Fig. 31.14**). The ELT fiber may be attached coaxially with an endoscope, or a second paracentesis endoscopic view may be utilized.

4. The fiber tip is centered on the pigmented TM and advanced to be in contact with the TM. The SC is targeted whenever visible, or surgeons are advised to alternate placement of the fiber to anterior, middle, and posterior TM regions to ensure some of the channels will, in fact, enter into the SC. The most common protocol consists of creating 10 ELT channels in the TM, spread over an area of 90 degrees.

5. The laser is activated, delivering laser pulses at 20 Hz per treatment site. Each pulse converts the tissue at the fiber tip into a gas. These gas bubbles may be seen

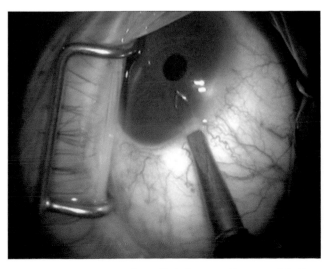

Fig. 31.11 Paracentesis in the perilimbal cornea. (Courtesy of U. Giers, Germany.)

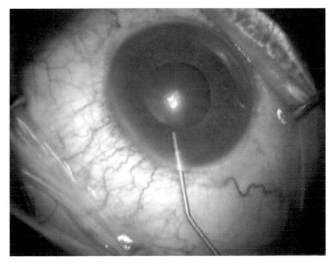

Fig. 31.12 Viscoelastic agent is introduced into the AC. (Courtesy of U. Giers, Germany.)

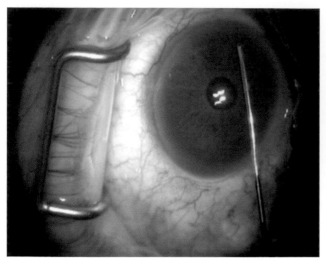

Fig. 31.13 Laser probe is inserted through the paracentesis crossing the AC to contact the TM in a region overlying the SC. (Courtesy of U. Giers, Germany.)

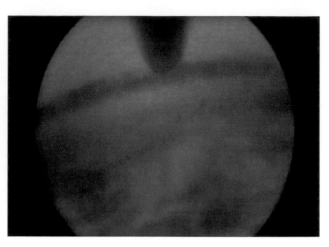

Fig. 31.14 Endoscopic view of the coaxial ELT probe. The SC may be visible when the IOP is lower than the episcleral venous pressure. (Courtesy of J. Funk, Switzerland.)

exiting around the fiber tip during each channel's ablation (**Fig. 31.15**).

6. Pulse by pulse, an opening is created, channeling aqueous humor from the AC into the SC, and bypassing the JCTM to the inner wall of the SC. Once the outflow obstruction is bypassed and the SC is entered, the pathway of gas, previously retrograde along the fiber, becomes anterograde, enabling the gas to enter the SC. This process of "pneumatic canaloplasty" potentiates dilation of both the SC and adjacent collector channels (see **Fig. 31.5**).

7. The probe tip is then repositioned such that additional channels are created.

8. The probe is removed from the anterior chamber.

9. The viscoelastic agent is exchanged with balanced salt solution (BSS) by coaxial or bimanual irrigation/aspiration (**Fig. 31.16**).

10. The patency of trabeculostomy sites can be confirmed during the viscoelastic/BSS exchange by inducing temporary iatrogenic hypotony to induce blood reflux from the SC, enabling visualization and confirming the patency of the ELT channels. (**Fig. 31.17**).

Combined with Cataract Extraction

For patients with OAG and cataracts, ELT can be easily combined with cataract surgery to generate an even greater reduction in IOP than either cataract surgery or ELT surgery alone. ELT is easy to perform during clear-corneal phacoemulsification. Surgery is prolonged for only 2 to 3 minutes and requires no additional

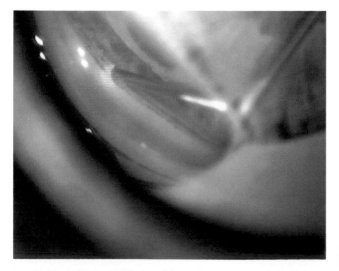

Fig. 31.15 Following positioning of the probe in contact and slightly compressing the TM over the SC, the laser is activated, delivering laser pulses at 20 Hz per treatment site. Each pulse converts the tissue at the fiber tip into a gas. These gas bubbles may be seen exiting around the fiber tip during each channel's creation.

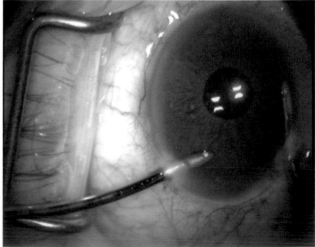

Fig. 31.16 Viscoelastic is exchanged for balanced salt solution (BSS) following completion of 10 ELT channels. (Courtesy of U. Giers, Germany.)

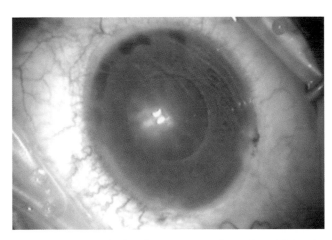

Fig. 31.17 Patency of trabeculostomy sites can be confirmed during the viscoelastic/BSS exchange by inducing temporary iatrogenic hypotony to produce blood reflux from SC, enabling visualization and confirming patency of the ELT channels. (Courtesy of U. Giers, Germany.)

corneal incision. A corneal tunnel of 2.4 mm or more is adequate for the combined endoscope handpiece and the laser fiber. Visualization is easier if the viscoelastic device (such as an OVD) is placed in the AC angle where the laser pores will be created. The other steps are similar to those for the gonioscopic approach. For an experienced cataract surgeon, the ELT can be readily learned. Cataract surgery alone lowers the IOP by ~ 4 mm Hg,[27] but the IOP-lowering efficacy is often compromised after 1 to 2 years.[28] Other surgeons have found that cataract surgery has no significant effect on IOP reduction.[29] A direct comparison of ELT alone versus ELT combined with cataract surgery documents the superior IOP-lowering efficacy of the combined procedure.[30] The advantage of the endoscopic procedure is that TM identification is simpler and that it can be performed even with poor corneal visibility (e.g., corneal scars, corneal edema).

Complications Specific to ELT as a Stand-Alone Procedure

Uncommon complications:
- Microhyphema (can lead to temporary IOP spikes during the early postoperative period)
- Anterior chamber flare and inflammation (similar to after cataract surgery)
- Inflammatory cells (mild, moderate, severe, very severe) (similar to after cataract surgery)

Rare complications:
- Hyphema and bleeding in the AC (can lead to temporary IOP spikes during the early postoperative period and must be treated with topical or systemic hypotensive medications)
- Corneal edema and/or opacifications (more so after endoscopic ELT, usually resolved within a few days)

Very rare complications:
- Contact with endothelium
- Iris damage
- Iritis
- Endophthalmitis (anterior and posterior segment inflammation; similar to after cataract surgery)
- Sterile hypopyon
- Cataract formation or worsening (when ELT procedure alone is performed in phakic eyes)

- IOL luxation, secondary cataract formation (when ELT is performed in pseudophakic eyes as a stand-alone procedure)
- Cystoid macular edema (similar to after cataract surgery)
- Infection (localized to external ocular surface including wound)
- Unplanned surgical reintervention (e.g., AC washout for persistent AC bleeding)

Postoperative Management

At the end of the procedure, topical prednisolone acetate 1% or dexamethasone 0.1% and topical antibiotics are administered to the operative eye. The eye is then shielded or patched, and the patient may be released once stable, similar to after phacoemulsification. The operative eye is treated with topical fixed steroid combination (prednisolone acetate 1% or dexamethasone 0.1%) and antibiotic eyedrops q.i.d. for 7 days, tapering medication over the following 3 weeks. In rare cases of an inflammatory reaction of the AC, mydriatic ophthalmic drops may be added and the topical steroid intensified at the surgeon's discretion.

Ideally, in addition to IOP measurement and anterior segment slit-lamp biomicroscopy, patients are monitored postoperatively with gonioscopy, and the number and location of patent trabeculostomy sites are documented. For cases that have been followed in this manner, channels have been documented to remain patent many years after the ELT procedure, and in some of these patients, goniolens "pumping" can induce blood to appear at the channels, further confirming the patency of these channels into the SC (**Fig. 31.18**).

Safety, Efficacy, and Clinical Trials

To date, the study with the largest sample size was published in 2006 by Pache et al.[30] Included were 135 eyes with OAG or ocular hypertension after ELT alone or ELT combined with phacoemulsification. Follow-up took place after 1 year. Two subgroups

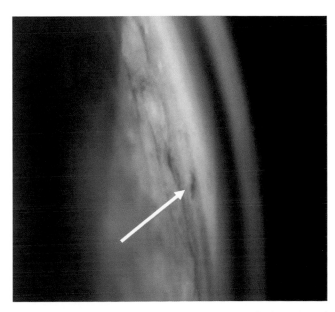

Fig. 31.18 Blood reflux visible at the patent opening of a laser channel *(white arrow)* from the SC induced by "pumping" the goniolens, 3 years after ELT. (Courtesy of U. Giers, Germany.)

(subgroup 1 with IOP > 22 mm Hg at baseline and subgroup 2 with IOP ≤ 21 mm Hg at baseline) were separately analyzed. Success was defined as a set of conditions including IOP ≤ 21 mm Hg, 20% reduction from baseline, anti-glaucoma medications (AGMs) ≤ baseline, and no subsequent IOP-lowering surgery. The baseline IOP for ELT alone subgroup 1 was 27.9 ± 3.9 mm Hg, and at 1-year follow-up it was 19.3 ± 5.5 mm Hg. For subgroup 2 the baseline IOP was 20.2 ± 1.1 mm Hg and at 1-year follow-up it was 17.6 ± 3.3 mm Hg. The Kaplan-Meier survival curve showed a success rate for ELT alone of 57% in subgroup 1 and 41% in subgroup 2. The baseline IOP for ELT combined with phacoemulsification was 26.4 ± 2.8 mm Hg and at 1-year follow-up it was 16.7 ± 2.8 mm Hg. For subgroup 2, the baseline IOP was 19.6 ± 1.1 mm Hg and at 1-year follow-up it was 16.3 ± 2.2 mm Hg. The Kaplan-Meier survival curve showed a success rate for ELT combined with phacoemulsification of 91% in subgroup 1 and 52% in subgroup 2. Hence, IOP reduction by ELT appears to be effective in both groups, but much more effective in eyes with higher baseline IOP.

Wilmsmeyer et al[31] investigated the outcome of ELT alone (70 eyes) versus ELT combined with phacoemulsification (60 eyes) after a follow-up of 2 years in patients with OAG or ocular hypertension. At 2 years, they found a higher reduction of IOP after the combined procedure; IOP was reduced from 24.1 ± 0.7 mm Hg to 16.8 ± 1.0 mm Hg for ELT alone versus 22.4 ± 0.6 mm Hg to 12.6 ± 1.5 for combined ELT. AGM use did not significantly change.

Babighian et al[32] found comparable results in an ELT study with 2 years follow-up of 21 eyes with OAG. Success (20% IOP decrease with no additional medication or surgery) rates were 54% and IOP was reduced from 24.8 ± 2.0 mm Hg at baseline by 7.9 ± 0.1 mm Hg at 2 years.

Töteberg-Harms et al[33] were the first to show simultaneous IOP reduction and reduction of AGM after combined ELT. At 1 year, IOP changed from 25.33 ± 2.85 mm Hg (baseline) to 16.54 ± 4.95 mm Hg while medications were reduced from 2.25 ± 1.26 (baseline) to 1.46 ± 1.38. Complete success was defined as IOP < 21 mm Hg, IOP reduction ≥ 20%, no AGM, and no subsequent IOP-lowering surgery in their study population. Complete success was 21.4% and qualified success (same as complete success but additional AGM were not excluded) was 64.3% at 1 year. The same group showed that IOP reduction depends on preoperative IOP with greater reduction in eyes with higher preoperative IOP.[34]

Berlin's group[35] investigated 37 eyes after combined ELT with a follow-up of 5 years. The authors reported that the IOP was lowered from 25.5 ± 6.3 mm Hg at baseline to 15.9 ± 3.0 mm Hg at 5 years, and AGMs were reduced from 1.93 ± 0.87 at baseline to 0.93 ± 1.12 at 5 year. The authors also investigated 46 eyes after ELT alone with a follow-up of 5 years.[36] Baseline IOP of 25.5 ± 6.3 mm Hg was reduced to 15.9 ± 3 mm Hg at 5 years. Preoperative AGM use was reduced by 72.5% at 12 months and by 51.8% at 5 years. The IOP and AGM lowering effect remained stable over the entire 5-year follow-up for the ELT combined patients and the ELT-alone patients (**Fig. 31.19**).

The ELT procedure has shown favorable outcomes in comparison to other outflow procedures (**Fig. 31.4**). When compared with office laser treatments, patients undergoing SLT achieved up to a 27% postoperative decrease in the IOP but a negligible decrease in medications. Patients undergoing ALT had similar results, with a maximum 23.5% postoperative decrease in the IOP and negligible decreases in medications.

Patients undergoing clear cornea phacoemulsification followed by ab interno gonioscopically guided implantation of one iStent (Glaukos Corp., Laguna Hills, CA) achieved a mean IOP

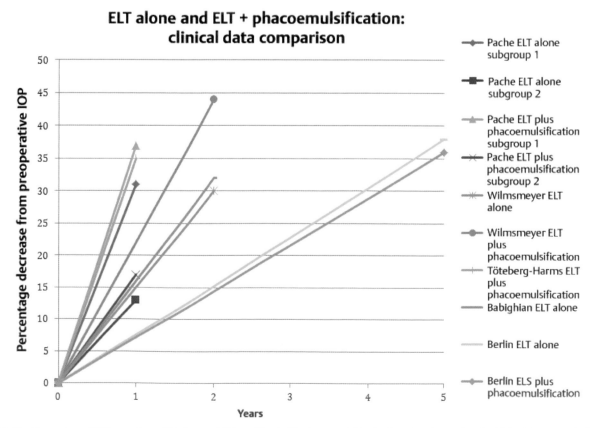

Fig. 31.19 Comparison of ELT procedures. ELT alone and ELT combined with phacoemulsification based on the results of published clinical study data.

decrease of 16% and a medication decrease of 0.5 at 5 years postoperative. Patients undergoing phacoemulsification cataract extraction combined with the Trabectome (NeoMedix, Tustin, CA) achieved IOP decreases of up to 31.1% and medication decreases of 41.7%.[36]

Conclusion

The ELT procedure as an invasive surgical procedure has shown favorable outcomes when compared with other MIGS procedures. Of most relevance is the finding that ELT has shown long-term IOP-lowering results (decrease of 38.6% after 5 years) comparable to those of significantly more invasive and risk-inherent surgeries (i.e., trabeculectomy and tube shunt procedures). In the Collaborative Initial Glaucoma Treatment Study (CIGTS) on trabeculectomy, patients demonstrated IOP decreases of 57.1% and medication decreases of up to 90%. However, the 5-year postoperative IOP measurements for ELT at all time points averaged only 1 mm Hg higher than those in the 300 patients who underwent trabeculectomy documented in CIGTS. In addition, the intraoperative complication rate of trabeculectomy was 12% and the 1-month postoperative complication rate was 50% versus ELT intraoperative and postoperative complication rates of 0%.[37,38]

The ELT procedure is a safe and effective method to reduce both IOP and medication use with minimal complications in most patients with OAG. It is less invasive than the methodologies currently being practiced and thus reduces many postoperative issues, including patient discomfort, the number of postoperative visits required to ensure adequacy and stability, and the long-term risks generally associated with filtering procedures. Due to the minimal tissue trauma associated with UV tissue photoablation and the subsequent minimal healing response, using only a few small channels into the SC has proven adequate to control the IOP and may facilitate the likelihood of long-term efficacy. Unlike trabeculectomy, ELT preserves the integrity of the TM and SC. Natural outflow may be restored without the creation of blebs or invasive foreign body implants. ELT is an important adjunct to cataract surgery, enabling physicians to address two pathologies in one surgical intervention without a conjunctival incision. ELT has been approved for use in the European Union and Switzerland since 1998. Thousands of ELT procedures have been successful in lowering and maintaining a lower IOP for years. Currently, clinical studies are pending in both Canada and the United States.

References

1. Maguen E, Martinez M, Grundfest W, Papaioannou T, Berlin M. Excimer laser ablation of the human lens at 308 nm with a fiber delivery system. In: XXVI World Congress of the International College of Surgeons, Milan, July 3–9, 1988
2. Krasnov MM. Laseropuncture of anterior chamber angle in glaucoma. Am J Ophthalmol 1973;75:674–678
3. Hager H. Besondere mikrochirurgische Eingriffe. 2. Erst Erfahrungen mid dem Argon-Laser-Gerät 800. Klin Monatsbl Augenheilkd 1973;162:437–450
4. van der Zypen E, Fankhauser F, Bebie H, Marshall J. Changes in the ultrastructure of the iris after irradiation with intense light. A study of long-term effects after irradiation with argon ion, Nd:YAG and Q-switched ruby lasers. Adv Ophthalmol 1979;39:59–180
5. Beckman H, Kinoshita A, Rota AN, Sugar HS. Transscleral ruby laser irradiation of the ciliary body in the treatment of intractable glaucoma. Trans Am Acad Ophthalmol Otolaryngol 1972;76:423–436
6. Beckman H, Sugar HS. Neodymium laser cyclocoagulation. Arch Ophthalmol 1973;90:27–28
7. Wise JB. Long-term control of adult open angle glaucoma by argon laser treatment. Ophthalmology 1981;88:197–202
8. Glaucoma Laser Trial Research Group. The Glaucoma Laser Trial (GLT) and glaucoma laser trial follow-up study: 7. Results. Am J Ophthalmol 1995; 120:718–731
9. Odberg T, Sandvik L. The medium and long-term efficacy of primary argon laser trabeculoplasty in avoiding topical medication in open angle glaucoma. Acta Ophthalmol Scand 1999;77:176–181
10. Heijl A, et al. Reduction of IOP and glaucoma progression: results from the early manifest glaucoma trial. Arch Ophthalmol 2002;120:1268
11. Shingleton BJ, Richter CU, Dharma SK, et al. Long-term efficacy of argon laser trabeculoplasty. A 10-year follow-up study. Ophthalmology 1993; 100:1324–1329
12. Jacobi PC, Dietlein TS, Krieglstein GK. Prospective study of ab externo erbium:YAG laser sclerostomy in humans. Am J Ophthalmol 1997;123:478–486
13. Iwach AG, Hoskins HD Jr, Mora JS, et al. Update on the subconjunctival THC:YAG (holmium) laser sclerostomy Ab externo clinical trial: a 4-year report. Ophthalmic Surg Lasers 1996;27:823–831
14. Latina MA, Park C. Selective targeting of trabecular meshwork cells: in vitro studies of pulsed and CW laser interactions. Exp Eye Res 1995;60:359–371
15. Tripathi RC. Ultrastructure of Schlemm's canal in relation to aqueous outflow. Exp Eye Res 1968;7:335–341
16. Holmberg A. Schlemm's canal and the trabecular meshwork. An electron microscopic study of the normal structure in man and monkey (*Cercopithecus aethiops*). Doc Ophthalmol 1965;19:339–373
17. Berlin MS. Excimer laser applications in glaucoma surgery. Ophthalmol Clin North Am 1988;1:255
18. Berlin MS, Rajacich G, Duffy M, Grundfest W, Goldenberg T. Excimer laser photoablation in glaucoma filtering surgery. Am J Ophthalmol 1987; 103:713 714
19. Huang S, Yu M, Feng G, Zhang P, Qiu C. Histopathological study of trabeculum after excimer laser trabeculectomy ab interno. Yan Ke Xue Bao 2001;17:11–15
20. Vogel M, Lauritzen K. [Selective excimer laser ablation of the trabecular meshwork. Clinical results]. Ophthalmologe 1997;94:665–667
21. Jahn R, Lierse W, Neu W, Jungbluth KH. Macroscopic and microscopic findings after excimer laser treatment of different tissue. J Clin Laser Med Surg 1992;10:413–418
22. Peterson WS, Jocson VL. Hyaluronidase effects on aqueous outflow resistance. Quantitative and localizing studies in the rhesus monkey eye. Am J Ophthalmol 1974;77:573–577
23. Neuhann T, Scharrer A, Haefliger E. Excimer laser trabecular ablation ab interno (ELT) in the treatment of chronic open-angle glaucoma, a pilot study. Ophthalmochirugie. 2001;13:3
24. Laurtizen K, Vogel M. Trabecular meshwork ablation with excimer laser – a new concept of therapy for glaucoma patients. Invest Ophthalmol Vis Sci 1997;38:826
25. Walker R, Specht H. [Theoretical and physical aspects of excimer laser trabeculotomy (ELT) ab interno with the AIDA laser with a wave length of 308 mm]. Biomed Tech (Berl) 2002;47:106–110
26. Kaufmann R, Hibst R. Pulsed Er:YAG- and 308 nm UV-excimer laser: an in vitro and in vivo study of skin-ablative effects. Lasers Surg Med 1989;9:132–140
27. Friedman DS, Jampel HD, Lubomski LH, et al. Surgical strategies for coexisting glaucoma and cataract: an evidence-based update. Ophthalmology 2002;109:1902–1913
28. Gimbel HV, Meyer D, DeBroff BM, Roux CW, Ferensowicz M. Intraocular pressure response to combined phacoemulsification and trabeculotomy ab externo versus phacoemulsification alone in primary open-angle glaucoma. J Cataract Refract Surg 1995;21:653–660
29. Shingleton BJ, Gamell LS, O'Donoghue MW, Baylus SL, King R. Long-term changes in intraocular pressure after clear corneal phacoemulsification: normal patients versus glaucoma suspect and glaucoma patients. J Cataract Refract Surg 1999;25:885–890
30. Pache M, Wilmsmeyer S, Funk J. [Laser surgery for glaucoma: excimer-laser trabeculotomy]. Klin Monatsbl Augenheilkd 2006;223:303–307
31. Wilmsmeyer S, Philippin H, Funk J. Excimer laser trabeculotomy: a new, minimally invasive procedure for patients with glaucoma. Graefes Arch Clin Exp Ophthalmol 2006;244:670–676
32. Babighian S, Rapizzi E, Galan A. Efficacy and safety of ab interno excimer laser trabeculotomy in primary open-angle glaucoma: two years of follow-up. Ophthalmologica 2006;220:285–290

33. Töteberg-Harms M, Ciechanowski PP, Hirn C, Funk J. [One-year results after combined cataract surgery and excimer laser trabeculotomy for elevated intraocular pressure]. Ophthalmologe 2011;108:733–738

34. Töteberg-Harms M, Hanson JV, Funk J. Cataract surgery combined with excimer laser trabeculotomy to lower intraocular pressure: effectiveness dependent on preoperative IOP. BMC Ophthalmol 2013;13:24

35. Stodtmeister R, Kleineberg L, Berlin M, Pillunat L, Giers U. Excimer laser trabeculostomy: five year post-op observations. Invest Ophthalmol Vis Sci 2013;54:2141–2141

36. Berlin MS, Kleinberg L, Stodtmeister R, Spitz J, Giers U. The IOP lowering efficacy of excimer-laser-trabeculostomy in open angle glaucoma patients remains consistent over 5 years. Poster session presented at the 23rd annual meeting of the American Glaucoma Society, San Francisco, March 1–3, 2013

37. Stodtmeister R, Kleinberg L, Berlin M, Pillunat L, Giers U. Excimer laser trabeculostomy: 5-year follow-up. Abstract submitted for the 111th congress of the German Association of Ophthalmologists, Berlin, September 19–22, 2013

38. Jampel HD, Musch DC, Gillespie BW, Lichter PR, Wright MM, Guire KE; Collaborative Initial Glaucoma Treatment Study Group. Perioperative complications of trabeculectomy in the collaborative initial glaucoma treatment study (CIGTS). Am J Ophthalmol 2005;140:16–22

IIB Uveoscleral Outflow Procedures

32 Canaloplasty

Mahmoud A. Khaimi and Andrew K. Bailey

Traditional glaucoma surgical procedures such as trabeculectomy, although very effective in lowering the intraocular pressure (IOP), may be associated with numerous complications, including bleb leaks, cataracts, blebitis, endophthalmitis, and vision loss. Consequently, many glaucoma specialists seek a safer and less invasive procedure that delivers the same IOP-lowering benefits as trabeculectomy. Canaloplasty is a bleb-free procedure that works by restoring the natural ocular outflow system. Published evidence indicates that canaloplasty may be used across the glaucoma treatment spectrum, as it is both safe and effective, it reduces the need for medical therapy, and it entails minimal postoperative care. Perhaps unsurprisingly, canaloplasty is gradually becoming the go-to treatment for glaucoma specialists seeking a minimally invasive, maximally effective solution for open-angle glaucoma.

Case Presentation

A 61-year-old African-American woman presented to the glaucoma service after referral from a local optometrist who had been treating her for many years. She had a long-standing diagnosis of primary open-angle glaucoma (POAG) and high myopia, and was recently diagnosed with visually significant cataracts by the referring optometrist.

Upon presentation, her best corrected visual acuity was 20/30 in the right eye and 20/50 in the left eye. Her current glasses were –14.25 +1.50 × 171 OD and –11.25 +1.50 × 040 OS. Subjective manifest refraction at our first visit was –14.00 +1.00 × 165 OD and –11.50 +1.50 × 044 OS. This yielded a visual acuity of 20/40 –2 OD and 20/60 OS.

Goldman applanation tonometry was 24 mm Hg in both eyes. She was compliant with instilling latanoprost in both eyes at bedtime and dorzolamide/timolol in both eyes b.i.d. Central corneal thickness was 478 µm OD and 492 µm OS. Gonioscopy exhibited an open angle to 40 degrees, and a flat iris approach with 1+ pigmentation to the trabecular meshwork. There were a few iris processes intermittently throughout each angle; 2+ nuclear sclerosis with cortical changes and central vacuoles were also observed. The remaining anterior segment was unremarkable. Posterior examination demonstrated tilted optic nerves with temporal sloping. Cup-to-disk ratios were 0.8 in both eyes. Peripapillary atrophy was noted bilaterally. The maculae were flat without evidence of degeneration. No posterior staphyloma was identified. The remaining posterior segment examination was unremarkable.

Ancillary testing included a Humphrey visual field, optical coherence tomography, and intraocular lens (IOL) calculations. The Humphrey visual field was reliable and demonstrated an early superior arcuate defect in the right eye and an early inferior arcuate defect in the left eye with superior nasal step changes. Optical coherence tomography demonstrated retinal nerve fiber layer thinning in both eyes. The superior and inferior nerve fiber layers were significantly thinned compared with age-matched controls.

The patient underwent uncomplicated cataract extraction with IOL implantation followed by successful canaloplasty surgery in the right eye. Approximately 6 weeks later, the same procedure was completed successfully in the left eye. No complications were encountered. Postoperatively, the patient has done very well. She is no longer using ocular medication to control her IOP and her vision is 20/20 in both eyes with a minimal need for corrective lenses. Her IOP has remained in the mid-teen range, and she has been off medications since the time of surgery.

The Procedure

Until relatively recently, treatment for POAG was restricted to medical therapy or traditional glaucoma surgeries such as aqueous shunts and trabeculectomy. Many physicians still regard trabeculectomy as the gold standard in glaucoma treatment because of its ability to effectively lower IOP and arrest disease progression, but it is also associated with numerous immediate and delayed postoperative complications.[1-6] Additionally, although we know that suboptimal ocular outflow is a key factor in the development of glaucoma, trabeculectomy works by circumventing, rather than restoring, natural ocular outflow. In contrast, canaloplasty, a modification of viscocanalostomy, restores the physiological outflow pathways, thus lowering IOP both safely and effectively.[7,8] Although canaloplasty is usually indicated for patients with POAG who have not undergone previous filtration surgery, growing evidence suggests it may also be considered in patients for whom other types of surgery have failed.[9] As the above case presentation demonstrates and as clinical data from literature indicate, canaloplasty may also be safely combined with cataract surgery.[10-12]

Rationale Behind the Procedure

Canaloplasty is a surgical procedure performed under local anesthesia. It entails circumferential viscodilation and tensioning of Schlemm's canal to restore natural aqueous outflow. Canaloplasty is performed with the iTrack™ 250 Canaloplasty Microcatheter System (Ellex Medical Lasers, Adelaide, Australia), a patented microcatheter with an inner lumen that is used to inject high viscosity sodium hyaluronate for safe and effective 360-degree dilation of Schlemm's canal, the trabecular meshwork, and the outflow collector channels, enabling aqueous humor to exit as normal. Canaloplasty often includes a tensioning device such as a suture /stent to assist in longer term canal patency. By addressing all aspects of the "traditional" or trabeculocanalicular outflow pathway including distal outflow system, canaloplasty helps to significantly lower the IOP.

139

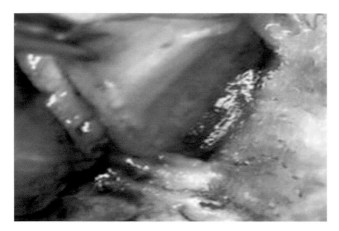

Fig. 32.1 Nonpenetrating, external dissection with exposure of Schlemm's canal.

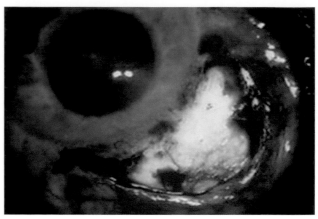

Fig. 32.2 Fornix-based conjunctival peritomy down to bare sclera following application of light cautery.

Surgical Technique

Canaloplasty is accomplished by exposing Schlemm's canal via nonpenetrating dissection and using the iTrack 250 microcatheter (**Fig. 32.1**) to circumferentially viscodilate and intubate Schlemm's canal with a tensioning suture. The microcatheter system is engineered specifically for safe and effective 360-degree viscodilation of Schlemm's canal. It has a 250-μm atraumatic bulbous tip that helps to bypass collector channel ostia as well as to minimize tissue trauma; the diameter of the working length is 200 μm. The iTrack also contains a fiber optic that enables illumination of the tip so that its passage through the canal can be monitored continuously, and it includes a support wire to enhance "push-ability" during catheterization. Additionally, the working length of the iTrack has the same lubricious coating as cardiac catheters, which facilitates circumferential passage throughout Schlemm's canal.

Typically, anesthesia and akinesia are achieved with a retrobulbar block. A corneal traction suture is placed superiorly next to the limbus. Next, a fornix-based conjunctival incision is created followed by careful dissection of the conjunctiva and Tenon's capsule down to bare sclera (**Fig. 32.2**). We prefer a superonasal approach during this step, as it leaves the superior and superotemporal conjunctiva undisturbed in case future incisional sur-

geries are necessary. Hemostasis is achieved with wet-field cautery. Antifibrotics, such as mitomycin C, are unnecessary.

Once the bare sclera is exposed, a superficial one-third to one-half thickness scleral flap is created at the limbus. A 3.5 mm × 3.5 mm parabolic shape may be used; however, individual surgeon preference dictates the shape of the scleral flap. Within the base of the superficial scleral flap a 3 mm × 3 mm deep scleral flap is created with a dissection plane just superficial to the choroid. The choroid may be slightly visible beneath the deep scleral flap. The deep scleral flap is dissected anteriorly to unroof Schlemm's canal (**Fig. 32.3**). While dissecting forward, the surgeon pays close attention to identifying the cross-striations of the scleral spur. This verifies that the surgeon has reached the correct depth and plane while fashioning the deep flap. Identifying the cross-striations of the scleral spur also anatomically orients the surgeon to the location of Schlemm's canal, which is immediately anterior.

At this point, a paracentesis is performed to lower the IOP to the middle to high single digits. This serves to decompress the eye and decrease the risk of perforating into the anterior chamber while isolating Schlemm's canal and creating Descemet's window. Once the canal is identified, the deep flap is carefully dissected further anteriorly to detach Schwalbe's line and to create an appropriately sized Descemet's window, which should

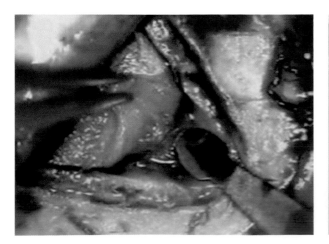

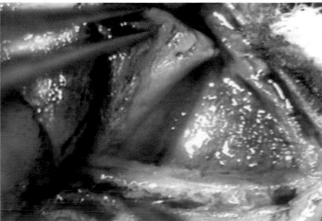

a   b

Fig. 32.3 Fashioning of the deep scleral flap. Note the depth of the dissection plane located just superficial to the underlying choroidal tissues (**a**). As the dissection is carried toward the limbus, the canal becomes visualized (**b**) just after cross-striations of the scleral spur are exposed.

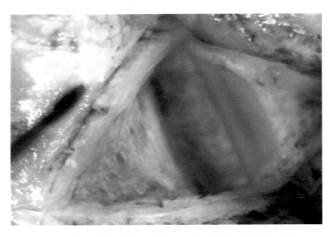

Fig. 32.4 Traditionally, a 500-μm Descemet's window is fashioned.

at minimum be 500 μm **(Fig. 32.4)**. Aqueous humor usually, but not always, percolates through the Descemet's window. The iTrack microcatheter is then inserted through one of the canal ostia. The lights on the microscope are dimmed to enable visualization of the lighted tip of the microcatheter as it is advanced through Schlemm's canal **(Fig. 32.5)**. If an obstruction is encountered during cannulation, the microcatheter may be retracted, inserted into the opposite ostia, and cannulated in the other direction to achieve successful passage. Once circumferential cannulation is completed, a 10-0 or 9-0 polypropylene (Prolene, Ethicon, Switzerland) suture is tied to the distal end of the catheter, which is retracted, introducing the suture into Schlemm's canal. As the suture is pulled through, ophthalmic viscosurgical device (OVD) is injected at a rate of 0.5 μL for each arc segment of two clock positions, that is, a 1/8th turn of the OVD injector for every two clock positions. The suture is tied, placing appropriate tension on the canal without inadvertently performing a trabeculotomy. Suture tensioning is important, as it enables tension to be transmitted 360 degrees on Schlemm's canal and keeping its long-term patency.

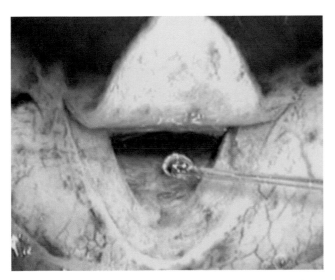

Fig. 32.5 A primed iTrack catheter about to enter Schlemm's canal and navigate 360-degrees in a clockwise fashion. The lighted beacon, located at the tip of the catheter, provides the surgeon with feedback by facilitating visualization of the catheter tip during advancement.

Creation of a scleral lake is accomplished by excising the deep scleral flap followed by watertight closure of the superficial scleral flap with interrupted 8-0 Vicryl sutures. The conjunctiva and Tenon's capsule is reapproximated with 8-0 Vicryl at the limbus, and finally subconjunctival antibiotics are given along with topical antibiotic-steroid ointment.[13]

Patient Selection

As with any surgical procedure, correct patient selection is a key factor in achieving optimal outcomes. Canaloplasty is primarily indicated for patients with mild-to-moderate open-angle glaucoma with an IOP target of the low to middle teens. It is also an ideal treatment option for patients with very thin conjunctiva and patients with uncontrolled ocular hypertension (OHT) on maximum tolerated medical therapy. However, the procedure may be unsuitable for patients with chronic angle closure, narrow angles, angle recession, or neovascular glaucoma.[14]

It is currently believed that canaloplasty is also unsuitable for, or at least is likely to have only limited success in, patients who have undergone previous filtering surgery. However, findings from a six-eye study by Paolo Brusini and Claudia Tosoni[9] suggest that canaloplasty can be considered as a possible surgical option in eyes with failed trabeculectomy. In this study, the mean preoperative IOP was 32.2 ± 9.6 mm Hg (range, 25 to 48 mm Hg). Postoperatively, the mean IOP at 6, 12, 18, and 24 months was 17.3, 15.4, 14.7, and 16.3 mm Hg, respectively. Additionally, the number of medications used preoperatively and at the 2-year follow-up was 3.2 ± 1.2 and 2.3 ± 0.5, respectively.[9] These findings suggest that, it may be possible to offer canaloplasty to patients across the entire treatment spectrum, from the newly diagnosed and previously untreated patient to the desperate patient for whom all other treatments have failed to deliver satisfactory outcomes.

Phaco-Canaloplasty

As noted earlier, canaloplasty may also be combined with cataract surgery, and is often referred to as "phaco-canaloplasty." Cataract surgery alone has been shown to lower IOP by up to 5 mm Hg.[15–17] Unsurprisingly, phaco-canaloplasty shows a lower IOP trend than canaloplasty alone.[18] Indeed, a 2-year study by Tetz and colleagues[10] compared 82 phakic eyes that received canaloplasty alone with 51 eyes that underwent cataract surgery before or during canaloplasty. The study found that the phakic eyes that were treated with a phaco-canaloplasty had a baseline IOP of 23.5 ± 5.2 mm Hg (mean ± standard deviation) and a mean number of glaucoma medications used of 1.5 ± 1.0 decreasing to a mean IOP of 13.6 ± 3.6 mm Hg on 0.3 ± 0.5 medications at 3 years postoperatively. Pseudophakic eyes undergoing canaloplasty alone had a mean baseline IOP of 23.9 ± 5.2 mm Hg on a mean number of glaucoma medications of 1.8 ± 0.8 decreasing to 15.6 ± 3.5 mm Hg on 1.1 ± 0.8 medications at 3 years. These differences between the two groups were significant.

During phaco-canaloplasty, clear corneal cataract extraction via phacoemulsification is performed using traditional methods. A side-port paracentesis is performed followed by introduction of OVD into the anterior chamber. Planning paracentesis placement is important when glaucoma surgery is expected to follow. The surgeon must position the side-port incision so that it will not intersect the anticipated corneal traction suture needed during canaloplasty. For example, if working on the right eye, a right-handed surgeon may place the side-port incision at about the 10 o'clock position and skew the clear corneal incision (CCI) inferotemporally. A continuous curvilinear capsulorrhexis follows, with subsequent hydrodissection and hydrodelineation.

Removing the nucleus may be achieved via divide-and-conquer, phaco-chop techniques or whatever the anterior chamber surgeon favors, keeping in mind certain risk factors present in glaucoma patients such as zonular weakness in pseudoexfoliates. Epinuclear material may be removed with the phacoemulsification handpiece, and the irrigation and aspiration handpiece is then used to remove remaining cortical material. After placing the IOL within the capsule and removing any remaining OVD, a suture may be placed through the CCI wound to promote anterior chamber stability during the canaloplasty portion of the combined procedure. Ensure that all remaining OVD is removed prior to suturing the wound as remaining OVD may cause unsafe IOP elevation postoperatively. The surgeon may then proceed with the canaloplasty.

Efficacy and Safety

The safety and efficacy of canaloplasty has been evaluated in more than 50 peer-reviewed clinical studies. Perhaps most notable are the results of a 3-year, nonrandomized multicenter, international study of 157 eyes with open-angle glaucoma that underwent canaloplasty or combined cataract-canaloplasty surgery. The study was reported in the *Journal of Cataract and Refractive Surgery* in 2011 by Lewis et al,[11] who found that canaloplasty produced a significant, sustained reduction in IOP with an excellent short- and long-term safety profile. At 3 years postoperative, all study eyes had a mean IOP of 15.2 ± 3.5 mm Hg and a mean number of medications used of 0.8 ± 0.9, compared with a baseline IOP of 23.8 ± 5.0 mm Hg on 1.8 ± 0.9 medications. When combined with phacoemulsification, canaloplasty reduced pressure and medication use from preoperative 23.5 ± 5.2 mm Hg

and 1.5 ± 1.0 medications used to 13.6 ± 3.6 mm Hg and 0.3 ± 0.5, respectively. Medication use and IOP in all eyes were significantly decreased from baseline at every follow-up time point (*p* < 0.001). Late postoperative complications included cataract (12.7%), transient IOP elevation (6.4%), and partial suture extrusion through the trabecular meshwork (0.6%).[11]

The safety and IOP-lowering effects of canaloplasty alone are also well reported. A comparative series study that included 15 eyes reported a mean IOP of 14.5 ± 2.6 mm Hg on 0.3 ± 0.5 medications at 18 months postoperatively as compared with preoperative levels of 26.5 ± 2.7 mm Hg on 2.1 ± 1.0 medications.[19] There were no significant complications.

A 3-year prospective, multicenter, interventional study of 109 eyes in open-angle glaucoma patients undergoing canaloplasty or phacocanaloplasty found that pressure and medication use results for all study eyes were significantly decreased from baseline in both groups.[7] Additional studies highlighting canaloplasty's ability to consistently lower IOP to the low to middle teens, both alone and in combination with phacoemulsification, are summarized in **Tables 32.1** and **32.2**.

Importantly, canaloplasty has been found to be as effective as trabeculectomy. In a consecutive case series study of 30 eyes, Brüggemann et al[20] demonstrated that canaloplasty reduced the mean IOP from 26.73 ± 6.4 mm Hg preoperatively to 13.21 ± 2.83 mm Hg at 12 months postoperative. Additionally, the number of glaucoma medications decreased from 2.5 preoperatively to 0 at 12 months. The authors reported that although canaloplasty and trabeculectomy were both effective in lowering IOP, canaloplasty patients required fewer follow-up visits and significantly fewer complications and interventions. Klink et al[21] also reported that compared with trabeculectomy, canaloplasty was associated with

Table 32.1 Reductions in Intraocular Pressure (IOP) and Use of Medical Therapy Following Canaloplasty

Author	Year	Number of Eyes	Follow-Up (Months)	IOP Reduction (mm Hg)	IOP Reduction (%)	Postoperative IOP (mm Hg)	Reduction in No. of Medications (%)
Lewis et al	2007	74	12	8.6 ± 0.5	35.8	16.2 ± 3.5	1.3 (68)
Lewis et al	2009	84	24	6.9 ± 0.1	29.3	16.3 ± 3.7	1.4 (70)
Lewis et al	2011	103	36	8.6 ± 1.5	34	15.5 ± 3.5	1.0 ± 0.1
Peckar and Koerber	2008	97	18	13.1 ± 5.2	48	14.1 ± 3.2	2.4 (76)
Grieshaber et al	2010	90	15	28.6 ± 7.2	36.4	16.2 ± 4.9	—
Grieshaber et al	2010	60	36	31.7 ± 6.7	65.8	13.3 ± 1.7	—
Grieshaber et al	2011	32	18	14.2 ± 2.1	47.2	13.1 ± 1.2	2.6
Koerber	2012	15	18	12.0 ± 0.1	45.3	14.5 ± 2.6	1.7 (85)
Matthaei et al	2011	46	12	5.6 ± 3.2	30.7	12.6 ± 2.4	1.3 (43)
Bull et al	2011	82	36	7.9 ± 1.3	34.3	15.1 ± 3.1	0.9 (53)
Fujita et al	2011	11	12	8.4 ± 1.8	35.9	15.0 ± 4.1	1.6 (25)
Ayyala et al	2011	33	12	7.4 ± 1.5	32	13.8.±4.9	2
Klink et al	2012	20	9	10.6 ± 4.2	32.5	13.3.±9.9	2.6 (82)
Brüggemann et al	2013	30	12	14.6 ± 4.5	50.3	13.2.±2.8	2.5 (100)

Source: Adapted from Brandão LM, Grieshaber MC. Update on minimally invasive glaucoma surgery (MIGS) and new implants. J Ophthalmol 2013;2013:705915.

Table 32.2   Reductions in IOP and Use of Medical Therapy Following Phacocanaloplasty

Author	Year	Number of Eyes	Follow-Up (Months)	IOP Reduction (mm Hg)	IOP Reduction (%)	Postoperative IOP (mm Hg)	Reduction in No. of Medications (%)
Lewis et al	2007	13	12	10.7 ± 1.8	45.5	12.8 ± 3.6	NA
Lewis et al	2011	54	36	9.8 ± 2.6	42.1	13.6 ± 3.6	1.0 ± 0.1
Bull et al	2011	16	36	10.5 ± 2.8	43.2	13.8 ± 3.2	1.0 (66)
Shingleton et al	2008	54	12	10.7 ± 1.7	43.8	13.7 ± 4.4	1.3 (86)

Source: Adapted from Brandão LM, Grieshaber MC. Update on minimally invasive glaucoma surgery (MIGS) and new implants. J Ophthalmol 2013;2013:705915.

less impairment of the quality of life and higher patient satisfaction after surgery.

Complications

Although published studies indicate that canaloplasty has an excellent safety profile, several complications have been reported. As noted previously, in the 3-year study by Lewis et al[11] the late postoperative complications included cataract (12.7%), transient IOP elevation (6.4%) and partial suture extrusion through the trabecular meshwork (0.6%). Earlier interim findings (2 years) by the same author found that common complications included microhyphema (< 1.0 mm layered blood, 7.9%), early-elevated IOP (0–3 months postop, 7.9%), and hyphema (≥ 1.0 mm layered blood, 6.3%). However, all hyphemas and microhyphemas resolved by 1 month postoperative; IOP elevation was also transient and resolved by the next follow-up visit.[22] Notably, the complication rate after canaloplasty has been reported to be much lower than that after trabeculectomy, particularly with regard to severe, sight-threatening complications such as choroidal effusion and hypotonus with maculopathy, neither of which has been reported with canaloplasty.[23]

Postoperative Management

Effective postoperative management is a key factor in optimizing outcomes. Canaloplasty postoperative care is typically straightforward—and much more so than that for trabeculectomy. Patients are usually assessed at 1 day, 1 week, and 3 to 4 weeks postoperatively. Patients are placed on eyedrops containing a low-dose steroid and a third- or fourth- generation fluoroquinolone, to be used three to four times daily. However, it is important to start weaning patients from treatment within 2 weeks so as to minimize the risk of steroid response.[24] It is also important to take the patient's lifestyle into account when devising a postoperative care plan. For example, highly active patients who lift weights or individuals who have strenuous work requirements may need to limit their activities for the first 2 weeks postoperatively.

If IOP remains elevated following an adequate postoperative steroid washout, neodymium:yttrium-aluminum-garnet (Nd:YAG) goniopuncture can be considered. This procedure consists of an initial application of topical aesthesia followed by placement of the gonioprism lens. The trabecular-Descemet's window is identified, and a photodisruptive laser, typically 10 to 50 bursts consisting of 3 to 10 mJ of power given at 1 pulse per burst, is applied. The IOP is measured 30 minutes after laser application. If the IOP has not decreased, ocular hypotensive medications are

initiated. All patients receive a topical nonsteroidal anti-inflammatory drug for 1 week, regardless of IOP responsiveness.[25]

Conclusion

Canaloplasty is a very effective treatment for POAG and a promising alternative to traditional glaucoma surgery. Although trabeculectomy is still the most frequently used glaucoma treatment, peer-reviewed studies suggest that canaloplasty is similarly effective but without the potential sight-threatening complications. Some surgeons may shy away from canaloplasty due to the perceived difficult learning curve. Although there is a learning curve for successful catheterization of Schlemm's canal, canaloplasty is a very forgiving procedure that fills an unmet need for glaucoma patients who wish to control their condition without medication or invasive filtering surgery. Consequently, canaloplasty has earned its place in the glaucoma treatment armamentarium.

References

1. Jones E, Clarke J, Khaw PT. Recent advances in trabeculectomy technique. Curr Opin Ophthalmol 2005;16:107–113
2. Borisuth NSC, Phillips B, Krupin T. The risk profile of glaucoma filtration surgery. Curr Opin Ophthalmol 1999;10:112–116
3. Gedde SJ, Herndon LW, Brandt JD, Budenz DL, Feuer WJ, Schiffman JC. Surgical complications in the Tube Versus Trabeculectomy Study during the first year of follow-up. Am J Ophthalmol 2007;143:23–31
4. Scott IU, Greenfield DS, Schiffman J, et al. Outcomes of primary trabeculectomy with the use of adjunctive mitomycin. Arch Ophthalmol 1998;116:286–291
5. Jampel HD, Musch DC, Gillespie BW, Lichter PR, Wright MM, Guire KE; Collaborative Initial Glaucoma Treatment Study Group. Perioperative complications of trabeculectomy in the collaborative initial glaucoma treatment study (CIGTS). Am J Ophthalmol 2005;140:16–22
6. Edmunds B, Thompson JR, Salmon JF, Wormald RP. The National Survey of Trabeculectomy. III. Early and late complications. Eye (Lond) 2002;16:297–303
7. Bull H, von Wolff K, Körber N, Tetz M. Three-year canaloplasty outcomes for the treatment of open-angle glaucoma: European study results. Graefes Arch Clin Exp Ophthalmol 2011;249:1537–1545
8. Grieshaber MC, Pienaar A, Olivier J, Stegmann R. Canaloplasty for primary open-angle glaucoma: long-term outcome. Br J Ophthalmol 2010;94:1478–1482
9. Brusini P, Tosoni C. Canaloplasty after failed trabeculectomy: a possible option. J Glaucoma 2014;23:33–34
10. Tetz M, Koerber H, Shingleton BJ, et al. Phacoemulsification and intraocular lens implantation before, during, or after canaloplasty in eyes with open-angle glaucoma: 3-year results. J Glaucoma 2013

11. Lewis RA, von Wolff K, Tetz M, et al. Canaloplasty: three-year results of circumferential viscodilation and tensioning of Schlemm canal using a microcatheter to treat open-angle glaucoma. J Cataract Refract Surg 2011;37:682–690

12. Lopes-Cardoso I, Esteves F, Amorim M, Calvão-Santos G, Freitas ML, Salgado-Borges J. [Circumferential viscocanalostomy with suture tensioning in Schlemm canal (canaloplasty)-one year experience]. Arch Soc Esp Oftalmol 2013;88:207–215

13. Khaimi MA. Canaloplasty. In: Kahook M, ed. Essentials of Glaucoma Surgery. Thorofare, NJ: SLACK Inc., 2012

14. Khaimi MA. Canaloplasty using iTrack 250 microcatheter with suture tensioning on Schlemm's canal. Middle East Afr J Ophthalmol 2009; 16:127–129

15. Shingleton BJ, Paternack JJ, Hung JW, O'Donoghue MW. Three and five year changes in intraocular pressure after clear corneal phacoemulsification in open angle glaucoma patients. J Glaucoma 2006;15:494–498

16. Hayashi K, Hayashi H, Nakao F, Hayashi F. Effect of cataract surgery on intraocular pressure control in glaucoma patients. J Cataract Refract Surg 2001;27:1779–1786

17. Mathalone N, Hyams M, Neiman S, Buckman G, Hod Y, Geyer O. Long-term intraocular pressure control after clear corneal phacoemulsification in glaucoma patients. J Cataract Refract Surg 2005;31:479–483

18. Azuara-Blanco A, Katz LJ. Dysfunctional filtering blebs. Surv Ophthalmol 1998;43:93–126

19. Koerber NJ. Canaloplasty in one eye compared with viscocanalostomy in the contralateral eye in patients with bilateral open-angle glaucoma. J Glaucoma 2012;21:129–134

20. Brüggemann A, Despouy JT, Wegent A, Müller M. Intraindividual comparison of canaloplasty versus trabeculectomy with mitomycin C in a single-surgeon series. J Glaucoma 2013;22:577–583

21. Klink T, Sauer J, Körber NJ, et al. Quality of life following glaucoma surgery: canaloplasty versus trabeculectomy. Clin Ophthalmol 2015;9:7–16

22. Lewis RA, von Wolff K, Tetz M, et al. Canaloplasty: circumferential viscodilation and tensioning of Schlemm canal using a flexible microcatheter for the treatment of open-angle glaucoma in adults: two-year interim clinical study results. J Cataract Refract Surg 2009;35:814–824

23. Brusini P. Canaloplasty in open-angle glaucoma surgery: a four-year follow-up. ScientificWorldJournal 2014;2014:469609

24. Harvey BJ, Khaimi MA. A review of canaloplasty. Saudi J Ophthalmol 2011;25:329–336

25. Tam DY, Barnebey HS, Ahmed II. Nd: YAG laser goniopuncture: indications and procedure. J Glaucoma 2013;22:620–625

33 Ab Interno Viscodilation of Schlemm's Canal: VISCO 360 and ABiC

Steven R. Sarkisian, Jr. and Mahmoud A. Khaimi

Case Presentation

A 75-year-old man presents with moderate primary open-angle glaucoma (POAG) and an intraocular pressure (IOP) of 30 in both eyes. He has been instilling latanoprost and fixed combination timolol and dorzolamide in both eyes. The patient has a target IOP in the mid-teens, and a laser trabeculoplasty was done 6 months ago. The patient had cataract extraction 3 years prior to presentation. The patient has a small but significant nasal step visual field defect in both eyes but does not want to worry about having the risks associated with trabeculectomy. He elects to have ab interno viscodilation of Schlemm's canal in both eyes. One year after surgery, his IOP is 12 mm Hg OD and 15 mm Hh OS on no medications.

Rationale Behind the Procedure

Canaloplasty has been performed for over a decade and is well described in Chapter 32. However, with the emergence of minimally invasive glaucoma surgery (MIGS), the utilization of canaloplasty with the placement of a retention suture in the canal has steadily declined, reserved for moderate to severe glaucoma patients. Studies have suggested that the most critical step of canaloplasty is the dilation of Schlemm's canal with viscoelastic delivered by a catheter.[1-4] In the MIGS era, the decline of canaloplasty is likely due to the fact that surgeons are hesitant to perform a surgery that creates an incision in the conjunctiva; however, the IOP lowering of the ab interno stenting procedures reported in other chapters has not been conventionally seen as able to reduce high IOPs (over 30 mm Hg) in patients on multiple (3+) medications to the mid-teens on one medication or none. Moreover, in the United States, insurance reimbursement for the only currently available trabecular stent requires that cataract surgery be performed. Therefore, there has been a need for a MIGS procedure to expand the treatment algorithm.

When one evaluates the original data for canaloplasty, it should be noted that there was a subset of patients for whom an obstruction in the canal caused no suture to be placed; however, viscodilation of the canal was performed. This subgroup of patients was not considered as failures, but the resulting IOP was in the mid-teens.[3] This led to the thinking that, if a viscodilation is required and a suture is not critical, then perhaps the canal can be dilated from an ab interno approach using either the same catheter, or in some other way, with the canal visualized intraoperatively by a surgical gonioprism.

Surgical Procedure

There are two methods of dilating Schlemm's canal in an ab interno fashion that are currently available. The first utilizes the same iTrack microcatheter described in the Chapter 32, and discussed in Chapter 25, and has been dubbed ABiC (for ab interno canaloplasty). The second uses what looks identical to the TRAB360 device described in Chapter 27, but rather than being used for an ab interno trabeculotomy, the device is filled with viscoelastic and when the probe is pulled back into the device, it injects viscoelastic into the canal. This latter technique has been called VISCO 360.

VISCO 360

This procedure is typically performed with the patient under topical anesthesia and the surgeon sitting on the temporal side. After a 1.5- to 2-mm incision is made in the clear cornea, with the surgeon ensuring that the incision is not so far posterior as to bleed and obstruct the gonioscopic view, the anterior chamber is filled with a cohesive viscoelastic. If the procedure is combined with cataract surgery, the main phaco wound can be used to do the procedure and it can be done after the lens is placed but before the viscoelastic is removed from the eye. With both the ABiC and VISCO 360 procedures, it may be advantageous to use a miotic medication after the lens is placed but before the procedure is performed. If the procedure is done without cataract surgery, pilocarpine should be placed preoperatively.

The TRAB360 device (**Fig. 33.1**), which is used for the VISCO 360 procedure, has a red stopper on the back of it. This stopper slides to the side, exposing the opening where a cohesive viscoelastic is injected gently until it is noted to be coming out of the tip of the device. The red stopper is then removed. The surgeon is careful not to remove the red stopper before the viscoelastic is injected, otherwise the device will be rendered inoperable.

Viscoelastic is then placed on the cornea and the gonioprism is placed on the eye after the microscope is tilted 30 degrees away from the surgeon and the patient's head is tilted 30 degrees away as well. The tip of the device is then placed in the eye, taking care not to hit the iris or the cornea. The tip is sharp and is used to puncture the trabecular meshwork. Once a small goniotomy is performed with the tip of the device, the blue wheel on the top of the device is turned toward the surgeon to release the nylon catheter into the canal. The wheel is turned until the catheter cannot be advanced further and the surgeon can no longer

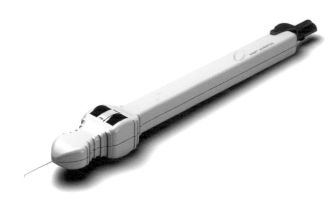

Fig. 33.1 The TRAB360 device, which is used for the VISCO 360 procedure. Note the blue "roller" on the surface and the metallic tip through which the blue nylon probe is guided. (Courtesy of Sight Sciences, Inc.)

turn the wheel. The wheel is then turned in the opposite direction, away from the surgeon, and the catheter is brought back through the metal guide, back into the device. While it is retracted, the catheter releases the viscoelastic into the canal. The device is then removed from the eye and the other 180 degrees of dilation is then performed in the same manner. Viscoelastic may be required between sides to improve the view, as transient hyphema is frequent at the site of entry. Saline is then used to flush the viscoelastic from the eye. If combined with cataract surgery, the usual irrigation/aspiration technique can be used to remove the viscoelastic.

The wound is sealed with hydration in the usual fashion, and a drop of antibiotic is placed on the eye.

ABiC

This procedure is almost identical to the gonioscopy-assisted transluminal trabeculotomy procedure (Chapter 25), except instead of using the iTrack microcatheter to do a trabeculotomy, the catheter is simply pulled out while injecting viscoelastic through the device and into the canal **(Fig. 33.2)**. The patient setup is the same as described above for VISCO 360. After a 1.5- to 2-mm incision is placed in the temporal clear cornea, a 1- to 2-mm incision is placed close to the nasal cornea angled so that the catheter can be passed smoothly into the nasal aspect of the canal. A 27-gauge needle is used to make a goniotomy incision in the nasal angle. The catheter is placed through the nasal wound and directed toward the goniotomy incision. A microforceps is then placed through the temporal wound and the surgical gonioprism is placed on the cornea to provide visualization of the surgery. The microforceps is then used to guide the catheter into the canal and pass the catheter around for 360 degrees. Once it is passed, the catheter is retracted and the viscoelastic is injected, turning the dial for 15 to 20 clicks for all 12 clock positions of the canal. The viscoelastic in the anterior chamber is then removed and the wounds are hydrated.

Results

Currently, there are no peer-reviewed publications using these devices in an ab interno manner; however, one can extrapolate the outcomes based on data from ab externo canaloplasty without suture. In fact, one would assume that the data for these ab interno techniques would be even better, due to the fact that the patients treated with an original ab externo canaloplasty without suture did not have the suture placed because of damaged or obstructed canals, not because they were in a specific arm of the study. This subgroup of patients without suture was only later

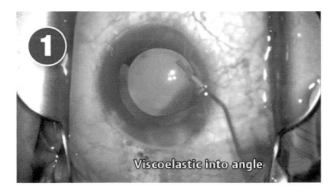

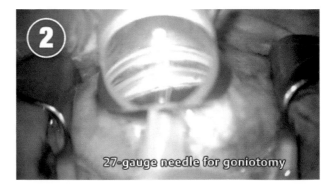

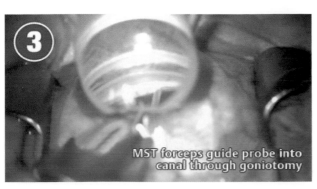

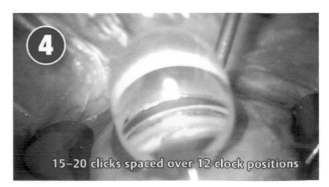

Fig. 33.2 The four treatment steps of the ab interno canaloplasty (ABiC). MST, MicroSurgical Technology (Redmond, WA).

Table 33.1   ABiC Case Series: Stand-Alone Procedure

Exam	Number	Mean Intraocular Pressure (IOP) (mm Hg) ± SD	Mean Medications (*n*) ± SD
Baseline	38	22.0 ± 8.2	2.0 ±1.0
3 Months	27	18.1 ± 4.6	1.0 ± 1.0
6 Months	26	15.7 ± 3.8	1.0 ± 1.0
12 Months	8	13.9 ± 1.6	1.0 ± 1.0

Notes: Reduction in mean IOP: 36.8% (at 12 months).
Reduction in number of medications: 50% (at 12 months).

evaluated to ascertain the effectiveness of canaloplasty with viscodilation alone.[1]

Khaimi[5] has presented his results of ABiC at the 2016 American Society of Cataract and Refractive Surgery (ASCRS) annual meeting **(Table 33.1)**. In patients treated with ABiC as a stand-alone procedure, he reported a 36.8% drop in IOP at 1 year and a 50% reduction in the number of medications, with a mean IOP of 13.9 at 12-month follow-up.

Conclusion

Ab interno viscodilation of Schlemm's canal has been shown to be safe and effective in achieving IOP reduction and reduced dependence on glaucoma medications.

The procedure has been shown to be effective as an adjunct to cataract surgery and also as a standalone procedure. It can be used to provide IOP reduction in uncontrolled glaucoma patients; the procedure can also effectively reduce the medication burden in controlled glaucoma patients.

The key advantages that distinguish ab interno canal viscodilation from other MIGS procedures are as follows: it preserves the conjunctiva; it can be performed in conjunction with, or before or after, cataract extraction; it restores natural outflow pathways with minimal tissue trauma; there is no permanent implant or stent; and it is a comprehensive treatment that addresses the trabecular meshwork, Schlemm's canal, and collector channels.

Further data are needed to more accurately determine where ab interno viscodilation of the canal fits in our treatment algorithm; however, all conventional glaucoma procedures can still be performed in the event that ab interno viscodilation of the canal does not result in the patient reaching the target IOP.

References

1. Lewis RA, von Wolff K, Tetz M, et al. Canaloplasty: circumferential viscodilation and tensioning of Schlemm canal using a flexible microcatheter for the treatment of open-angle glaucoma in adults: two-year interim clinical study results. J Cataract Refract Surg 2009;35:814–824

2. Smit BA, Johnstone MA. Effects of viscoelastic injection into Schlemm's canal in primate and human eyes: potential relevance to viscocanalostomy. Ophthalmology 2002;109:786–792

3. Tamm ER, Carassa RG, Albert DM, et al. Viscocanalostomy in rhesus monkeys. Arch Ophthalmol 2004;122:1826–1838

4. Khaimi MA. Safety and efficacy of ab externo canaloplasty to treat open-angle glaucoma: 3-year results of a large patient cohort. Presented at the American Society of Cataract and Refractive Surgery annual meeting, New Orleans, May 7, 2016

5. Khaimi MA. Ab interno canaloplasty for open angle glaucoma. Presented at the America n Society of Cataract and Refractive Surgery annual meeting, New Orleans, May 7, 2016

34 Suprachoroidal Shunt: SOLX Gold Shunt

Jessica E. Chan and Peter A. Netland

Case Presentation

A 72-year-old woman with advanced primary open-angle glaucoma was referred after placement of an EX-PRESS Glaucoma Filtration Device (Alcon, Fort Worth, TX) under the conjunctiva, without a partial-thickness scleral flap. The patient had noted blurry vision and discomfort in the left eye. She was functionally monocular, having lost central vision in the right eye due to glaucoma.

On examination, the vision was CF (counts fingers) OD and 20/200 OS. The intraocular pressure (IOP) was 15 mm Hg OD and 32 mm Hg OS. She had been using brinzolamide in both eyes b.i.d., bimatoprost in both eyes at bedtime, and Combigan in both eyes b.i.d., and was previously treated with a laser trabeculoplasty. The EX-PRESS implant had eroded through the conjunctiva, but there was no aqueous leak. The superior conjunctiva surrounding the device was immobile. There was focal hyperemia around the device. There was mild corneal edema, the anterior chamber was deep, the posterior chamber intraocular lens was centered, and there was advanced cupping of the disk with a grossly normal macula. Previous automated perimetry (Humphrey visual field, Swedish Interactive Threshold Algorithm [SITA] Standard, 30–2) had shown apparent loss of central fixation in the right eye with a central island of vision in the left eye, and a mean defect of –31.11 OD and –26.74 OS. Her previous best-corrected vision was 20/40 OS.

Because of the conjunctival scarring and erosion, the options for transscleral filtration were limited. The patient was treated with removal of the EX-PRESS device, closure of the fistula, debridement of the area, and closure of the conjunctiva, followed by implantation of a SOLX Gold Shunt (SOLX Inc., Waltham, MA) in the temporal quadrant. The IOP was 4 to 6 mm Hg in the immediate postoperative period, with no formation of choroidal effusions. After the first week, the IOP increased to the low teens. After several months, the IOP increased to the high teens and the patient was treated with digital massage and medical therapy. Over a period of several months, her best-corrected vision in the left eye returned to 20/40, which was her baseline vision (**Fig. 34.1**).

The Procedure

The above case is an example of the use of the SOLX Gold Shunt in a patient with advanced open-angle glaucoma refractory to primary glaucoma surgery. In addition to use as a secondary or tertiary procedure for glaucoma, the device potentially may be used for primary surgical treatment of glaucoma not responsive to medical or laser therapy. The SOLX Gold Shunt is a suprachoroidal shunt, designed to drain aqueous humor from the anterior chamber into the suprachoroidal space, with eventual drainage through the uveoscleral outflow pathway, obviating the need for a bleb. It has been approved for usage in Canada and CE Mark countries in Europe, and is currently under investigation in a Food and Drug Administration (FDA) multicenter clinical trial in the United States. It is a 24-karat-gold, nonvalved, flat-plate drainage device that has been found to be biocompatible and inert in the eye.[1]

The current model of the SOLX Gold Shunt is the third generation of the device; it became commercially available in 2010. The device is ~ 80 µm thick, weighs 9.2 mg, and is 5.5 mm long, with a 3.2-mm anterior width and a 2.1-mm posterior width. Previous versions of the device contained channels to direct aqueous flow and were primarily used to study safety. Previous versions of the device were called GMS (Gold Micro Shunt) and GMS+, whereas the current commercial device is simply called the SOLX Gold Shunt. The device has 100 internal posts, which enhance structural support while enabling aqueous humor to flow from the anterior entry point of the shunt in the anterior chamber to the posterior exit point of the shunt in the suprachoroidal space. The aqueous can flow freely around the posts and does not run through channels. Aqueous humor drains from the anterior side of the shunt placed in the anterior chamber, draining out the posterior side of the shunt in the suprachoroidal space. The free flow of aqueous around the internal posts in the SOLX Gold Shunt creates less flow resistance compared with prior generations of the device. Other improvements in this model include central fixation holes for easier implantation, increased tensile strength, and a preloaded inserter to improve handling (**Fig. 34.2**).

Rationale Behind the Procedure

Filtering procedures such as trabeculectomy and glaucoma drainage implants are currently the standard surgical approaches in the treatment of glaucoma. Both procedures are dependent on the formation of a filtering bleb, which has several well-known potential complications, including leakage with hypotony, subconjunctival fibrosis, bleb encapsulation, blebitis, and endophthalmitis.[2] A bleb-less surgical approach that uses an alternative pathway for aqueous outflow would potentially avoid complications that can lead to poor outcomes.

A natural pressure gradient of 1 to 5 mm has been found to exist between the anterior chamber and the suprachoroidal space.[3] Using a cynomolgus monkey model, Emi et al[3] found that this pressure differential correspondingly increased with higher IOP levels when the anterior chamber and the suprachoroidal space was directly cannulated. It could then be inferred that a device connecting these two spaces could take advantage of the pressure gradient to directly lower the IOP, with subsequent flow of aqueous humor through the uveoscleral pathway. The SOLX Gold Shunt uses this approach to augment uveoscleral outflow from the anterior chamber to the suprachoroidal space, without bleb formation.

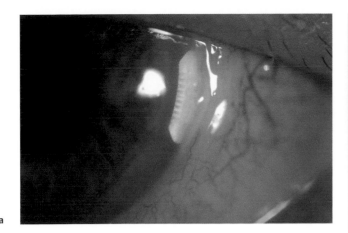

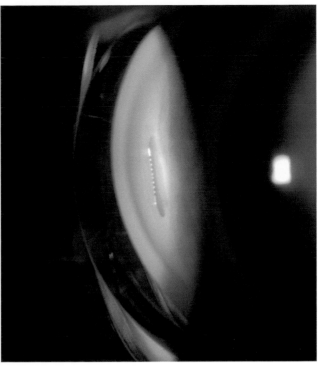

Fig. 34.1 Clinical appearance of the patient described in the case presentation after implantation of the SOLX Gold Shunt. **(a)** Slit-lamp biomicroscopic image of the SOLX Gold Shunt positioned in the temporal quadrant. **(b)** Gonioscopic view of the anterior end of the SOLX Gold Shunt positioned in the anterior chamber.

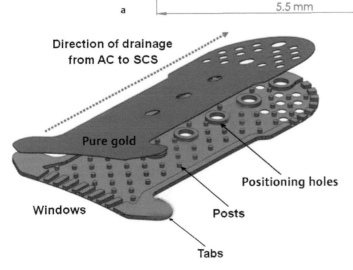

Fig. 34.2 SOLX Gold Shunt. **(a)** The device is 80 μm thick, with the other dimensions as shown. The wider end of the device is placed in the anterior chamber, with the narrower end in the suprachoroidal space. **(b)** Structural support is provided by 100 posts, providing openings for aqueous flow from the anterior chamber (AC) into the suprachoroidal space (SCS). (Courtesy of SOLX Inc.)

An observational case series of patients after Gold Shunt implantation by Mastropasqua et al[4] confirmed the lack of formation of a filtering bleb in all patients after SOLX Gold Shunt model-GMS implantation with anterior segment optical coherence tomography (AS-OCT). In addition, using in vivo confocal microscopy, these investigators examined the conjunctiva of the patients, who were divided into two groups: successful Gold Shunt implantations (defined as a third reduction in preoperative IOP with or without antiglaucoma treatment) and failed implantations (defined as a less than a third reduction in preoperative IOP). There was a statistically significant difference in the number of both mean conjunctival microcysts density (cysts/mm²) and area (μm^2) between the two groups, with the group of successful implantations exhibiting an approximately fivefold or sixfold increase in both numbers versus the failed implantation group. Epithelial microcysts have been previously identified as a marker for aqueous humor filtration through the conjunctiva in the bleb wall of successful trabeculectomies.[5] The presence of microcysts in patients with successful Gold Shunt implantation could be interpreted as a sign of aqueous humor filtration across the sclera, providing evidence that this may be one of the possible outflow pathways used by the shunt.[4]

Patient Selection

Previous studies have examined the efficacy of the SOLX Gold Shunt in patients with refractory glaucoma, with uncontrolled IOPs on maximal medical therapy, or with a history of prior failed glaucoma surgery.[6-9] Even in such a challenging patient population, the SOLX Gold Shunt appears to be efficacious and safe.[6-8] Patients should have at least one quadrant of healthy scleral tissue for implantation, but otherwise it does not appear that a history of prior glaucoma surgery prevents performing subsequent SOLX Gold Shunt implantation. Likewise, SOLX Gold Shunt implantation itself does not seem to preclude further glaucoma surgery.[9]

Complication rates have been low after implantation of the SOLX Gold Shunt.[6-9] This low rate of complications, along with the straightforward surgical procedure and the potential benefits of bleb-less surgery, suggest that there is a future role for the SOLX Gold Shunt in primary surgical treatment of glaucoma. In a clinical case series outside the United States of 103 patients with uncontrolled glaucoma (defined as baseline IOP > 21 mm Hg on maximum tolerated medications), the mean IOP reduction at 12 months was similar in subjects with a prior history of glaucoma surgery (n = 59) as compared with subjects with no prior history of glaucoma surgery (n = 44), with reduction rates of 31.6% and 34.5%, respectively (SOLX Inc., unpublished data). Successful treatment, defined as achieving an IOP ≤ 21 mm Hg, was achieved in 70.7% of patients with a prior history of glaucoma surgery, and in 93.9% of patients with no prior history of glaucoma surgery (SOLX Inc., unpublished data). For patients who have glaucoma not adequately controlled on maximal medical therapy, the SOLX Gold Shunt may be a useful primary surgical option in the future.

Surgical Technique

SOLX Gold Shunt Alone

Local anesthesia including retrobulbar, sub-Tenon, or peribulbar injection is usually sufficient. Either a corneal traction suture or a superior rectus bridle suture can be used for fixation.

The chosen quadrant for Gold Shunt placement should be in an area of healthy scleral tissue, with an open angle without

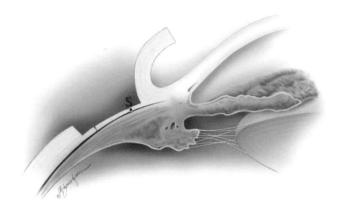

Fig. 34.3 Technique for implantation of the SOLX Gold Shunt. Under a deep scleral flap, a 3.5-mm long incision is made into the suprachoroidal space, with the incision located ~ 2 mm posterior to the scleral spur. (Courtesy of SOLX Inc.)

any peripheral anterior synechiae.[10] A fornix-based conjunctival flap is created, and episcleral vessels are cauterized. Either an anterior chamber maintainer or a cohesive viscoelastic should be placed via a paracentesis to maintain the anterior chamber. A 4-mm base by 3- to 4-mm-long scleral flap is created, with 80 to 90% scleral depth. A full-thickness scleral incision, 3.5 mm in length, is made 2 to 2.5 mm posterior to the scleral spur (**Fig. 34.3**). A second full-thickness scleral incision, again 3.5 mm in length, is made 1 mm posterior to the scleral spur leaving a 1-mm belt of scleral tissue between the two incisions (**Fig. 34.4**). A small amount of viscoelastic can be injected into both choroidal incisions. A 3.0-mm keratome is utilized to enter the supraciliary space through the anterior full-thickness incision (**Fig. 34.5**), gently advancing anteriorly to the entry point into the anterior chamber (**Fig. 34.6**). The incision is made into the anterior chamber with the keratome along the same plane as the supraciliary space (**Fig. 34.7**). The location and angulation of the anterior chamber entrance is an important step, with too anterior an entry leading to shunt-corneal touch, and too posterior an entry possibly leading to bleeding or iris touch.[10] The Gold Shunt is placed underneath the scleral flap, using the included preloaded inserter, with the anterior end positioned into the anterior chamber using the positioning holes, and the posterior end placed over the 1-mm belt of sclera into the supracho-

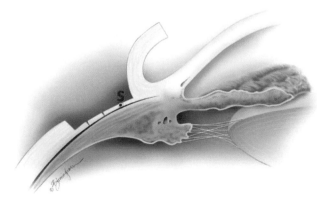

Fig. 34.4 Technique for implantation of the SOLX Gold Shunt (continued). A second 3.5-mm-long incision into the supraciliary space is made ~ 1 mm posterior to the scleral spur. (Courtesy of SOLX Inc.)

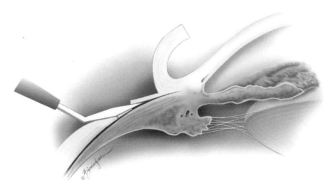

Fig. 34.5 Technique for implantation of the SOLX Gold Shunt (continued). The anterior incision is entered with the blade, which is advanced slowly in the supraciliary space toward the anterior chamber. (Courtesy of SOLX Inc.)

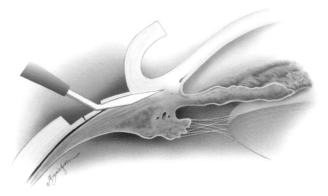

Fig. 34.6 Technique for implantation of the SOLX Gold Shunt (continued). The supraciliary space is followed until it ends at the entry point into the anterior chamber. (Courtesy of SOLX Inc.)

roidal space through the more posterior full-thickness incision (**Fig. 34.8**).

This insertion technique enables safe and reproducible placement of the anterior end of the device into the anterior chamber. Additionally, entering the suprachoroidal space through the more posterior incision enables the midsection of the shunt to rest on the scleral belt. This positioning gives support to the weight of the device and helps lock the device in place, minimizing the risk of shunt migration. Approximately 1 mm of the shunt should be visible in the anterior chamber. The scleral flap is sutured with interrupted 10-0 nylon sutures to ensure tight wound closure and checked for leakage. The overlying conjunctiva is closed using 9-0 or 10-0 Vicryl. Some clinicians use Ologen (Aeon Astron B.V., Leiden, the Netherlands) in the suprachoroidal space, in the area for drainage of aqueous at the posterior end of the device (Gabriel Simone, personal communication). When Ologen is used, a 4 mm × 4 mm piece is placed in the suprachoroidal space in the posterior scleral incision. After SOLX Gold Shunt placement, a second piece of Ologen collagen matrix can be placed over the top of the implant in the suprachoroidal space. The use of collagen matrix may reduce the fibrosis around the posterior end of the implant in the suprachoroidal space, but the influence of this adjunctive technique on the outcome after Gold Shunt placement is unknown at this time.

Combined with Cataract Extraction

Most surgeons perform cataract surgery first, followed by Gold Shunt implantation. The procedure is identical to the procedure performed without cataract surgery. Placement of the Gold Shunt in a different quadrant than used for cataract surgery is recommended.

Complications

The majority of complications associated with SOLX Gold Shunt implantation occur in the immediate postoperative period and are usually self-limited (**Table 34.1**), with hyphema reported as the most common complication. The other common complications in the early postoperative period (≤ 3 months) include hypotony, anterior chamber cell/flare, and blurred vision (SOLX Inc., unpublished data), which generally resolved by 3 months after surgery. Melamed et al[6] found minimal anterior chamber cell and flare, conjunctival congestion over the surgical site, slight discomfort (mild stinging and burning), and mild-to-moderate hyphema to be the most common complications in the immediate postoperative period, all of which resolved in a few days. Other complications in their study included shunt exposure in one patient, synechia formation in one patient, and exudative

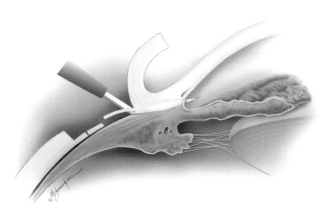

Fig. 34.7 Technique for implantation of the SOLX Gold Shunt (continued). The entry incision into the anterior chamber is parallel to the iris plane. (Courtesy of SOLX Inc.)

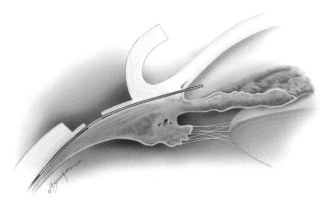

Fig. 34.8 Technique for implantation of the SOLX Gold Shunt (conclusion). The Gold Shunt is positioned with the anterior end 1 mm into the anterior chamber, and the posterior end in the suprachoroidal space. (Courtesy of SOLX Inc.)

Table 34.1 Complications After Implantation of the SOLX Gold Shunt

Complication	Melamed et al[6] (n = 38) % (n)	Figus et al[7] (n = 55) % (n)	Skaat et al[8] (n = 20) % (n)
Mild-to-moderate hyphema	21% (8)	22% (12)	15% (3)
Corneal edema	0	4% (2)	0
Shallow anterior chamber	0	0	15% (3)
Choroidal effusions	0	11% (6)	5% (1)
Exudative inferior retinal detachment	3% (1)	2% (1)	0
Shunt exposure	3% (1)	0	0

inferior retinal detachment in one patient. Similarly, Figus et al[7] identified mild-to-moderate hyphema and minimal anterior chamber inflammation to be the most common postoperative complications. Less common postoperative complications included bullous choroidal detachment (in six eyes, all of which resolved spontaneously), corneal edema (in two eyes), and exudative inferior retinal detachment (in one eye). None of the patients in a study by Skaat et al[8] experienced any major postoperative complications (such as endophthalmitis, retinal detachment, or suprachoroidal hemorrhage), with complications being limited to injection, hyphema, choroidals, and shallow anterior chamber, all of which resolved on their own. Hueber et al[9] reported low-grade chronic inflammation or newly developed rubeosis iridis in a total of four patients.

Recognition and Management of Complications

As the majority of complications appear to occur in the early postoperative period, a careful anterior and posterior examination should be performed at each postoperative visit. Judicious monitoring and medical therapy appear to be sufficient in the majority of cases, with resolution of most complications occurring within a short period of time as discussed in the aforementioned studies.[6–8] Removal of the SOLX Gold Shunt may be necessary in a minority of cases. Melamed et al[6] removed one

shunt due to exposure. In their case series, Figus et al[7] explanted the SOLX Gold Shunt (model GMS) in three patients, two of whom had corneal edema due to endothelial contact with the shunt, and one patient with an exudative inferior retinal detachment due to excessive filtration, all of whom returned to their initial preoperative clinical condition after explantation. SOLX Gold Shunt (model GMS+) removal was deemed necessary in six of 31 eyes in the study reported by Hueber and coworkers.[9]

Postoperative Management

After surgery, patients are treated with topical antibiotics and steroids (four to six times per day) for 1 week, followed by tapering of the steroid over a 6-week period. Postoperative visits are usually scheduled for day 1, the end of week 1, the end of month 1, and the end of month 2, followed by routine visits after the month-2 visit. Additional visits are scheduled as needed. Patients with increased inflammation may be treated with increased frequency of topical steroids, or Tenon's injection of corticosteroid.

Safety, Efficacy, and Clinical Results

Summary results are shown for mean IOP **(Fig. 34.9)** and surgical success **(Table 34.2)**. Mean IOP after SOLX Gold Shunt is in the

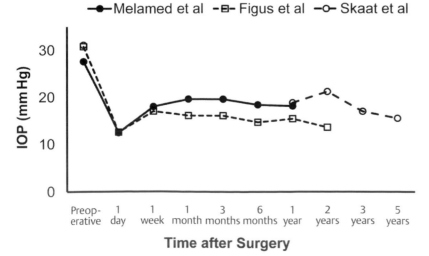

Fig. 34.9 Mean intraocular pressure (IOP) over time after SOLX Gold Shunt implantation in patients with refractory glaucoma in three studies. In all three studies, mean IOP was in the mid- to high teens during the postoperative period. (Data from Melamed et al,[6] Figus et al,[7] and Skaat et al.[8])

Table 34.2   Surgical Success After Implantation of the SOLX Gold Shunt

Study	Definition of Success	Study End Point	Success at End Point % (n)
Melamed et al[6]	Surgical success: IOP > 5 mm Hg and < 22 mm Hg with or without glaucoma medications at the last follow-up	1 year	79% (30)
Figus et al[7]	Qualified success: IOP < 21 mm Hg with a reduction of baseline IOP by 33% with or without any topical medications	2 years	67% (37)
Skaat et al[8]	IOP > 5 mm Hg and < 22 mm Hg, with at least 20% reduction from preoperative IOP with or without medications	5 years	77.8% (7) with 24-μm GMS 72.7% (8) with 48-μm GMS

Abbreviation: IOP, intraocular pressure.

ranges of the mid- to high teens. Surgical success has ranged from 70 to 80%.

To date, there have only been a few published studies on the efficacy of the SOLX Gold Shunt. The first prospective study of the SOLX Gold Shunt was reported by Melamed et al,[6] in which 38 patients with uncontrolled glaucoma were implanted with the GMS model of the SOLX Gold Shunt. All patients had a baseline IOP of ≥ 22 mm Hg on maximally tolerated medical therapy, and 20 patients (53%) had previous glaucoma surgery or a glaucoma drainage device. The IOP decreased by a mean of 9 ± 7.5 mm Hg from 27.6 ± 4.7 mm Hg to 18.2 ± 4.6 mm Hg in the last follow-up visit, which represented an average decrease of 32.6% from baseline. Surgical success, which was defined as an IOP > 5 mm Hg and < 22 mm Hg with or without glaucoma medications at the last follow-up, was achieved in 79%, or 30 patients. Complete success, which was defined as an IOP > 5 mm Hg and < 22 mm Hg without glaucoma medications at last follow-up, was obtained in 13.2%, or five patients.

Mastropasqua et al[4] published an observational case series of 14 eyes that underwent GMS implantation after multiple failed previous glaucoma surgeries. Patients were divided into two groups: successful implantations (33% reduction in preoperative IOP with or without glaucoma medications) and failed implantations (reduction < 33% in preoperative IOP on maximal tolerated medical therapy). Eight of 14 patients (57%) were deemed successes, and six (43%) were deemed failures. The mean overall postoperative IOP reduction was 22.5% across both groups, from 28.8 ± 3.9 mm Hg to 22.1 ± 10.6 mm Hg.

A prospective uncontrolled case series by Figus et al[7] examined the results of the GMS model of the SOLX Gold Shunt implantation in 55 patients with refractory glaucoma (defined as IOP > 21 mm Hg despite maximal medical therapy and/or previously failed surgical treatment). Patients had undergone an average of 1.9 previous filtrations or cyclodestructive surgical treatments (range 1–5). At 2 years of follow-up, a qualified success, defined as a lowering of IOP to < 21 mm Hg with a reduction of baseline IOP by 33% with or without any topical medications, was reached in 67% of cases, or 37 eyes. These eyes had a mean IOP decrease of 50.4%, or 13.9 mm Hg. Only 5.5%, or three eyes, obtained a complete surgical success, which was a lowering of IOP to < 21 mm Hg with a reduction of 33% of the baseline IOP without any topical medications. Eighteen eyes (32.7%) were in the failure group. Ultrasound biomicroscopy (UBM) and gonioscopy identified the causes of failure as follows: anterior block of the GMS lumen due to a thin inflammatory membrane in 12 eyes (66.7%), posterior blockage due to scarring in the suprachoroidal space in three eyes (16.7%), and the absence of shunt posterior bending in the remaining three eyes (16.7%).

A histopathological study by Agnifili et al,[11] of five GMS-model SOLX Gold Shunts that were unsuccessfully placed in five

eyes and then subsequently removed, confirmed that connective tissue in the device likely led to failure. Connective tissue was found filling all of the inner spaces of the GMS, with a thick fibrotic capsule surrounding the ends of the device. Similarly, Rękas et al[12] examined four explanted Gold Micro Shunts, two cases of GMS and two of GMS+ removal. In all four cases, connective tissue was found in the channels and around the implant. Fibrosis appears to be the main etiology of failure of the Gold Shunt. Fibrosis in the anterior chamber blocking aqueous entry into the device can be treated with 1- to 2-mJ pulses of the neodymium:yttrium-aluminum-garnet (Nd:YAG) laser, which can reestablish aqueous flow (Peter A. Netland, personal communication).

Hueber et al[9] found high rates of failure in a retrospective study of 31 eyes with severe glaucoma with uncontrolled IOP that underwent SOLX Gold Shunt (model GMS+) placement. Surgical success was defined as an IOP < 21 mm Hg and > 5 mm Hg, and at least a 20% reduction of IOP from baseline at least 6 months after GMS+ implantation. Criteria for failure included (1) an IOP outside the success range on one visit at least 6 months after GMS+ implantation; (2) serious complications (including retinal detachment, endophthalmitis, suprachoroidal hemorrhage, low-grade inflammation, and newly developed rubeosis iridis) at any time, and (3) need for additional glaucoma surgery (except GMS+ repositioning) at any time. Thirty of the 31 eyes met at least one of the three criteria for failure, with a 1-year failure rate of 71% and a 2-year failure rate of 90%. A secondary surgery was performed due to elevated IOP in 24 (77%) of eyes, and two eyes (6%) required a secondary surgery (GMS+ explantation) due to low-grade inflammation and rubeosis iridis without elevated IOP. A total of six GMS+ shunts were explanted. The results of this short-term study (6 months) differed significantly from prior published studies. Hueber et al hypothesized that the differences may have stemmed from a different surgical technique (full-thickness scleral flap versus simple scleral incision), different device (GMS+ versus GMS), or failure to check and control for bending of the device in all eyes. It should be noted that the criteria for success were more stringent in this study, and that the definition of failure was broader. In addition, patients with a poor prognosis were enrolled, including those with uveitic or neovascular glaucoma.

A study by Skaat et al[8] compared the outcomes of the Ahmed glaucoma valve (AGV) with the results from two different models of the SOLX Gold Shunt (24-μm GMS and 48-μm GMS). In this randomized interventional prospective clinical trial, a total of 29 eyes with refractory glaucoma (defined as a mean baseline IOP ≥ 22 mm Hg on maximal medications, with a history of at least one failed trabeculectomy, and a defined visual field defect) were randomized to receive either AGV (Ahmed FP7 glaucoma valve), 24-μm GMS, or 48-μm GMS implantation. There were nine patients in the AGV group, nine in the 24-µm GMS group, and 11 in the 48-µm GMS group. Across all groups, the final IOP was statistically significantly lower than the preoperative IOP, with no statistically significant difference between groups in mean reduction of IOP. With a definition of success as an IOP > 5 mm Hg, < 22 mm Hg, and at least a 20% reduction from the preoperative IOP with or without glaucoma medications, cumulative probabilities of success at 5 years were 77.8%, 77.8%, and 72.7% for the AGV, 24-µm GMS, and 48-µm GMS groups, respectively. Failure was defined as an IOP < 5 mm Hg or > 22 mm Hg on at least two consecutive follow-up visits, the need for additional glaucoma surgery to control IOP, or loss of light perception. All failures (two in the AGV group, two in the 24-µm GMS group, and three in the 48-µm GMS group) were due to elevated IOP.

Further studies are certainly warranted to fully determine the safety and efficacy of the SOLX Gold Shunt. However, the majority of the data thus far seems to indicate good safety and efficacy profiles, making it a promising potential option for primary and secondary glaucoma surgery.

References

1. Sen SC, Ghosh A. Gold as an intraocular foreign body. Br J Ophthalmol 1983;67:398–399

2. Allingham RR, Schuman JS, Sofinski SJ, et al. Glaucoma filtration surgery. In: Albert DM, Jakobiec FA, eds. Principles and Practice of Ophthalmology. Philadelphia: WB Saunders; 1994:1623–1640

3. Emi K, Pederson JE, Toris CB. Hydrostatic pressure of the suprachoroidal space. Invest Ophthalmol Vis Sci 1989;30:233–238

4. Mastropasqua L, Agnifili L, Ciancaglini M, et al. In vivo analysis of conjunctiva in gold micro shunt implantation for glaucoma. Br J Ophthalmol 2010;94:1592–1596

5. Labbé A, Dupas B, Hamard P, Baudouin C. In vivo confocal microscopy study of blebs after filtering surgery. Ophthalmology 2005;112:1979

6. Melamed S, Ben Simon GJ, Goldenfeld M, Simon G. Efficacy and safety of gold micro shunt implantation to the supraciliary space in patients with glaucoma: a pilot study. Arch Ophthalmol 2009;127:264–269

7. Figus M, Lazzeri S, Fogagnolo P, Iester M, Martinelli P, Nardi M. Supraciliary shunt in refractory glaucoma. Br J Ophthalmol 2011;95:1537–1541

8. Skaat A, Sagiv O, Kinori M, Ben Simon GJ, Goldenfeld M, Melamed S. Gold Micro-Shunt Implants versus Ahmed glaucoma valve: long-term outcomes of a prospective randomized clinical trial. J Glaucoma 2016;25: 155–161

9. Hueber A, Roters S, Jordan JF, Konen W. Retrospective analysis of the success and safety of Gold Micro Shunt implantation in glaucoma. BMC Ophthalmol 2013;13:35

10. Tam DY, Ahmed IK. The SOLX® Gold Shunt Device for glaucoma. Eur Ophthalmic Rev 2009;2:39–41

11. Agnifili L, Costagliola C, Figus M, et al. Histological findings of failed gold micro shunts in primary open-angle glaucoma. Graefes Arch Clin Exp Ophthalmol 2012;250:143–149

12. Rękas M, Pawlik B, Grala B, Kozłowski W. Clinical and morphological evaluation of gold micro shunt after unsuccessful surgical treatment of patients with primary open-angle glaucoma. Eye (Lond) 2013;27:1214–1217

35 Ab Interno Suprachoroidal Shunts: CyPass and iStent Supra

Steven D. Vold and Steven R. Sarkisian, Jr.

Case Presentation

A 70-year-old man is referred for evaluation of his cataracts and glaucoma. A combined procedure is recommended by his referring physician. The patient frequently travels from the United States to the Middle East and France, and often forgets to take his eyedrops. His vision is 20/40 OD and 20/30 OS and his visual fields demonstrate an early superior nasal step defect in the right eye and are full in the left eye. *Optical coherence tomography* (OCT) shows mild thinning inferiorly in the left eye and inferior temporal thinning consistent with his visual field defect in the right eye. The patient's intraocular pressure (IOP) is 18 mm Hg OD and 15 mm Hg OS on latanoprost in both eyes and brinzolamide in the right eye.

The patient's goal is to have a lower IOP in the right eye and to perhaps get off at least one medication in each eye; however, he does not wish to have the long-term risk of infection associated with conventional trabeculectomy. He chooses to undergo cataract extraction with intraocular lens placement combined with a suprachoroidal stent, first in the right eye and then in the left.

Four to 6 weeks after surgery in both eyes, his visual acuity is 20/20 OU without correction and the IOP is 14 mm Hg OU. He is on latanoprost in the right eye only, and he is considered to be at target IOP.

The Procedure

In the past there has been a significant disparity identified for the timeline of transitioning from glaucoma medications to the incorporation of incisional procedures in the treatment of glaucoma. Often conventional procedures, such as trabeculectomy and shunt implants, must be reserved for more severe and end-stage glaucoma patients who have reached the point of being intractable to medication management. The reason for such restraint has come about as a result of research on the risk profile that is associated with these invasive procedures, reporting case complication rates of 39 to 60%.[1] Given this knowledge, recent research efforts have focused on the need to develop a minimally invasive intervention for providing effective IOP control in patients with mild to moderate glaucoma.

Supraciliary implants have been an area of intensive study within minimally invasive glaucoma surgery (MIGS) and provided great improvements in the efficacy of glaucoma treatment. These implants are among a variety of such devices currently being investigated in U.S. Food and Drug Administration (FDA) trials for safety and effectiveness. The underlying mechanism of such a device lies in accessing the suprachoroidal space and capitalizing on the uveoscleral flow as a means of reducing the IOP. This chapter provides a framework for understanding the research into this device and that prospective benefits that it has the potential to offer as a modality for future MIGS treatment.

Device Description

The CyPass micro-stent (Transcend Medical Inc., Menlo Park, CA) is a tube-shaped, supraciliary implant that acts as a conduit to the suprachoroidal space. It is made of biocompatible, nondegradable polyimide material. The device size measures 0.51 mm in external diameter and 0.30 mm in internal diameter, and 6.35 mm in length. The surface of the device distal to a prominent collar marking on the proximal end is accented by a fenestrated surface of 76-μm diameter pores along this length that aid in longitudinal and circumferential dispersal of drained aqueous humor from the anterior chamber into the suprachoroidal space.[2–4]

A similar suprachoroidal micro-stent currently undergoing evaluation is the iStent Supra (**Fig. 35.1**), (Glaukos, Laguna Hills, CA), which is implanted in much the same manner that the CyPass is placed. Both of these ab interno supraciliary micro-stents are currently under investigation in the United States in eyes with mild-to-moderate primary open-angle glaucoma at the time of cataract surgery. These devices potentially offer benefit in more advanced glaucomatous disease and may eventually play a role in angle-closure glaucomas.

Rationale Behind the Procedure

Uveoscleral outflow is estimated to account for roughly half of the aqueous drainage in normal human eyes.[3] Physiology studies have identified a gradient of negative pressure within the suprachoroidal space that serves as the conduit for this aqueous flow pathway.[2,3] This gradient has been measured at -0.8 ± 0.5 mm Hg between the anterior chamber and the perilimbal portion of the suprachoroidal space with deeper compartmental sections near the optic nerve decreasing to around -3.7 ± 0.4 mm Hg.[2] An understanding of the potential for this physiological pathway as a diversion for aqueous flow release in situations of elevated IOP is not new to the field of glaucoma surgery. Yet the minimally invasive ab interno approach offered by devices such as the iStent Supra or the CyPass micro-stent is a softer approach than has previously been attempted. The ab interno technique has permitted minimization of trauma to tissues during device implantation and has helped to avoid the detrimental fibroblastic proliferative response that had plagued the long-term results of earlier ab externo techniques.[2]

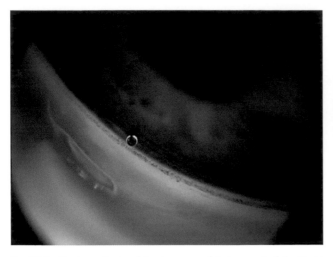

Fig. 35.1 Gonioscopic view following successful placement of the iStent Supra. (Courtesy of Steven Vold, MD.)

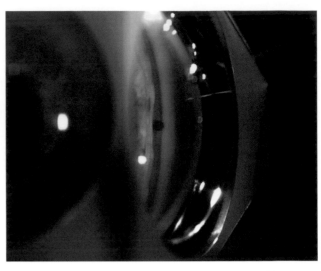

Fig. 35.2 Anatomic illustration for the proper placement of the CyPass micro-stent. (Courtesy of Steven Vold, MD.)

Patient Selection

Studies thus far examining the safety and efficacy of the suprachoroidal stenting have selected patients based on criteria of uncontrolled (IOP ≥ 21 mm Hg) open-angle glaucoma (OAG) in contexts both with and without medication use.[1,3] CyPass has also been implemented in studies of patients who desired to reduce dependency on medications for already-controlled IOP.[1] Performing the CyPass procedure in patients concomitantly undergoing phacoemulsification has also been implemented and demonstrated great success (COMPASS, unpublished data). A patient history of prior glaucoma surgery does not preclude the possibility of utilizing a CyPass implant for further pressure control, nor does CyPass implantation prohibit performing further surgery, if needed, for IOP control.[1] Studies of the iStent Supra are currently ongoing, but it is expected that the results will be similar.

Surgical Technique

The supraciliary implant is inserted via an ab interno approach that is facilitated through a 1.5- to 2.0-mm clear corneal incision. A standard clear corneal cataract incision may also be utilized.[1,2] Obtaining the correct insertion angle for this micro-stenting procedure is assisted by the use of an ophthalmic viscosurgical device to slightly overfill and thereby deepen the anterior chamber.[2,5] The use of viscoelastic further serves the purpose of protecting the corneal endothelium during micro-stent delivery.[2] Device insertion is aided by the use of a curved delivery tool with a retractable guidewire.[2] The base of the scleral spur serves as a critical landmark in targeting the device for successfully accessing the suprachoroidal space. To perform this, the tip of the guidewire must be engaged with the iris root and subsequently passed into the suprachoroidal space.[1]

In addition to proper intracameral preparation and insertion technique, the appropriate positioning of the operating microscope, aided by using a gonioprism, is necessary for visualization of the implant site. By rotating the microscope 30 to 40 degrees away from the operator as well as a tilting the patient's head an equivalent angle away, the best possible view of the operating site is achieved. The addition of viscoelastic to the surface of the cornea further serves as an interface for improvement of the image quality provided by the approximated goniolens.[2]

The final appearance of the micro-stent after device insertion should demonstrate a single ring exposed at the proximal end of the device resulting in 1.0 mm of exposed implant (**Fig. 35.2**). To determine proper positioning, the device should be observed with its exposed end residing between the pigmented trabecular meshwork and Schwalbe's line.[2] Once ascertainment of final positioning is made, an evacuation of viscoelastic should be performed using irrigation and aspiration followed by corneal wound closure by either the hydration technique or the use of a single interrupted suture.[2,3]

Postoperative assessment of device placement can be performed by gonioscopy (**Fig. 35.3**), optical coherence tomography, or ultrasound bimicroscopy.[3,4]

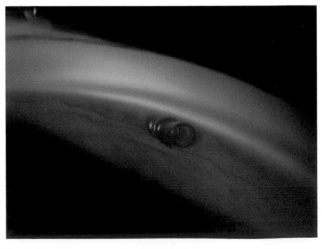

Fig. 35.3 Gonioscope examination of the CyPass micro-stent after implantation. (From Glaucoma Today Supplement: Innovations in Ophthalmology. Wayne, PA: Bryn Mawr Communications; 2011:56–57. http://bmctoday.net/innovations2011/digital_supplement/article.asp?f=inno-2011-transcend. Accessed October 14, 2015. Reproduced with permission.)

Postoperative Management

The minimally invasive nature of the suprachoroidal stent insertion is much less traumatic to tissues and permits a shorter recovery time than is achievable by traditional full-thickness penetration procedures such as trabeculectomy.[1] The follow-up for patients receiving these implants uses assessment parameters similar to those used in patients undergoing isolated cataract procedures.[2] A typical follow-up schedule has consisted of patient office visits for examination at 1 day, 1 week, and 1 month in the postoperative timeframe. Prophylaxis for infection is still performed in the perioperative period through the use of topical antibiotics. Additionally, 1 month of topical anti-inflammatory medication postoperatively is recommended. Medications used for this purpose of stemming inflammation associated with this procedure have included prednisolone acetate 1.0% and loteprednol 0.5%.[2]

Complications

In examining patients in the postoperative period following CyPass micro-stent placement, investigators have observed improved safety profiles over traditional glaucoma surgical procedures, including tube shunts and trabeculectomy.[3] In studies examining the long-term safety at 1 and 2 years postintervention, there have been no serious or vision-threatening ocular adverse events (endophthalmitis, hypopyon, suprachoroidal hemorrhage, flat anterior chamber, encapsulated bleb, wound leak choroidal effusion, or retinal detachment) observed.[2-4] The most common minimal adverse events observed in the postoperative period have been transient, with the majority resolving spontaneously within 1 month and almost all completely resolving within 6 months. The most common minimal adverse events observed following CyPass micro-stenting include transient early hypotony (IOP ≤ 6 mm Hg), transient IOP increases, hyphema, cataract progression, and iritis. Iatrogenic events related to malpositioning of the device included 5.4% of cases in a study by Hoeh et al.[1] These incidents, resulting in device occlusion, were identified as predominantly occurring because of the operator advancing the device too far within the supraciliary space.

Safety, Efficacy, and Clinical Results

Evidence obtained for examining both the safety and effectiveness of the CyPass micro-stent for the treatment of glaucoma has been accumulated in studies ranging from smaller scale prospective cohorts to large FDA randomized controlled trials (RCTs).

García-Feijoo et al[3] performed a multicenter clinical study in Europe and found that CyPass micro-stenting effectively lowered the IOP in > 80% of cases. This study followed 55 subjects designated to have uncontrolled (IOP > 21 mm Hg) and medicated OAG for 1 year after CyPass intervention was performed. The results demonstrated a 32% reduction in mean IOP from baseline coupled with a 30% reduction in the mean number of medications for eyes that did not require any additional surgery for IOP control after Cypass implant, which included 70% of cases. No serious intraoperative events or major adverse events (retinal or choroidal detachment, persistent uveitis, persistent hyphema, hypotony maculopathy) occurred over the course of this study. Minor adverse events reported in the study were transient IOP elevation (IOP ≥ 30 mm Hg that resolved spontaneously or with medication) in 10.8% of cases. Transient hyphema was observed in 6.2% of cases and resolved within the first month after surgery for all patients affected. Progression of cataracts was observed in 12.2% of cases.

Low rates of surgical complications were identified in a prospective interventional case study excerpted from an ongoing open-label, interventional, multicenter study known as CyCLE (CyPass Clinical Experience) performed by Hoeh et al.[1] In this study the safety and efficacy of the CyPass micro-stent for the treatment of OAG concomitant with cataract surgery was assessed postoperatively after 6 months. This study divided patients into two cohorts. Cohort 1 consisted of patients with uncontrolled (IOP ≥ 21 mm Hg) primary or secondary OAG, having failed topical or surgical treatment previously. Cohort 2 consisted of patients with controlled IOP (< 20 mm Hg) who want to reduce their dependence on glaucoma medications. At the 6-month follow-up, 57 patients were available from cohort 1 for assessment and 41 patients from cohort 2. Both cohorts experienced a reduction in the mean number of medications used. Between baseline to 6 months, 55% and 71.4% of patients experienced a medication reduction for cohort 1 and 2, respectively. Additionally, mean IOP for cohort 1 demonstrated a significant 10 mm Hg (37%) sustained reduction from baseline to a mean of 15.6 ± 0.53 mm Hg, whereas the IOP for cohort 2 remained controlled (< 21 mm Hg). The most common postoperative complications experienced were early hypotony (13.8%) and transient IOP increase. The majority of the hypotony cases resolved spontaneously within 1 month, and a single patient remaining with hypotony resolved spontaneously at 6 months. No removal of any micro-stent was required.

CyPass micro-stenting augmented with supraciliary viscoexpansion of the suprachoroidal space has also been conducted and shown to successfully reduce IOP and decrease glaucoma medication usage. Results obtained in a multicenter, randomized controlled, pilot study examined 63 primary OAG cases. Patient criteria for inclusion were an OAG of Shaffer grade 3 to 4 with uncontrolled IOP (IOP ≥ 21 mm Hg with or without glaucoma medication use). Subjects were followed for 1 year postoperatively. Three groups were generated and included a stent-only group, group V30 (30 μL of Healon-5 injected with stent), and group V60 (60 μL of Healon-5 injected with stent). Primary outcomes for efficacy were measured by observing a reduced IOP and decreased medication use. The safety of the procedure was evaluated by the number and type of adverse events recorded. The mean IOP baseline was similar for each group after medication washout, being recorded at 22.2 ± 5.8 mm Hg (stent-only group), 22.5 ± 6.5 mm Hg (V30), and 22.4 ± 5.7 mm Hg (V60). At 12 months postintervention, all study groups stained statistically significant mean decreases in IOP by 28% (stent-only group), 32% (V30), and 37% (V60). Topical antihypertensive medication use was found to be sustained at a remarkably declined level from baseline in all groups (Ianchulev et al, unpublished data). The safety profile results of this study were noted to be similar to those of other studies examining the CyPass micro-stent.[1,3] This is beneficial, as it is understood that the patient numbers evaluated within this study were not large enough to support assertions of safety and efficacy over a broader patient demographic alone. Yet the results do serve to demonstrate the feasibility and potential benefits that viscoelastic expansion coupled to CyPass stenting may have to offer as a future modality of treatment.

Findings of efficacy and safety for the CyPass micro-stent have been further expanded to treatment in mild-to-moderate glaucoma patients by a recent and pivotal multicenter, interventional RCT known as the COMPASS study. This study has been working to examine the long-term (2-year) efficacy of CyPass micro-stenting. It represents the first study ever to examine long-term clinical benefit and efficacy for micro-interventional treatment in mild-to-moderate OAG patients. In this study, 505 patients were randomized to a control group (n = 131) and a stent group (n = 374). Groups were divided between those undergoing CyPass micro-stenting in combination with phacoemulsification (stent group) versus phacoemulsification alone (control group). A primary efficacy outcome measure of this study looked at subjects achieving a ≥ 20% reduction in nonmedicated IOP reduction from the mean total cohort baseline (24.4 ± 2 mm Hg) after medication washout. It was discovered that this outcome was sustained within a significantly greater proportion of the stent (76%) versus control (61%) subjects at 24 months.

A secondary efficacy outcome was the mean unmedicated IOP changes at 24 months between groups. Results measuring this outcome showed a decrease of 30% and 22% for the stent and control groups, respectively (COMPASS, unpublished data). Safety-related secondary outcomes examined during the study revealed no serious or vision-threatening ocular adverse events in either group. The four most frequently observed minor adverse events were best corrected visual acuity loss ≥ 10 letters (8% stent group/13.7% control group), visual field loss (5.1% stent/ 7.6% control), iritis (7.8% stent/3.8% control), and corneal edema (3.2% stent/1.5% control) (COMPASS, unpublished data). The researchers observed these minor adverse events as being transient and indicate that they would be unlikely to affect the success of future surgical interventions. Overall, the results obtained from this large-scale RCT examining the CyPass micro-stent have demonstrated that the ab interno MIGS approach offered by this new modality provides an improved safety profile over conventional glaucoma surgery.

Conclusion

The cultivation of evidence on the efficacy and safety achievable by supraciliary access of the suprachoroidal space substantiates the incredible advancements in the capabilities offered by ab interno MIGS treatment. With results from large RCT studies such as the COMPASS and the international randomized trial on visco-augmented micro-stenting, level 1 clinical evidence for CyPass micro-stenting has now been provided. The results of pending studies for the other suprachoroidal stent, the iStent Supra, are expected to be similar. The potential that this technology demonstrates for providing an effective approach to addressing a wide range of severity in glaucoma holds a promising future in minimally invasive treatments.

References

1. Hoeh H, Ahmed IIK, Grisanti S, et al. Early postoperative safety and surgical outcomes after implantation of a suprachoroidal micro-stent for the treatment of open-angle glaucoma concomitant with cataract surgery. J Cataract Refract Surg 2013;39:431–437

2. Bailey AK, Sarkisian SR Jr, Vold SD. Ab interno approach to the suprachoroidal space. J Cataract Refract Surg 2014;40:1291–1294

3. García-Feijoo J, Rau M, Grisanti S, et al. Supraciliary micro-stent implantation for open-angle glaucoma failing topical therapy: 1-year results of a multicenter study. Am J Ophthalmol 2015;159:1075–1081

4. Saheb H, Ianchulev T, Ahmed II. Optical coherence tomography of the suprachoroid after CyPass Micro-Stent implantation for the treatment of open-angle glaucoma. Br J Ophthalmol 2014;98:19–23

36   Endoscopic Cyclophotocoagulation

Ramya N. Swamy, Vikas Chopra, and Brian A. Francis

The Procedure

The objective of most glaucoma surgery is to improve aqueous outflow. Treatments to reduce aqueous inflow by treating the ciliary body have existed since the 1950s.[1] Cyclodestruction can be achieved through various means including cryotherapy and laser, but cyclophotocoagulation has been the most commonly employed process. Transscleral cyclophotocoagulation (TCP) was introduced in the 1970s as a way to treat intractable end-stage glaucoma.[2] However, because TCP application is nontargeted and can have significant collateral tissue damage, a more tissue-specific application to decrease aqueous production was needed. The diode laser employed in the transscleral method was modified by Martin Uram[3] for use through an endoscopic system to perform endoscopic cyclophotocoagulation (ECP), which allowed visualization and tissue-targeted application of laser energy.[4,5]

Rationale Behind the Procedure

The ciliary processes consist of pigmented ciliary epithelium (PCE) and nonpigmented ciliary epithelium (NPCE), which in concert produce the aqueous humor. Histopathologically, Pantcheva et al[6] found that eyes that have been treated with ECP demonstrate less histopathological damage compared with eyes that had undergone TCP. Other histopathological studies have demonstrated that ECP-treated eyes showed loss of melanin granules in the treated areas when compared with relative preservation of the ciliary stroma and blood vessels in the untreated areas.[7] An animal study by Lin[8] in rabbits using fluorescein angiography demonstrated disrupted blood flow to the ciliary processes immediately following treatment with TCP and ECP. However, 1 month later, the ECP-treated ciliary processes showed some degree of reperfusion, demonstrating that the effects were somewhat reversible and might enable retreatment and fewer side effects such as hypotony. This is likely due to the fact that ECP enables guided delivery of laser energy because it permits direct visualization of the treatment. This has expanded the use of ECP from recalcitrant glaucoma to eyes with better visual potential.

In addition, ECP is the only minimally invasive glaucoma surgery (MIGS) procedure that targets aqueous production and thus offers an alternative mechanism of action to lower the intraocular pressure (IOP). Therefore, it can be performed after other angle-based surgeries have failed, and it can be combined easily with other glaucoma surgeries or phacoemulsification utilizing the same clear-corneal incision. Because ECP does not involve disruption of the conjunctiva or sclera, it spares those tissues for future trabeculectomy ab externo or aqueous tube shunt implantation. This makes ECP one of the few procedures that can be performed at any stage of glaucoma ranging from mild to refractory.

Patient Selection

Since ECP was first introduced, the patient population that might benefit from this procedure has expanded to include a range from mild glaucoma to end-stage glaucoma, as well as in combination with other procedures. The following patient populations can be treated with this procedure[9]:

- Patients with both cataracts and ocular hypertension who can benefit from cataract surgery combined with ECP, with the goal of reducing the number of glaucoma medications, thus reducing costs and eliminating compliance issues
- Patients with mild-to-moderate open-angle glaucoma (primary open angle, pigmentary, pseudoexfoliation) who are undergoing concomitant cataract surgery or as a stand-alone ECP procedure
- Patients at potentially increased risk of complications from filtering surgery (postvitrectomy, aphakia, history of suprachoroidal hemorrhage)
- Patients who require surgical treatment to lower the IOP but do not want to undergo more invasive procedures. In these patients, ECP may also be combined with angle-based MIGS procedures such as trabecular bypass stent (iStent) or trabeculotomy ab interno (Trabectome) along with cataract extraction if needed.
- Patients who have had complications from filtering surgery (trabeculectomy) in the contralateral eye
- Patients who have previously undergone filtering surgery or aqueous drainage implantation but continue to have an elevated IOP
- Patients on anticoagulant therapy for systemic diseases at increased risk of intraocular bleeding with filtering surgery or aqueous shunt implantation
- Patients with anatomic narrow angles with plateau iris configuration
- Patients with corneal opacification with limited view of the anterior and posterior chambers
- Patients with angle-closure glaucoma who are not candidates for angle-based surgeries (trabecular bypass)
- Pediatric patients with congenital glaucoma who have failed traditional surgeries such as goniotomy and trabeculotomy

Surgical Technique

The only endoscopic system that is currently approved for use in the United States by the Food and Drug Administration is the E2 system by Beaver Visitec (originally EndoOptiks, Waltham, MA).

This machine involves a single probe that combines an 810-nm diode laser, a helium-neon aiming beam, a 175 W xenon light source, and a camera for video imaging (**Fig. 36.1**). These elements are combined in a 20-gauge probe, which offers a 110-degree field of view and depth of focus of 1 to 30 mm. The endoprobes are available in the straight or curved configurations.

The typical settings that are used on the machine include the following:

- Aiming beam set at 20 to 40
- Power of 0.25 to 0.40 W
- Continuous ablation time, which can be controlled by the surgeon via the foot pedal
- The intensity of the light source is adjusted based on surgeon preference to lightly illuminate the ciliary processes while still being able to appreciate their whitening and shrinkage, which are the end points of treatment.

While performing the procedure, the surgeon sits temporally or superiorly for the best approach. To perform ECP using the anterior-segment approach, a 2- to 2.4-mm clear corneal incision is typically created, or the main incision from the concurrent cataract extraction can be utilized. A cohesive viscoelastic is used to deepen the anterior chamber as well as to inflate the sulcus space to create room between the iris and the lens. The endoprobe is then positioned outside the incision and the camera probe is rotated to align the view and to bring the image into focus. The endoprobe is then inserted into the anterior chamber and guided toward the sulcus space while being visualized through the operating microscope. The surgeon then directs her/his view toward the monitor. The endoprobe is advanced until six to eight ciliary processes are visualized on the monitor with the proper illumination setting (**Fig. 36.2**). The aiming beam is then placed on a single process, and laser energy is applied via the foot pedal until whitening and shrinkage of the ciliary process is seen. The epithelium in between each process should also be treated. Care must be taken to ensure that the ciliary process is treated and not the adjacent iris tissue (**Fig. 36.3**). In contrast to performing the TCP, the surgeon should use the visible whitening and shrinkage of the ciliary processes as the end point of treatment and avoid any inadvertent "pops" or explosion of the ciliary processes. At the end of the procedure, all the viscoelastic

must be thoroughly removed using either automated or manual irrigation and aspiration methods to prevent postoperative IOP spikes.

When ECP is performed through a posterior pars plana approach, the technique is modified. This approach can only be performed in aphakic and pseudophakic eyes. The surgeon sits superiorly and a conjunctival peritomy is made nasally and temporally. Sclerostomies are then made 3 to 3.5 mm posterior to the limbus using a 20-gauge myringovitreoretinal (MVR) blade or keratome. An anterior chamber maintainer supplies infusion during the procedure. Endoscope-guided vitrectomy is then typically performed prior to the ECP using the same sclerotomies. After the completion of the vitrectomy, the ECP probe is placed through one of the sclerotomies and advanced until the ciliary processes are visualized. This approach typically facilitates visualization of all of the ciliary processes as well as the pars plana, which enables greater and more effective treatment. Treatment, therefore, needs to be titrated to ensure the patient does not develop hypotony.

Additional Considerations and Surgical Tips

- The amount of energy delivered to an individual ciliary process is determined by the proximity of the probe to the tissue target as well as the duration of treatment and the power level.
- The ciliary sulcus must be widely expanded with a viscoelastic that pushes the iris anteriorly to the cornea and the lens posteriorly. A poorly inflated sulcus will result in inadequate treatment and trauma to the iris (**Fig. 36.4**).
- While treating the ciliary processes, it is recommended to let the laser "soak in" after the initial whitening and shrinkage of the process to achieve a greater reduction in the IOP. However, be careful not to overtreat, which results in the process exploding with a "pop" and causing greater postoperative inflammation.
- In unicameral or fully vitrectomized eyes with aphakia, an anterior chamber maintainer is typically needed to keep the eye pressurized during the procedure (**Fig. 36.5**).

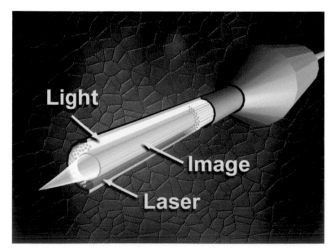

a

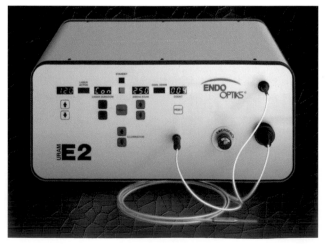

b

Fig. 36.1 **(a)** Illustration of the endoprobe with fiberoptic light source, camera, treating diode laser, and aiming beam. **(b)** Photograph of the endolaser console with display, showing *(left to right)* laser power, laser duration set to continuous, activation indicator, aiming beam power, and number of spots. There are three ports for the illumination, camera, and laser.

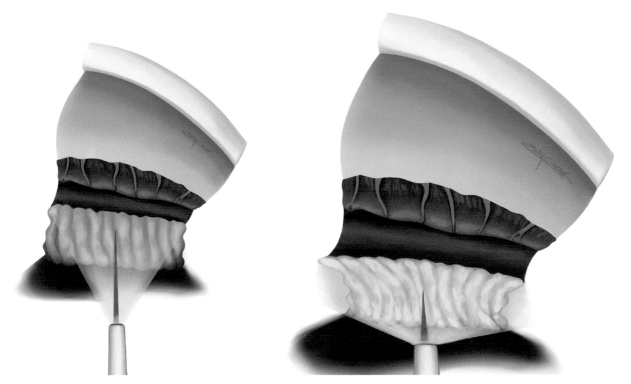

Fig. 36.2 Photograph of the endoscopic view of the ciliary processes illustrating the correct orientation and distance for treatment. Note the posterior iris superiorly with ciliary processes below followed by pars plana and intraocular lens.

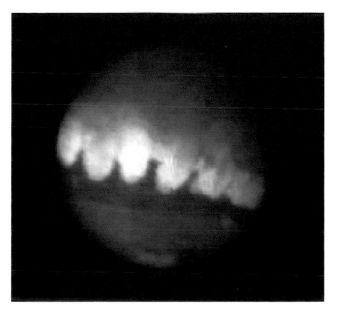

Fig. 36.3 Photograph of the endoscopic view of overaggressive treatment that includes the posterior surface of the iris. This will result in more postoperative inflammation and may cause pupil irregularity.

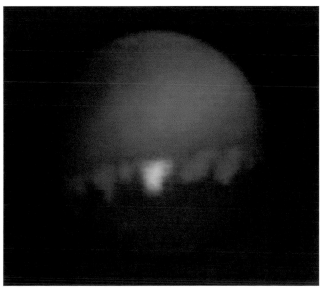

Fig. 36.4 Photograph of the endoscopic view of a poorly inflated sulcus that results in inadequate visualization and treatment of the ciliary processes.

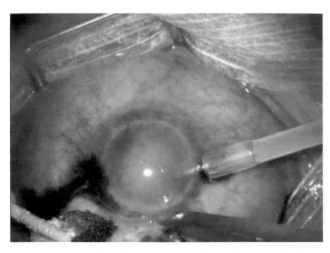

Fig. 36.5 Anterior chamber maintainer used in endoscopic cyclophotocoagulation (ECP) via a pars plana approach or in ECP in post-vitrectomized aphakic or unicameral eyes.

- When treating greater than 270 degrees, a second incision placed 90 to 180 degrees away from the first incision is helpful for accessing all the ciliary processes. In situations where phacoemulsification cataract surgery is combined with ECP, the second incision could be a previously placed paracentesis that can then be enlarged to accommodate the endoscope.
- The endoscope tip should be wiped cleaned each time it is withdrawn from the eye, and additional viscoelastic should be added to the anterior chamber and sulcus space to improve the view and access to the ciliary processes.
- Scleral depression may facilitate a more complete treatment during an anterior approach by providing greater access to the ciliary processes and the areas in between that contain ciliary epithelium.
- Anesthetic placement using a retrobulbar, peribulbar, or sub-Tenon's approach is typically needed to provide adequate anesthesia for the procedure and to keep the patient from feeling discomfort.
- If intracameral anesthetic is used, it should be flushed directly into the ciliary sulcus space. This may be inadequate for anything greater than a light treatment.

Complications

Endoscopic cyclophotocoagulation has been shown to have a good safety profile, especially in comparison with transscleral cyclophotocoagulation or cryoablation.

A retrospective study by Chen et al[10] in patients with refractory glaucoma who underwent ECP found that the most common complications with the procedure were fibrin exudates (24%), hyphema (12%), cystoid macular edema (10%), and vision loss of more than two Snellen lines (6%). Most of these complications were amenable to treatment in the postoperative period, especially with aggressive postoperative steroids as well as anti-inflammatory treatment. In addition, it is important to identify patients at higher risk of inflammation (diabetics, patients with angle-closure glaucoma or uveitis) and treat them more aggressively with anti-inflammatory medications in the postoperative period to minimize these complications.

Other potential complications include risk of damage to the iris either through mechanical trauma or inappropriate application of laser energy to the iris.[11] This can usually be avoided by adequate inflation of the ciliary sulcus. Choroidal effusions have also been noted.[12] These may be a result of intraoperative hypotony, especially in aphakic or unicameral patients. Using an anterior chamber maintainer can help minimize this complication. Another potential cause is uveal inflammation following the procedure, which should be treated with aggressive but short-term anti-inflammatory medications. In phakic patients, there is always a risk of violating the lens capsule. It is recommended that only the most experienced surgeons perform ECP on phakic patients, and only on those patients with a deep anterior chamber that allows good inflation of the sulcus space. Because the ECP probe cannot be visualized via the microscopy during the treatment, there is the possibility of the probe causing damage to the iris or corneal endothelium without the surgeon being aware of it. A case report in the literature presents a patient whose iris adhesion to the treatment probe resulted in aniridia.[13]

A theoretical complication is sympathetic ophthalmia because there is a breakdown of the blood–aqueous barrier while performing the procedure. However, there have been no reported cases of this occurring in the ECP literature, although cases have been reported with TCP. In a retrospective case series, a total of six patients were noted to present with sympathetic ophthalmia, an incidence rate of 0.001% following transscleral cyclophotocoagulation. However, all of these eyes had previously undergone at least one other surgical procedure, and two eyes had also experienced prior trauma.[14] Hypotony and phthisis bulbi are also potential complications of ECP that the surgeon needs to aware of, especially in patients who are undergoing more aggressive treatment using the posterior-segment approach. Studies of TCP patients have shown that there is a dose–response relationship with the degree of energy applied and hypotony.[15] In high-risk patients undergoing ECP, care must be taken to ensure that one to three clock positions of ciliary processes are left untreated so that some aqueous production remains. The case of a patient with underlying rheumatologic disorder who undergoes TCP and subsequently develops necrotizing scleritis has been reported,[16] and the risk of similar complications likely exists in similar patient populations.

Postoperative Management

Depending on the level of treatment and the patient's ocular status, ECP can induce variable but significant degrees of inflammation. Aggressive management of this inflammation plays a key role in postoperative care to achieve success while minimizing inflammation-related complications. Typically, patients receive intracameral steroids and optionally systemic steroids at the time of the procedure. Frequent use of topical steroids administered every hour may be necessary for the first few days after the procedure. On occasion, patients may also benefit from a short course of oral steroids.

Management of steroid use, however, needs to be tailored to the degree of inflammation that is noted postoperatively. This is important because many of the patients who have glaucoma can be steroid responders, and use of steroids can mask the IOP-lowering effects of ECP. Therefore, once inflammation is under control, steroids should be tapered. This can be done with the concurrent use of nonsteroidal anti-inflammatory drugs to prevent rebound inflammation.

Safety, Efficacy, and Clinical Results

There are reports in the literature of ECP being successfully utilized across various patient populations, either as a stand-alone procedure or as an adjunct to phacoemulsification or filtering surgeries in mild, moderate, and refractory glaucomas. When ECP was first introduced, it was used primarily for refractive cases or end-stage cases. In the initial study utilizing ECP, Uram[3] demonstrated its efficacy in 10 patients with neovascular glaucoma.

Advanced Glaucoma Treatment

Chen et al[10] performed a retrospective study of ECP in 68 eyes with refractory glaucoma (defined as elevated IOP despite maximally tolerated medical therapy, and a history of failed filtering procedure or previous TCP). They reported a 90% success rate (as defined by IOP < 21 mm Hg) at 1-year follow-up. These eyes underwent 180 to 360 degrees of endoscopic cyclophotocoagulation, with the majority through a limbal incision but a few through a pars plana approach. The ECP-treated eyes demonstrated a reduction in mean IOP from 27.7 mm Hg to 17.0 mm Hg over a 12-month follow-up period. In addition, there was a statistically significant reduction in the number of glaucoma medications (an average of one less glaucoma mediation). More importantly, none of the treated eyes suffered major complications such as hypotony or phthisis.

An early randomized study by Gayton et al[11] compared the effectiveness of cataract surgery combined with trabeculectomy versus cataract surgery combined with ECP as the primary surgical treatment for glaucoma. Fifty-eight eyes were randomized to the two groups and were followed over a 2-year period. IOP control was defined as < 19 mm Hg. The two groups achieved comparable success in IOP reduction without the need for additional medications (40% of eyes treated with combined cataract surgery and trabeculectomy versus 30% of eyes treated with combined cataract surgery and ECP). Additionally, rates of treatment failure between the two groups were also comparable, with three eyes in the trabeculectomy group and four eyes in the ECP group needing additional surgical intervention at the end of the study period.

A prospective study by Lima et al[12] compared Ahmed drainage implantation versus ECP in eyes with prior failed trabeculectomy with antimetabolite. The two groups achieved equivalent IOP lowering, with the IOP in the Ahmed group lowered from a preoperative average of 41.3 mm Hg to 14.7 mm Hg postoperative, and in the ECP group from a preoperative average of 41.6 mm Hg to 14.1 mm Hg postoperative. However, compared with the ECP group, the Ahmed group had a higher rate of postoperative complications (choroidal detachment, shallow anterior chamber, hyphema).

The ECP procedure has also been studied in patients with refractory glaucoma following previously implanted aqueous drainage implant. Francis et al[17] conducted a prospective study in 25 eyes with uncontrolled IOP despite maximally tolerated medical therapy and a previously implanted, functional Baerveldt 350-mm^2 aqueous shunt. All eyes underwent 360-degree ECP treatment and were followed for up to 2 years. At 1-year follow-up, the mean IOP decreased by 30.8% from the preoperative 24.0 mm Hg to 15.7 mm Hg postoperative. There was a significant reduction in the number of topical medications needed to control IOP from 3.2 preoperative to 1.5 postoperative. Again, similar to the other studies mentioned thus far, no major complications were noted. Transscleral diode laser has been successfully utilized to treat refractory glaucoma and pseudoexfoliation glaucoma, even as primary therapy,[18] and ECP likely will be just as successful with likely fewer side effects and complications.

ECP Plus

The ECP-plus procedure entails a pars plana approach with treatment of the pars plana (**Fig. 36.6**). Its use in ultra-refractory glaucoma was reported in 20165 by Tan et al[19] in a retrospective, noncomparative, interventional case series . The patient population included 53 eyes of 53 consecutive patients who had failed multiple glaucoma surgeries, including trabeculectomy and aqueous tube shunt. The mean preoperative IOP dropped from 27.9 to 10.2 at 6 months and 10.7 at 12 months. The cumulative treatment success was 81% at 6 months and 78% at 12 months. The number of medications fell from 3.4 ± 1.2 pretreatment to 0.8 ± 1.0 at 1 to 6 months and 0.7 ± 1.2 at 12 months postoperatively. Early complications included hypotony, fibrinous uveitis, and cystoid macular edema. Late complications occurred in 16% of subjects and included hypotony, choroidal detachment, cystoid macular edema (CME) without hypotony, and failed corneal graft.[19]

Endoscopic Cycloplasty and Lens Extraction for Plateau Iris Syndrome

The treatment of severe plateau iris syndrome with lens extraction and endoscopic cycloplasty (ECPL) (**Fig. 36.7**) was described in a prospective case series by Francis et al[20] of 12 eyes of

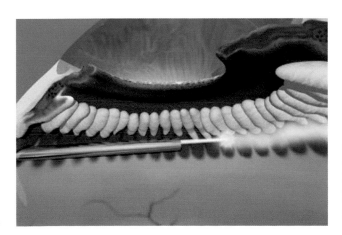

a

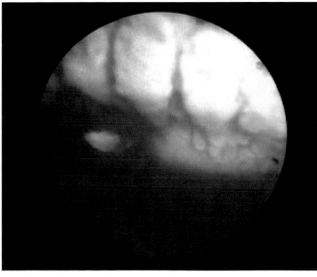

b

Fig. 36.6 ECP-plus procedure. **(a)** Endoscopic treatment of the ciliary processes and pars plana. **(b)** Image as viewed through the monitor.

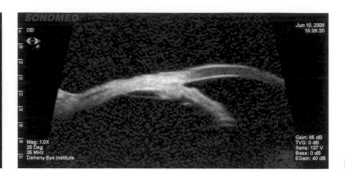

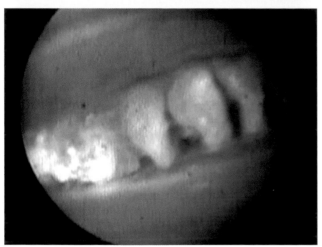

Fig. 36.7 Endoscopic cycloplasty and lens extraction for plateau iris syndrome. **(a)** Preoperative ultrasound biomicroscopy of the shallow anterior chamber angle with appositional closure. Note the prominent and anteriorly rotated ciliary process pushing the peripheral iris anteriorly. **(b)** Postoperative ultrasound biomicroscopy showing a greatly widened anterior chamber angle with no appositional closure. The treated ciliary process has been flattened and shrunken. **(c)** Photograph through the endoscope showing treatment of the large, anteriorly rotated processes in severe plateau iris syndrome. Note the treated processes *(left)* and the untreated processes *(right)*.

six patients with plateau iris refractory to laser iridotomy and iridoplasty, miotic and other glaucoma medical treatment, with appositional angle closure in at least three quadrants. The surgery consisted of lens extraction and ECPL, and an endoscopic diode laser treatment of the ciliary processes in the superior, nasal, and inferior quadrants. Ultrasound biomicroscopy (UBM) measurement parameters included anterior chamber depth (ACD), angle opening distance (AOD 500), trabecular ciliary process distance (TCPD), iris ciliary process distance (ICPD), iris depth (ID), iridocorneal angle (ICA), and sulcus angle (SA). Four novel measurements included ciliary process thickness (CPT), ciliary process width (CPW), ciliary process area (CPA), and iris ciliary process contact length (ICPCL). The ACD, AOD 500, and ICA all increased significantly ($p < 0.001$). ICPD, CPT, CPW, CPA, and ICPL all decreased significantly ($p < 0.01$). Parameters remaining unchanged were the TCPD, ID, and SA. The untreated quadrants showed measurements similar to the preoperative measurements, supporting the assertion that the effect seems to be mostly from the laser treatment rather than from the lens extraction alone. Similar results have also been demonstrated by Ahmed et al.[21]

ECP and Cataract Extraction in Mild-to-Moderate Glaucoma

The ECP procedure has been used successfully in combination with phacoemulsification for management of mild-to-moderate glaucoma, and this has been demonstrated in various studies. In patients undergoing phacoemulsification cataract surgery combined with ECP, Kahook et al[22] compared the effectiveness of 240- to 300-degree ECP treatment using one-site corneal incision versus 360-degree ECP treatment using two-site corneal incision. Both treatments were very effective in lowering IOP,

but greater ECP treatment (360 degrees) yielded greater IOP reduction. This study demonstrated that two-site 360-degree ECP treatment resulted in a 47% decrease in mean IOP (to 13 mm Hg) compared with the single-site 240- to 300-degree ECP treatment, which showed a 32% decrease in mean IOP (to 16 mm Hg). Even though larger treatment area yielded more significant IOP lowering, there were no differences in the rate of complications (including hypotony) between the two groups.

A recent study by Francis et al[23] compared phacoemulsification combined with ECP versus phacoemulsification alone in patients with medically controlled glaucoma. Eighty patients were matched in both groups in this prospective nonrandomized study and followed for a 2-year period. Patients in the ECP group had a decrease in mean IOP from 18.1 mm Hg to 16.0 mm Hg at 1 and 2 years postoperative compared with the phacoemulsification-alone group, which demonstrated a decrease from 18.1 mm Hg to 17.5 mm Hg at 1 year and to 17.3 mm Hg at 2 years. In addition to achieving greater IOP reduction, the phaco plus ECP group also needed fewer glaucoma medications for IOP control at both 1- and 2-year follow-up.

The TCP procedure has been shown to be effective in the treatment of chronic angle-closure glaucoma that is medically uncontrolled,[24] and ECP can be an equally effective option in such cases and in other glaucoma cases where filtration surgery is not an easy option.[25]

Overall, the clinical data demonstrate that ECP can be applied to treat all stages of glaucoma from mild to refractory in a safe and effective manner. Additionally, it can be performed through a small incision in stand-alone cases, or through the phacoemulsification cataract incision in combined cases. ECP does not involve manipulation of the sclera or conjunctiva, allowing these tissues to be preserved for future surgical procedures.

Pediatric Glaucoma

In addition to treatment in adults, ECP has also been utilized successfully in the pediatric population. Although the primary treatment of congenital glaucoma is often successful using either goniotomy or trabeculotomy, refractory cases of glaucoma can be difficult to manage in this patient population.

One of the earliest reports, by Neely and Plager[26] in 2001, studied 36 eyes of pediatric patients who had undergone ECP for uncontrolled IOP. At an average of 19 months following treatment, patients were noted to have a 30% decrease in IOP from 35.1 mm Hg to 23.6 mm Hg. Many of the patients had undergone more than one treatment with an average of 260 degrees. Complications included hypotony and retinal detachment, all of which occurred in patients who were aphakic.

Another retrospective study by Carter et al[27] evaluated the safety and efficacy of ECP in children with glaucoma who were aphakic or pseudophakic. Thirty-four eyes of patients who developed glaucoma following cataract extraction were included in the study and underwent ECP for IOP control. Of note, patients with congenital glaucoma or anterior segment dysgenesis were excluded from the study. The average number of interventions per eye was 1.5, and over the mean follow-up period of 44.4 months the IOP was lowered by 9.7 mm Hg (29.7%). The main complication that was noted was retinal detachment in the aphakic eyes, with two eyes developing detachments within the first month of treatment. The study also demonstrated that ECP could be safely repeated in this population without risk of hypotony.

The ECP procedure has been utilized effectively in the pediatric population with concurrent glaucoma and corneal opacities. Al-Haddad and Freedman[28] performed ECP on 12 eyes with glaucoma and corneal opacities (including Peters anomaly, anterior segment dysgenesis with corneal scar, and failed corneal transplants). Ten of the 12 eyes had previously received external cycloablation for IOP control. Approximately six clock positions were treated with ECP, and the IOP was lowered from a baseline of 36.8 mm Hg to 28.2 mm Hg and was not found to be statistically significant. However, in four patients who failed treatment, defined as IOP > 21 mm Hg with or without medications, tube shunt surgery was performed, and the endoscope of the ECP unit was utilized to guide tube placement/positioning in three of those cases.

A recent study by Kraus et al[29] compared the safety and effectiveness of TCP and ECP in pediatric glaucoma. This retrospective study found similar rates of IOP reduction between the two procedures, 28.6% in TCP compared with 33.2% in ECP without significant differences in rates of complications. A case report by Barkana et al[30] highlighted one of the main advantages of ECP, which is that it enables real-time visualization and tissue-specific treatment compared with lack of visualization leading to nonspecific treatment with TCP. In a patient who had previously been treated with TCP unsuccessfully, direct visualization using the endoscope during the subsequent ECP procedure demonstrated that the previous TCP treatment had been inadvertently directed at the pars plana instead of at the ciliary processes.

Other Anterior Segment Endoscopic Procedures

In addition to the ECP procedure, the endoscope surgical system can be used for internal ocular viewing to assist a variety of anterior segment surgeries, as summarized in a review paper.[9] In the anterior chamber angle, the endoscope can be used to perform cyclodialysis cleft repair, lysis of goniosynechiae, goniot-

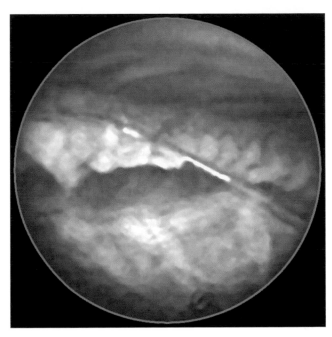

Fig. 36.8 Secondary intraocular lens (IOL) implantation. Endoscopic view of the IOL haptic in the ciliary sulcus space. The endoscope facilitates viewing the haptic position, the amount of posterior and anterior capsule remaining, and the integrity of the zonular support. (Reproduced with permission from Francis BA, Kwon J, Fellman R, et al. Endoscopic ophthalmic surgery of the anterior segment. Surv Ophthalmol 2014;59:217–231.)

omy in pediatric glaucoma, and goniopuncture or trabeculotomy in adult open-angle glaucoma. In the ciliary sulcus space, it can be helpful in the evaluation and treatment of hypotony to view the ciliary processes, and remove any cyclitic membranes that can cause ciliary body detachment and hyposecretion of aqueous. When placing an aqueous tube shunt in the ciliary sulcus, the endoscope can view the entry site and verify positioning of the tube and if the tip is clear. During complex cataract extraction or secondary intraocular lens (IOL) implantation, the endoscope provides direct viewing of the IOL position and verification of capsular support and zonular compromise (**Fig. 36.8**). In uveitis glaucoma hyphema syndrome, the endoscope can aid in viewing the position of the IOL and its contact with the iris or uveal tissue in the sulcus. If abnormal blood vessels are seen, they can be coagulated with the laser (**Fig. 36.9**). Additionally, a case report demonstrated that ECP can be an effective treatment for malignant glaucoma that has failed standard medical and laser treatments.[31]

Cost-Effectiveness

In addition to the clinical effectiveness, ECP has been shown to be one of the most cost-effective minimally invasive procedures for treatment of glaucoma. A study by Iordanous et al[32] compared the cost savings associated with Trabectome ab interno trabeculotomy (NeoMedix, CA), iStent micro-bypass stent (Glaukos, CA), and ECP versus monodrug, bi-drug, and tri-drug glaucoma therapy over a 6-year period in Canada. ECP had a total cost savings of $779.23, $2072.55, and $2924.71 per patient versus monodrug, bi-drug, and tri-drug therapy, respectively. This cost savings was greater for each group when compared with the Trabectome and iStent groups. The study was also able to demonstrate that when successful, ECP could provide a per-patient cost reduction at as early as 2 years. In addition to its cost-effectiveness,

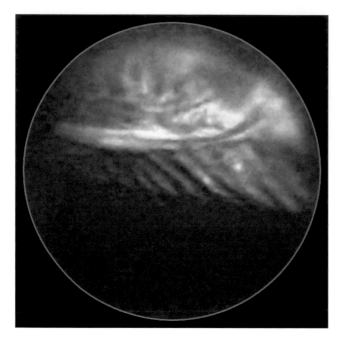

Fig. 36.9 Uveitis glaucoma hyphema syndrome. This endoscopic illustration of a pars plana approach shows the IOL in the sulcus space surrounded by a fibrovascular membrane. Recent bleeding is seen anterior to the lens haptic. To prevent further bleeding, the membrane must be removed and the lens may need to be removed or suture fixated more posteriorly. (Reproduced with permission from Francis BA, Kwon J, Fellman R, et al. Endoscopic ophthalmic surgery of the anterior segment. Surv Ophthalmol 2014;59: 217–231.)

ECP also helps eliminate the issue of patient compliance, and may also provide other indirect benefits to patients such as reduced side effects from medication use and overall improvement in quality of life.[32]

Case Presentations

Case 1: Combined Cataract Extraction and ECP in Mild-to-Moderate Glaucoma

A 74-year-old Caucasian man presented with mild-to-moderate primary open-angle glaucoma. His best corrected visual acuity is 20/50 OU with visually significant nuclear sclerotic and cortical cataracts bilaterally. His IOP is 15 mm Hg OU on two topical agents. His optic nerve cup-to-disk ratio is 0.7–0.75 OU. He is mostly compliant with his medications, but forgets to take them occasionally.

The patient undergoes surgery with combined cataract extraction, placement of IOLs, and endocyclophotocoagulation. Following surgery, the glaucoma medications were continued until the first month and then stopped sequentially after the topical steroid was discontinued. The best corrected visual acuity is 20/20 in both eyes. IOP remains 15 to 17 mm Hg on no glaucoma medications.

Case 2: ECP-Plus Procedure in Severe Refractory Glaucoma

A 66-year-old African-American woman presents with a prior history of corneal ulcer with two subsequent, failed penetrating keratoplasties in the right eye. The current graft is opacified with corneal neovascularization. She is pseudophakic and has previously undergone two aqueous drainage implants. Her vision is hand-motions only, and the IOP is uncontrolled at 46 mm Hg on maximum tolerated glaucoma medications, including oral carbonic anhydrase inhibitors. There is no view through the opacified cornea.

The patient undergoes a pars plana vitrectomy via the endoscopic approach combined with a pars plana ECP plus for her refractory glaucoma. Following surgery, she is able to discontinue the oral carbonic anhydrase inhibitors and the IOP drops to 14 mm Hg on two topical glaucoma medications. The vision remains hand-motions only with the opacified cornea. She is now undergoing evaluation for repeat corneal transplant versus keratoprosthesis procedure.

Case 3: Endoscopic Cycloplasty and Cataract Extraction in Severe Plateau Iris Syndrome

A 56-year-old Chinese American hyperopic woman presents with occludable narrow angles with evidence of plateau iris configuration and appositional angle closure confirmed on ultrasound biomicroscopy. She has previously undergone laser peripheral iridotomy as well as laser iridoplasty in both eyes, which have failed to open her narrow angles, placing her at continued risk of primary angle-closure glaucoma. Her visual acuity is 20/30 with a moderate combined nuclear and cortical cataract. She is currently not on any glaucoma medications and her IOP is 15 mm Hg OU. Additionally, her optic nerves have a cup-to-disk ratio of 0.5 without notching or rim thinning.

The patient undergoes combined cataract extraction in each eye with placement of an IOL (to address her pupillary block component of narrow angles) combined with ECPL to help treat the recalcitrant plateau iris component. After surgery, the IOP remains in the mid-teens on no glaucoma medications. Her vision improves to 20/20 best corrected. Her anterior chambers are now deep and the angle is open to grade 3 to 4 without apposition.

References

1. Bietti G. Surgical intervention on the ciliary body; new trends for the relief of glaucoma. J Am Med Assoc 1950;142:889–897
2. Beckman H, Kinoshita A, Rota AN, Sugar HS. Transscleral ruby laser irradiation of the ciliary body in the treatment of intractable glaucoma. Trans Am Acad Ophthalmol Otolaryngol 1972;76:423–436
3. Uram M. Combined phacoemulsification, endoscopic ciliary process photocoagulation, and intraocular lens implantation in glaucoma management. Ophthalmic Surg 1995;26:346–352
4. Lin SC, Chen MJ, Lin MS, Howes E, Stamper RL. Vascular effects on ciliary tissue from endoscopic versus trans-scleral cyclophotocoagulation. Br J Ophthalmol 2006;90:496–500
5. Uram M. Endoscopic cyclophotocoagulation in glaucoma management. Curr Opin Ophthalmol 1995;6:19–29
6. Pantcheva MB, Kahook MY, Schuman JS, Noecker RJ. Comparison of acute structural and histopathological changes in human autopsy eyes after endoscopic cyclophotocoagulation and trans-scleral cyclophotocoagulation. Br J Ophthalmol 2007;91:248–252
7. Alvarado J, Francis B. Characteristics of ciliary body lesions after endoscopic and transscleral laser cyclophotocoagulation. Poster presented at the American Academy of Ophthalmology meeting, New Orleans, November 1998
8. Lin SC. Endoscopic and transscleral cyclophotocoagulation for the treatment of refractory glaucoma. J Glaucoma 2008;17:238–247
9. Francis BA, Kwon J, Fellman R, et al. Endoscopic ophthalmic surgery of the anterior segment. Surv Ophthalmol 2014;59:217–231
10. Chen J, Cohn RA, Lin SC, Cortes AE, Alvarado JA. Endoscopic photocoagulation of the ciliary body for treatment of refractory glaucomas. Am J Ophthalmol 1997;124:787–796

11. Gayton JL, Van Der Karr M, Sanders V. Combined cataract and glaucoma surgery: trabeculectomy versus endoscopic laser cycloablation. J Cataract Refract Surg 1999;25:1214–1219

12. Lima FE, Magacho L, Carvalho DM, Susanna R Jr, Avila MP. A prospective, comparative study between endoscopic cyclophotocoagulation and the Ahmed drainage implant in refractory glaucoma. J Glaucoma 2004;13:233–237

13. Gayton JL. Traumatic aniridia during endoscopic laser cycloablation. J Cataract Refract Surg 1998;24:134–135

14. Albahlal A, Al Dhibi H, Al Shahwan S, Khandekar R, Edward DP. Sympathetic ophthalmia following diode laser cyclophotocoagulation. Br J Ophthalmol 2014;98:1101–1106

15. Murphy CC, Burnett CA, Spry PG, Broadway DC, Diamond JP. A two centre study of the dose-response relation for transscleral diode laser cyclophotocoagulation in refractory glaucoma. Br J Ophthalmol 2003;87:1252–1257

16. Shen SY, Lai JS, Lam DS. Necrotizing scleritis following diode laser transscleral cyclophotocoagulation. Ophthalmic Surg Lasers Imaging 2004;35:251–253

17. Francis BA, Kawji AS, Vo NT, Dustin L, Chopra V. Endoscopic cyclophotocoagulation (ECP) in the management of uncontrolled glaucoma with prior aqueous tube shunt. J Glaucoma 2011;20:523–527

18. Grueb M, Rohrbach JM, Bartz-Schmidt KU, Schlote T. Transscleral diode laser cyclophotocoagulation as primary and secondary surgical treatment in primary open-angle and pseudoexfoliative glaucoma. Long-term clinical outcomes. Graefes Arch Clin Exp Ophthalmol 2006;244:1293–1299

19. Tan JC, Francis BA, Noecker R, Uram M, Dustin L, Chopra V. Endoscopic cyclophotocoagulation and pars plana ablation (ECP-Plus) to treat refractory glaucoma. J Glaucoma 2016;25:e117–e122

20. Francis BA, Pouw A, Jenkins D, et al. Endoscopic cycloplasty (ECPL) and lens extraction in the treatment of severe plateau iris syndrome. J Glaucoma 2015; 2016;25:e128–e133

21. Ahmed IK, Podbielski DW, Naqi A, et al. Endoscopic cycloplasty in angle closure glaucoma secondary to plateau iris. Poster presentation at the American Glaucoma Society annual meeting, San Diego, March 5–8, 2009

22. Kahook MY, Lathrop KL, Noecker RJ. One-site versus two-site endoscopic cyclophotocoagulation. J Glaucoma 2007;16:527–530

23. Francis BA, Berke SJ, Dustin L, Noecker R. Endoscopic cyclophotocoagulation combined with phacoemulsification alone in medically controlled glaucoma. J Cataract Refract Surg 2014;40:1313–1321

24. Lai JS, Tham CC, Chan JC, Lam DS. Diode laser transscleral cyclophotocoagulation as primary surgical treatment for medically uncontrolled chronic angle closure glaucoma: long-term clinical outcomes. J Glaucoma 2005;14:114–119

25. Huang G, Lin SC. When should we give up filtration surgery: indications, techniques and results of cyclodestruction. Dev Ophthalmol 2012;50:173–183

26. Neely DE, Plager DA. Endocyclophotocoagulation for management of difficult pediatric glaucomas. J AAPOS 2001;5:221–229

27. Carter BC, Plager DA, Neely DE, Sprunger DT, Sondhi N, Roberts GJ. Endoscopic diode laser cyclophotocoagulation in the management of aphakic and pseudophakic glaucoma in children. J AAPOS 2007;11:34–40

28. Al-Haddad CE, Freedman SF. Endoscopic laser cyclophotocoagulation in pediatric glaucoma with corneal opacities. J AAPOS 2007;11:23–28

29. Kraus CL, Tychsen L, Lueder GT, Culican SM. Comparison of the effectiveness and safety of transscleral cyclophotocoagulation and endoscopic cyclophotocoagulation in pediatric glaucoma. J Pediatr Ophthalmol Strabismus 2014;51:120–127

30. Barkana Y, Morad Y, Ben-nun J. Endoscopic photocoagulation of the ciliary body after repeated failure of trans-scleral diode-laser cyclophotocoagulation. Am J Ophthalmol 2002;133:405–407

31. Muqit MM, Menage MJ. Malignant glaucoma after phacoemulsification: treatment with diode laser cyclophotocoagulation. J Cataract Refract Surg 2007;33:130–132

32. Iordanous Y, Kent JS, Hutnik CML, Malvankar-Mehta MS. Projected cost comparison of Trabectome, iStent, and endoscopic cyclophotocoagulation versus glaucoma medication in the Ontario Health Insurance Plan. J Glaucoma 2014;23.e112–e110

37   Translimbal Collagen Implant: AqueSys XEN Gel Stent

Herbert A. Reitsamer, Markus Lenzhofer, Melchior Hohensinn, Arsham Sheybani, Iqbal Ike K. Ahmed, and Vanessa Vera

Case Presentation

A 58-year-old Caucasian man with progressive primary open-angle glaucoma treated with topical prostaglandin analogue and a beta-blocker presented with increasing intraocular pressure (IOP) in his left eye with questionable adherence to the therapy. The decision to recommend surgery was supported by the patient's increasing discomfort with various prostaglandin analogues. Preoperative IOPs were 19 mm Hg OD and 26 mm Hg OS. Gonioscopy revealed a medium deep anterior chamber with a Shaffer angle grade 2 (**Fig. 37.1a [bottom]**), and visual acuity was 20/20 in both eyes. **Fig. 37.2** shows the visual field data and the optic disk topography both preoperatively and 5 years after surgery for both eyes.

In a day-clinic setting, surgery with the XEN Gel Stent (AqueSys Inc., Aliso Viejo, CA) was performed with local anesthesia. Two weeks before the surgery, the patient started treatment with preservative-free topical corticosteroids t.i.d. and topical glaucoma therapy was replaced by systemic carbonic anhydrase inhibitor (250 mg o.d.). Before implantation of the XEN Gel Stent, an off-target-site injection of 10 µg mitomycin C (0.1 mL solution) into the sub-Tenon's space was performed. To remain as nontraumatic as possible, the mitomycin depot was repositioned from the injection site into the target zone by directional massage with a cotton swab. The stent was then implanted into the superior nasal quadrant without complications (**Fig. 37.1b–d**). The patient was released on the same day of surgery and returned the next day for the first follow-up visit. No cycloplegia/pupil dilation was used in the postsurgical regimen. The day after surgery, the visual acuity was 18/20 and the IOP was 8 mm Hg. During the first 3 months, the highest IOP value was 14 mm Hg, which was followed by a consistent decrease until month 12. Final pressure after 5 years was between 11 and 12 mm Hg, with a beta-blocker (preservative free) and stable visual fields in both eyes. Visual acuity was stable at 20/20 from the first week after surgery on (**Fig. 37.1**).

The Procedure

The AqueSys XEN Gel Stent was introduced to provide a new form of filtration surgery for lowering IOP that meets the highest standards of safety and efficacy for the treatment of early as well as advanced glaucoma. Both glaucoma only as well as combined cataract–glaucoma procedures are within the field of application of the XEN Gel Stent. At present, more than 2,000 stents were implanted in patients with early to advanced glaucoma and the results are promising. Postsurgical follow-up is available up to 5 years with excellent safety and efficacy data.[1,2] So far, the XEN Gel Stent is the only ab interno device available that utilizes subconjunctival filtration for aqueous drainage.

Rationale Behind the Procedure

The XEN Gel Stent is a hydrophilic tube composed of a porcine gelatin and cross-linked with glutaraldehyde (**Fig. 37.3**). It decreases the IOP by creating a permanent outflow pathway from the anterior chamber to the subconjunctival space through which the aqueous humor can flow. From the subconjunctival space, the aqueous humor has numerous potential drainage pathways, including diffusion through the conjunctiva, diffusion into the venous system of the sclera and conjunctiva, as well as potential lymphatic pathways (**Fig. 37.3**).

During the implantation procedure, the stent is rigid and retains its straight form (which allows it to be implanted into sub-Tenon's space). Once in place, the stent immediately hydrates to become soft and highly flexible. As aqueous humor is introduced, the implant also swells to its final dimensions. This causes an increase in diameter, which prevents migration inside the implantation channel. Clinical findings demonstrate that the stent retains its position after implantation. The cross-linked collagen is durable and permanent, which provides a variety of desirable characteristics. The material has an extensive track record for medical use in a variety of geographic regions, including the European Union, the United States, Japan, and Canada. The XEN Gel Stent is made with gelatin that meets the compendium requirements of the European Pharmacopeia. The biocompatibility properties of gelatin are well established, and early clinical trials of the XEN Gel Stent also show a remarkable lack of foreign-body reactions in the human eye.[3]

The XEN Gel Stent has several key advantages when compared with other minimally invasive glaucoma therapies, as well as when compared with more traditional filtration procedures:

- The stent is implanted with a minimally invasive procedure with an excellent safety profile that reduces risk to the patient and minimizes damage from the surgery.
- The ab interno approach eliminates the need to surgically opening the conjunctiva and the need to perform scleral flap, thereby reducing postoperative inflammation and scarring.
- The procedure entails minimal damage to the conjunctiva and tissues, and multiple and repeatable implantations over the lifetime of the patient are feasible, if necessary.
- The procedure bypasses the trabecular meshwork, Schlemm's canal, and the collector channels entirely, thus avoiding the major structures of resistance for aqueous humor.
- The procedure entails low and diffuse outflow into intact tissue anatomy and drainage pathways in the

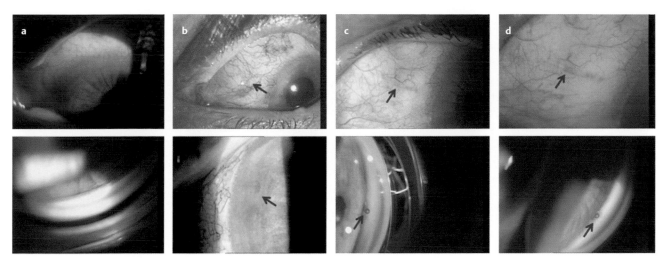

Fig. 37.1 Pre- and postoperative photographs of the area of implantation *(top row)* and the chamber angle *(bottom row)*. **(a)** Preoperative. **(b)** Postoperative day 1. **(c)** One year postoperative. **(d)** Five years postoperative. The stent *(arrows)* is clearly visible in the anterior chamber **(b)** as well as under the conjunctiva/Tenon's capsule and at the angle **(c,d)**. Even after 5 years, no biomicroscopical visible decay of the stent occurred. The bleb is not high and microcysts impose on its surface. Despite the small and flat conformation, sufficient efficacy of the bleb is observed in patients after XEN Gel Stent implantation.

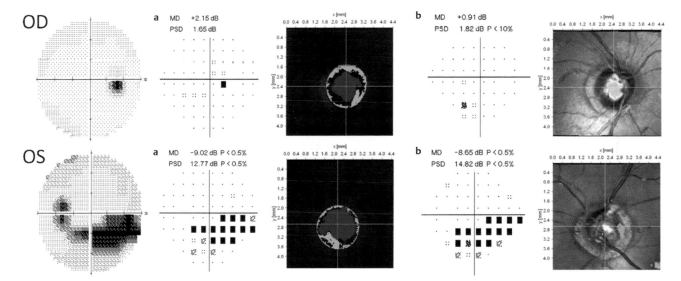

Fig. 37.2 Visual field with standard automated perimetry (Swedish Interactive Threshold Algorithms [SITA] standard) and Heidelberg Retina Tomograph II (HRTII) documentation of the right eye (OD, *top row*) and the left eye (OS, *bottom row*). **(a)** Preoperative exam with normal visual field parameters in the right eye and a typical Bjerrum scotoma in the left eye with corresponding loss of the neuroretinal rim in the optic disk tomography. **(b)** Five-year follow-up of the same patient. Mean deviation of the visual fields was stable over the follow-up period, which was confirmed by regression analysis. Pattern standard deviation increased from 12.77 to 14.82 dB (= 0.4 dB per year), but this increase was not statistically significant.

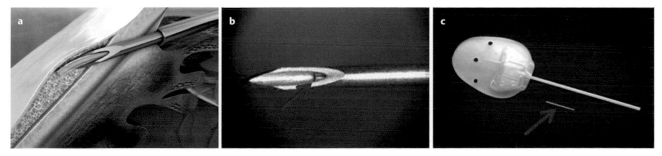

Fig. 37.3 **(a)** Drawing of a XEN 45 Gel Stent emerging from the XEN injector with 27-gauge cannula. **(b)** Photo of the injector cannula with the XEN 45 Gel Stent visible at the proximal end of the bevel. **(c)** The XEN 45 Gel Stent compared with the Ahmed valve, which uses a silicon tube as the connector to the anterior chamber.

conjunctiva, giving maximum efficacy pressure reduction.
- The current model, which has an inner diameter of 45 to 55 µm, avoids postoperative hypotony.

The laminar flow through a tube is calculated using the Hagen–Poiseuille equation. Using this equation, AqueSys has created three different versions of the XEN Gel Stent. The equation is as follows:

$$\Phi = \frac{dV}{dt} = v\pi R^2 = \frac{\pi R^4}{8\eta}\left(\frac{-\Delta P}{\Delta x}\right) = \frac{\pi R^4}{8\eta}\frac{|\Delta P|}{L}$$

where Φ = volumetric flow rate; ΔP = pressure difference between the two ends of the tube; η = dynamic fluid viscosity; L = length of the tube; R = internal radius of the lumen of the tube.

The Hagen-Poiseuille equation describes the relationship between the diameter and length of a tube and the resistance it develops when a fluid with certain properties passes through. This formula describes the hydrodynamic principle that the XEN Gel Stent's design is based on.

Table 37.1 shows different versions of the XEN Gel Stent. The XEN 140 and XEN 63 models entailed postoperative episodes of hypotony, but this does not occur with the latest version of the stent—the XEN 45.

Patient Selection

There are two important selection criteria for patients being considered for XEN Gel Stent implantation: (1) a chamber angle of Schaffer grade 2 or wider; and (2) the conjunctiva can accommodate bleb formation, which means that target zones with conjunctival scarring are not suitable for implantation. In combined cataract–glaucoma surgeries, the chamber angle is less of an issue because the lens is extracted before the XEN Gel Stent is implanted. A prospective clinical trial with narrow-angle patients has not yet been performed. However, patients with narrow angles have been implanted, and the early results suggest that the stent may be indicated in such cases; further studies will be required to confirm this. Until now, not many patients with uveitic glaucoma were treated with the XEN Gel Stent, and further experience with this group of patients also needs to be gained.

With the exception of the considerations mentioned above, any patient with a conjunctiva allowing for bleb formation is well suited for surgery with the XEN Gel Stent. This essentially means that if the conjunctiva and/or Tenon's capsule is scarred over due to previous surgeries or missing due to chemical burns or other trauma, the patient is not a candidate for filtration surgery. However, because the XEN Gel Stent gives rise to smaller blebs than does classic trabeculectomy, the exclusion criteria might be less strict.

The XEN implantation is performed in a day-clinic setting, and patients are discharged the same day of surgery. It is recommended that patients come in for a follow-up visit the next day, either at the day clinic or at their physician's office.

Surgical Technique

The implantation is performed from the inside of the anterior chamber (ab interno approach). This surgical approach is fundamentally different from other filtration surgeries currently used. The major advantage of an ab interno approach is conjunctiva preservation compared with approaches from outside the eye (ab externo), in which the conjunctiva needs to be dissected and displaced. The expectation from the minimally invasive XEN procedure is reduced scarring and reduced numbers of bleb failures.

The mechanism of action of the XEN procedure is fundamentally consistent with other full-thickness surgical treatments

Table 37.1 XEN Implant Model Variations by Internal Lumen Size

Name and Inner Diameter (ID)	Stent Length	Photo of the Stent
XEN 140 (~ 140 µm ID)	6 mm	
XEN 63 (~ 63 µm ID)	6 mm	
XEN 45 (~ 45 µm ID)	6 mm	

Note: During the development of the XEN Gel Stent, three different designs were used in clinical studies. Originally it was thought that higher diameters might serve better in advanced glaucoma, delivering lower intraocular pressures due to larger openings. The major disadvantage of the larger diameters (140 µm and 63 µm) is that over an implant length of 6 mm, the larger diameters do not add enough resistance to aqueous humor flow to avoid postoperative hypotony. For this reason, the two models were replaced by the XEN 45 Gel Stent, which is currently implanted worldwide. The XEN 45 adds enough resistance to aqueous flow to avoid hypotony after implantation in patients with roughly normal aqueous humor production (2–2.5 µL/min). Any local therapy that decreases aqueous production consequently lowers the pressure drop along the XEN Gel Stent, hence lowering intraocular pressure even further.

for glaucoma such as valved and nonvalved tube shunts and trabeculectomies (which, like XEN, bypass all potential outflow obstructions). However, it also mitigates several of the limitations of those technologies. The XEN Gel Stent maintains a microfistula between the anterior chamber and the subconjunctival space while the tissues surrounding the implant heal naturally. There is no need to create an iridotomy, and by introducing only a minimal amount of trauma, subsequent inflammation and fibrosis is minimized and many of the complications associated with more invasive procedures such as trabeculectomy and tube shunt implantation can be avoided.

During the course of development, the injector of the XEN Gel Stent underwent several changes in function and design; the current version is shown in **Fig. 37.4**. It can be operated with a single hand and the implantation can be performed with the surgeon positioned temporally **(Fig. 37.4a)** or superiorly **(Fig. 37.4b)** to the patient's head. A sliding mechanism moves various internal parts including the implantation needle to provide proper placement and handling of the implant. The device utilizes a small 27-gauge needle, and the injector is designed to both protect the XEN stent and to accurately place the implant into the correct anatomic location. It reaches from the anterior chamber (0.5 to 1.0 mm), through the angle, exits the sclera 2.5 to 3.5 mm posterior to the limbus, and extends into the subconjunctival and sub-Tenon's space (2.0 to 2.5 mm).

The preloaded/single-use injector comes individually packaged and sterile. After standard ophthalmic preparation is completed, the surgeon inserts the injector into the peripheral cornea and directs the needle across the anterior chamber to the angle to achieve the ideal scleral length of 3 mm **(Fig. 37.5a)**. The entry zone of the angle is a broad and forgiving area, giving the surgeon the flexibility of deciding whether to use gonioscopy during the procedure, in contrast to other minimally invasive glaucoma surgery (MIGS) procedures in which a specific target tissue landmark in the angle must be achieved. The needle can enter the

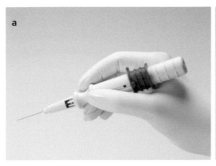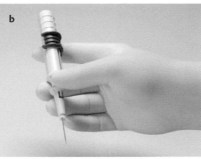

Fig. 37.4 Two ways of holding the XEN injector. **(a)** Handling of the injector with the surgeon's position temporal to the head of the patient (right eye). **(b)** Handling with the surgeon's position superior to the head of the patient (right eye). In both cases, the stent is advanced from temporal inferior toward superior. The stent is released by moving the blue slider toward the front of the implanter.

angle anywhere from the Schwalbe's line to the scleral spur **(Fig. 37.5b)**. The needle then goes through the sclera and into the sub-conjunctival/sub-Tenon's space, creating a slit as it cuts through the tissue.

As the needle bevel exits the sclera (~ 3 mm behind the limbus), the bevel angle is close to parallel with the conjunctiva tissue. This enables the Tenon and conjunctiva layers above the needle bevel to be pushed up versus being engaged in a penetrating fashion. As a result, perforating the conjunctiva with the needle bevel can be easily and consistently avoided. The surgeon is able to directly visualize the entire needle's bevel in the sub-conjunctival space through the surgical microscope **(Fig. 37.5c)**.

The physician then deploys the XEN Gel Stent, by actuating the slider on the single-handed injector, similar to an intraocular

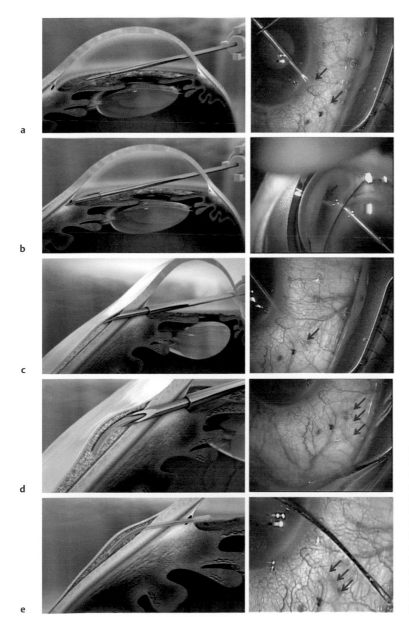

Fig. 37.5 Illustrations and photographs of the steps of the XEN implantation. **(a)** The injector tip is introduced into the anterior chamber via a 1-mm paracentesis. **(b)** The tip is aimed and introduced into the sclera at the height of the pigmented trabecular meshwork, and **(c)** advanced until the bevel can be seen emerging in the conjunctival/Tenon's side of the sclera *(arrow)*. The exit site should be roughly 3 mm behind the limbus. Step **b** can be performed with or without gonioscopy. After rotating the cannula of the implanter 60-degrees to the side, **(d)** the XEN Gel Stent is released into sub-Tenon's space *(arrows)*. **(e)** An automated withdrawal mechanism of the injector guarantees the correct proportions between the sub-Tenon's and the anterior chamber part of the XEN Gel Stent *(arrow)*: 1 mm in the anterior chamber, 3 mm intrascleral, 2 mm sub-Tenon's.

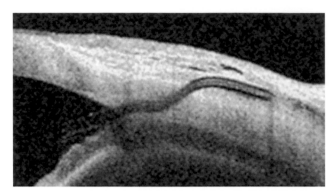

Fig. 37.6 Anterior-segment *optical coherence tomography* (OCT) of an in situ XEN 45 Gel Stent. Before and during implantation, the implant is rather rigid, which allows it to be directed into and through sub-Tenon's tissue backward from the limbus. Immediately after retraction of the implanter, hydration of the implant increases its flexibility and diameter, which prevents migration in the implantation canal. It also prevents erosions of the overlying conjunctival tissue, which can be a problem when using less flexible silicon tubing for implantation. Due to its high flexibility, the XEN Gel Stent adapts well to the distortion of the tissue during the implantation process, but sometimes these changes in pathway are caused on purpose. By lowering or lifting the tip of the implantation cannula, the surgeon can correct for deviations from the aimed exit site. The distortion of the tissue during implantation forms an S-shaped path that can nicely be observed in the computed tomography (CT) image.

lens (IOL) insertion procedure. During this step, the implant is slowly deployed into position by the internal mechanism of the implanter (**Fig. 37.5d**). Once the slider has been fully actuated, the procedure is complete and the needle is fully withdrawn into a sleeve, and the surgeon simply removes this blunt sleeve from the patient's eye (**Fig. 37.5e**). The stent immediately begins shunting fluid from the anterior chamber to the subconjunctival space after viscoelastic is removed (**Figs. 37.4** and **37.6**).

As body fluids come into contact with the XEN Gel Stent, the gelatin material becomes hydrated, soft, and flexible, and it expands; by the time the implant is placed in the final position, this swelling process is mostly complete. **Fig. 37.6** shows an anterior segment *optical coherence tomography* (OCT) demonstrating the location and flexibility of the implant. The expansion of the outer wall of the implant, as described in **Table 37.1**, in combination with the elastic nature of the tissue separated by the needle, holds the implant in position once the needle has been removed from the eye. A subconjunctival bleb forms upon implantation. Initially a classic bleb of the conjunctiva can be observed, but over the course of the first week, this bleb gradu-

ally reduces in volume as drainage pathways form from the subconjunctival space to the various outflow channels.[4,5]

Due to the small dimensions and mechanical attributes of the implant material, a gentle and diffuse dispersion of aqueous into Tenon's space and the subconjunctival space makes the morphology of an established, functioning bleb created by the XEN Gel Stent different from the blebs seen after filtering surgeries. The long-term appearance of the bleb is different from the bleb appearance after trabeculectomy.[1] Compared with blebs after trabeculectomy, XEN blebs are more uniform (with microcysts and generally no large cysts). The XEN blebs do not cover as much area, hence they are conjunctiva sparing, and, with little elevation, they cause less discomfort compared with larger and higher blebs.[1,2] The presence of microcysts throughout the epithelium adds further anatomic evidence to the fact that the aqueous humor moves transconjunctivally after filtration surgery, following the mechanism of filtration.[6,7]

In the majority of cases, the stent has been shown to create long-term effective IOP lowering without the use of antimetabolites such as mitomycin C at the time of surgery. Early glaucoma patients, without a long history of glaucoma drug usage, show remarkably low fibrosis rates and have great long-term function without the use of antimetabolites. However, the use of antimetabolites has shown better results, and the vast majority of implantations are now performed using pre-injections of mitomycin C (8 to 20 µg). The injection is performed before the implantation surgery starts. A mitomycin C depot is placed off the target site (**Fig. 37.7a,b**) and, using a cotton swab (**Fig. 37.7c**), is massaged into the region chosen for implantation (**Fig. 37.7d**). Mitomycin C or 5-fluorouracil (5-FU) can also be used as an adjuvant for postoperative needling procedures to improve the performance of the stent. This ability to tune the implant performance in the postoperative phase is another benefit of the XEN procedure (**Figs. 37.5** and **37.7**).

Glaucoma Surgery Only: Stand-Alone Procedure

The XEN Gel Stent was not designed as an add-on procedure to cataract surgery. The goal was to develop a safe, efficient, user-friendly, easy to implant and easy to revisit procedure for surgical reduction of IOP. Prospective studies were made in open-angle glaucoma patients, and in these studies it was recommended that the patients have angles of Schaffer grade 2 or higher to provide enough space to perform the surgery. However, due to the high flexibility and small diameter of the stent, the XEN procedure may allow for implantations in rather narrow angles. These observations in this and other centers led to the decision to perform further studies in narrow-angle and closed-angle glaucoma

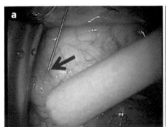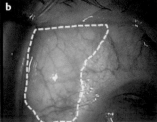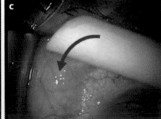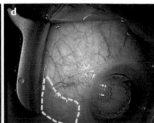

Fig. 37.7 **(a)** Preoperative injection of mitomycin C (MMC). *Arrow* points to the injection site. **(b)** The needle is placed under or within Tenon's capsule and 0.1 mL (8–20 µg) of MMC solution is injected separating **(c)** Tenon's capsule. *Dashed outline* show the extent of subconjunctival injection fluid. *Arrow* shows direction and technique of fluid massage. The depot is

shifted to the target zone by soft massage with a cotton swab. In the target zone, the MMC solution loosens up **(d)** Tenon's capsule from the sclera which creates the space the stent is delivered into. *Dashed outline* shows the target area of stent injection.

patients. The steps for successfully perform a stand-alone implantation of the XEN 45 Gel Stent are described above (see Surgical Technique).

Glaucoma–Cataract Surgery: Combined Procedure

The XEN Gel Stent procedure can be easily performed after cataract extraction. Combined surgery of cataract and glaucoma (phaco-trabeculectomy) has always been desirable for surgeons because they can accomplish two goals in a single surgery. However, numerous reports in the scientific literature suggest that combined procedures are less effective in lowering the IOP, and long-term follow-up indicates that there is 40% less efficacy 4 to 5 years after surgery. The most dramatic drop in efficacy occurs between months 3 and 10, but it continues to decline until the end of follow-up.[8] In the combined analysis of all surgeries, with all versions of the XEN Gel Stent (XEN 140, XEN 63, XEN 45), no significant differences in efficacy between XEN stand-alone and XEN–cataract combined procedures were identified. In the combined data both procedures seem to be equally efficient in lowering the IOP over the course of 3 years. However, patients from the XEN 45 phase 4 trial in Europe are still being followed, and the final analysis will provide more information on this topic.

Managing Complications

The procedure provides excellent safety for the patient and the surgeon. Despite the fact that the procedure is forgiving during the process of implantation, careful planning of the surgery is necessary. The following steps during implantation are important for successful delivery of the XEN Gel Stent and should be considered by every surgeon. Not all of these precautions are specific to the XEN Gel Stent procedure. Some of them are considerations related to ab interno procedures in general:

- The surgeon needs to avoid touching the lens in phakic eyes. This is especially important in eyes with shallow anterior chambers.
- The surgeon should mark the target exit site of the stent 3 mm posterior to the limbus. The surgeon can correct the implantation path by elevating or lowering the injector cannula on its way through the tissue. The position of the needle tip and the bevel can be observed through the sclera, as the needle is pushed through the tissue and comes closer to the surface. If the bevel would exit the sclera early and close to the limbus, retract the needle and angle down the injector while further pushing the cannula through the sclera. This will keep the tip inside the sclera and lengthen the implantation channel. If the bevel would exit the sclera posterior to the target site, pull back slightly, but stay inside the sclera channel. Then angle up the injector and proceed with the implantation process. This will result in a more anterior and on-target exit of the cannula tip.
- Intrascleral vessels or vessels at the exit site, if hit, can cause subconjunctival bleeding. In such cases, it depends on whether the blood obscures the visibility of crucial structures, which are essential to see for the successful performance of an implantation. In case of an anterior chamber bleeding before the needle is inserted into the sclera, the implantation needs to be suspended and the anterior chamber cleared of blood before a new attempt can be made. In cases in which severe subconjunctival bleeding cannot be cleared, the surgeon needs to go to a different target spot.

- If a gonioscope is not used for implantation, the surgeon needs to be aware that viscoelastic can displace the iris plane posteriorly. Orientation relative to the limbus is important in these cases, to avoid posterior implantations through the iris root. This can cause blockage of the inner opening of the stent by the iris tissue once the anterior chamber goes back to the original position.
- If the cannula exits the sclera close to the limbus, it enters an area with low conjunctival mobility. This is the only danger for perforations of the conjunctiva (0.4%, see **Table 37.2**) and delivery of the stent above Tenon's capsule. If the exit site is 2.5 to 3 mm behind the limbus, perforations of the conjunctiva are much less likely to happen because the conjunctiva there is free to move. The sleeve of the injector also does not allow for deeper implantations, thus limiting the length of the cannula that can subconjunctivally be exposed from the sclera.
- Surgeons need to make sure the bevel clears the sclera completely before the implantation is triggered with the slider on the injector. This is important to provide easy release of the XEN Gel Stent under or within Tenon's capsule. If the stent is released early, fibers of the episcleral or Tenon's capsule might hinder the straight delivery of the stent. In this case, stents can be straightened after implantation without injuring the conjunctiva.
- The surgeon should avoid forces transversal to the implantation axis during retrieval of the injector after implantation of the XEN Gel Stent is completed.
- The procedure is less prone to fibrotic closure and encapsulation than are average trabeculectomies in our patient population. In case of fibrosis or encapsulation, management according to the AqueSys standard operating procedures is recommended (see below).
- If for any reason the stent needs to be adjusted in position within the implantation channel, this is also possible by manipulation through the conjunctiva with a blunt forceps.
- In the case of an irregularly positioned stent, it is possible to remove the stent. Small-gauge vitreoretinal instruments can be used to extract the stent from its channel and remove it from the anterior chamber. An immediate replacement stent can be implanted next to primary implantation site. It has not been evaluated yet how many implantations in an eye can be performed. From the current point of experience, the amount of undisturbed conjunctiva seems to be the limiting factor.

Postoperative Management

The patient can be discharged the same day of implantation and is provided with a topical regimen of an antibiotic and a steroid. The antibiotic is discontinued after 1 week, and the steroid is given four times daily and tapered after week 6. The speed of tapering steroids in general depends on the visual and functional evaluation of the filtration bleb.

Postoperative hypotony is not an issue when the XEN 45 Gel Stent is used. Its inner diameter exerts enough resistance to avoid pressures under 6 mm Hg during the early postoperative period under normal aqueous humor production rates.

Evaluation of the filtration blebs after implantation of the XEN Gel Stent is easy and straightforward. It needs some adaptation of the surgeon to adjust to the small appearance of a bleb when compared with a classic bleb after trabeculectomy. Sometimes it is hard to tell if the stent is functioning from only visual

Table 37.2 Safety Data from the Combined XEN Gel Stent Study

XEN Gel Stent (all models, n = 505)	Stent Alone		Combo Cataract		Combined	
	Number	Rate	Number	Rate	Number	Rate
Subconjunctival bleeding obscuring view of implant	2	0.8%	4	1.7%	6	1.2%
Intraoperative AC bleeding	1	0.4%	5	2.1%	6	1.2%
Vitreous bulge or loss	0	0.0%	0	0.0%	0	0.0%
Shallow AC	3	1.1%	1	0.4%	4	0.8%
Choroidal effusion (self-limited, lasting < 30 days)	4	1.5%	1	0.4%	5	1.0%
Conjunctival perforation	2	0.8%	0	0.0%	2	0.4%
AC viscoelastic injection	2	0.8%	1	0.4%	3	0.6%
Hyphema	8	3.0%	5	2.1%	13	2.6%
Subconjunctival hemorrhage (occurring > 30 days postoperative)	1	0.4%	0	0.0%	1	0.2%
IOL subluxation	1	0.4%	0	0.0%	1	0.2%
Blebitis (bleb infection)	0	0.0%	0	0.0%	0	0.0%
Large bleb associated with ocular surface symptoms	1	0.4%	1	0.4%	2	0.4%
Stent blockage	3	1.1%	1	0.4%	4	0.8%
Explantation	0	0.0%	1	0.4%	1	0.2%
Converted to another IOP lowering procedure	3	1.1%	1	0.4%	4	0.8%

Abbreviations: AC, anterior chamber; IOL, intraocular lens; IOP, intraocular pressure.
Note: The table shows the most frequently seen complications. All other problems that can be seen in filtration procedures occurred either seldom or not at all, such as temporal visual loss and reduced visual acuity. This makes the implantation of the XEN Gel Stent a very safe surgery. The most commonly seen adverse event was a hyphema the next day after surgery in 13 of 505 treated patients. No patient had to undergo anterior chamber flushing due to unresolved hyphema.

examination through the slit lamp. It is currently not clear why the bleb appears shallower than after classic trabeculectomy, but the causes of failure are similar—fibrosis and encapsulation. In the case of high IOP, either fibrosis or encapsulation of the stent has occurred. Fibrosis is recognized if no bleb elevation is visible after ocular digital massage (**Fig. 37.8**).

In the case of fibrosis, needling of the bleb can be performed. In general, these needlings are performed with the adjuvant usage of mitomycin C or 5-FU. In the case of cystic encapsulation, it is recommended not to perform a needling. Instead, the patient is treated early with aqueous suppressants. Cystic encapsulation may resolve with this treatment, resulting in a normal functioning bleb, and needling can be avoided. If this treatment

is not successful after 3 months, it is recommended to switch strategy and perform a needling with adjuvant antimetabolites.

Safety, Efficacy, and Clinical Results

The safety and efficacy of the XEN Gel Stent are remarkable. **Fig. 37.9** shows the analysis of 638 implantations with three different models lumped together. Over 36 months, the XEN stent provides substantial reduction of the IOP. Although the analysis does not show complete follow-up of all patients over the entire evaluation period, it shows an impressive reduction of 41% after

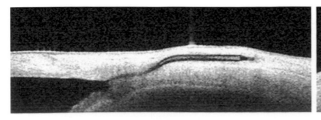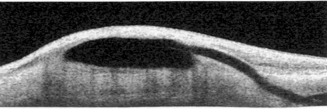

a b

Fig. 37.8 Two cases of high intraocular pressure 2 months after implantation. **(a)** Fibrosis of a XEN 45 Gel Stent, which was subsequently subjected to needling. **(b)** Encapsulation of a XEN 45 Gel Stent bleb with a cyst. This patient did not receive needling treatment; instead topical aqueous suppressants were utilized.

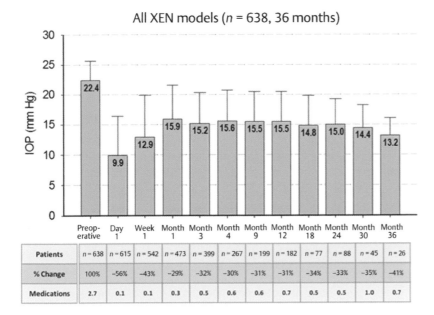

All XEN models (*n* = 638, 36 months)

Patients	*n* = 638	*n* = 615	*n* = 542	*n* = 473	*n* = 399	*n* = 267	*n* = 199	*n* = 182	*n* = 77	*n* = 88	*n* = 45	*n* = 26
% Change	100%	−56%	−43%	−29%	−32%	−30%	−31%	−31%	−34%	−33%	−35%	−41%
Medications	2.7	0.1	0.1	0.3	0.5	0.6	0.6	0.7	0.5	0.5	1.0	0.7

Fig. 37.9 The intraocular pressure (IOP)-lowering effect of all XEN Gel Stent models taken together. The observation period is up to 36 months. After 36 months, 26 patients were followed at a pressure reduction of 41% with an average reduction from 2.7 to 0.7 medications.

3 years of follow-up with a reduction in the number of glaucoma medications by 74% from 2.7 to 0.7 medications. But 5% of the patients analyzed in this sample had to undergo a different surgical procedure to reduce the IOP to therapeutic levels. The needling rate was between 15% and 20% when mitomycin C injections were used before implantation of the stent.

Table 37.2 shows the efficacy data of 505 analyzed implantations. The most common complications of the XEN Gel Stent procedure are bleedings. The choroidal effusions shown in this table are typical for the older models with larger inner diameter (XEN 140 and XEN 63) due to early postoperative hypotony. By switching over to the XEN 45 stent, this complication did not occur in our patient samples.

Conclusion

The XEN Gel Stent procedure is a safe and efficient procedure for the treatment of glaucoma alone as well as for the combined treatment of glaucoma and cataract. Future developments might include drug release systems and stents with nonhomogeneously cross-linked portions of the stent; that is, changes in the diameter of the stent might be possible. This could facilitate completely new postoperative management protocols, and efficacy and safety might be driven to even higher levels. We are using the XEN 45 Gel Stent in many of our patients with early or advanced glaucoma, replacing medications as well as traditional procedures such as trabeculectomy and valve implants.

References

1. Reitsamer HA, Lenzhofer M, Hohensinn M, et al. Ab interno approach to subconjunctival space: first 567 eyes treated with new minimally invasive gel stent for treating glaucoma. Presented at the American Society of Cataract and Refractive Surgeons annual meeting, San Diego, 2015

2. Reitsamer HA. Early results of a minimally-invasive, ab-interno gelatin stent in combination with a preoperative Mitomycin C injection for the treatment of glaucoma. Presented at the European Society of Cataract and Refractive Surgeons annual meeting, London, 2014

3. Lewis RA. Ab interno approach to the subconjunctival space using a collagen glaucoma stent. J Cataract Refract Surg 2014;40:1301–1306

4. Benedikt O. [The mode of action of trabeculectomy (author's transl)]. Klin Monatsbl Augenheilkd 1975;167:679–685

5. Yu DY, Morgan WH, Sun X, et al. The critical role of the conjunctiva in glaucoma filtration surgery. Prog Retin Eye Res 2009;28:303–328

6. Singh M, Chew PT, Friedman DS, et al. Imaging of trabeculectomy blebs using anterior segment optical coherence tomography. Ophthalmology 2007;114:47–53

7. Picht G, Grehn F. [Development of the filtering bleb after trabeculectomy. Classification, histopathology, wound healing process]. Ophthalmologe 1998;95:W380-7

8. Lochhead J, Casson RJ, Salmon JF. Long term effect on intraocular pressure of phacotrabeculectomy compared to trabeculectomy. Br J Ophthalmol 2003;87:850–852

38 Translimbal SIBS Shunt: The InnFocus MicroShunt

Juan F. Batlle Pichardo, Francisco Fantes, Isabelle Riss, Leonard Pinchuk, Rachel Alburquerque, Yasushi P. Kato, Esdras Arrieta, Adalgisa Corona Peralta, Paul Palmberg, Richard K. Parrish II, Bruce A. Weber, Jean-Marie Parel, Brian A. Francis, and Iqbal Ike K. Ahmed

Case Presentation: InnFocus Microshunt for Juvenile Open Angle Glaucoma

A 12-year-old Asian-American girl with mild-to-moderate juvenile primary open-angle glaucoma (POAG) presented for a surgical consultation. Her initial baseline intraocular pressure (IOP) was 25 mm Hg OD and 30 mm Hg OS. She was started on topical latanoprost 0.005% at bedtime in both eyes, and fixed combination brinzolamide 2% and timolol 0.5% twice daily in both eyes. Her medical history is positive for nail-patella syndrome (also known as hereditary onycho-osteodysplasia [HOOD] syndrome), an autosomal dominant syndrome characterized by abnormalities of the nails, knees, elbows, and pelvis. It is also associated with elevated IOP and renal disease.

Her best corrected visual acuity was 20/20 OU with myopic correction −5.25 D OD and −5.75 D OS. The IOP was 14 mm Hg OD and 11 mm Hg OS on medication. She had a mild posterior subcapsular cataract in both eyes. Her optic nerve cup-to-disk ratio was 0.75 OD with a superior notch, and 0.85 OS with superior rim thinning. The visual fields revealed a superior and inferior nasal defect in the right eye (−3.09 mean deviation) and an inferior nasal defect in the left eye (−3.61 mean deviation). The corneal thickness was 612 μm OD and 619 μm OS. Three months later, the IOP rose to 26 mm Hg OU, with some question as to patient compliance with medication. Over the next 6 months, different topical glaucoma medications were used, including bimatoprost 0.01%, the fixed combination brimonidine 0.2%–timolol 0.5%, and the fixed combination dorzolamide 2%–timolol 0.5%. Despite this, IOP the remained in the range of 21 to 26 mm Hg.

The patient underwent trabeculotomy ab interno with the Trabectome in the left eye, which initially controlled the IOP in the mid-teens, but it quickly rose to preoperative levels within 2 months. Alternative glaucoma surgeries were discussed, including trabeculectomy, glaucoma aqueous tube shunt, and the newer investigational subconjunctival filtration techniques.

The patient underwent transconjunctival gel implant with the XEN implant (AqueSys Inc., Aliso Viejo, CA; Allergan, Irvine, CA) in the left eye, but with conjunctival dissection and partial tenonectomy and application of mitomycin due to concerns about scarring. After initial hypotony, the IOP rose to the mid-20s after 2 months, with peripheral anterior synechiae covering the internal portion of the implant. The synechiae were lysed with neodymium:yttrium-aluminum-garnet (Nd:YAG) laser and the IOP stabilized to the low teens with dorzolamide-timolol twice a day.

Because of these issues in the left eye, the right eye underwent surgery with the InnFocus MicroShunt® (InnFocus, Miami, FL), also with partial tenonectomy and application of mitomycin. After hypotony in the range of 3 to 5 mm Hg for the first 6 weeks, the IOP stabilized at 8 to 11 mm Hg on no glaucoma medications. At the 5-month postoperative visit, the topical steroid was tapered off, with an IOP of 10 mm Hg, visual acuity 20/25, and a low diffuse bleb.

The Development of SIBS

The InnFocus MicroShunt is one of several products that originated from a 10-year quest to develop a novel synthetic biomaterial that would resist biodegradation, inflammation, and encapsulation in the body.

The key feature in the material used in this stent is a base co-polymer called polyisobutylene, shown in the central block of the tri-block polymer in **Fig. 38.1**. Polyisobutylene itself is a gum resembling chewing gum. The triblock polymer, poly(styrene-*block*-isobutylene-*block*-styrene) or "SIBS" is shown in **Fig. 38.1** where *N* is an integer greater than *M*.[1–4]

The first medical use of SIBS was for Boston Scientific Corporation's (Natick, MA) TAXUS® stent.[5,6] TAXUS is a small balloon-expandable metallic stent (2 to 3 mm in diameter and 10 to 20 mm long), with a SIBS coating that slowly releases the antiproliferative drug paclitaxel into the wall of the coronary artery to prevent restenosis. Data collected from studies of TAXUS confirmed no biodegradation and minimal tissue reaction.[7]

The Development of the Glaucoma Device

Histopathology results 2 months after implantation of rabbit studies with the first generation were reported by Parel et al[8] and Acosta et al.[9] They found that there were no myofibroblasts or angiogenesis in the vicinity of the SIBS disks, nor were there integral capsules surrounding the disks. In contrast, the silicone rubber controls showed angiogenesis, myofibroblasts, and significant capsules attached to the disks. In summary, SIBS was found to be totally innocuous in the eye.

Shortly thereafter, it was decided that a glaucoma drainage device without a plate might be achievable if the tube did not occlude. This would require that the lumen of the tube be larger than the diameter of a sloughed endothelial cell, which is about 40 to 50 μm, while at the same time sufficiently small to prevent hypotony. The lumen size was approximated from the Hagan-Poiseuille equation, and a series of rabbit eye implants by Arrieta et al[10] confirmed that a lumen diameter of approximately 70 μm would satisfy these requirements.[11]

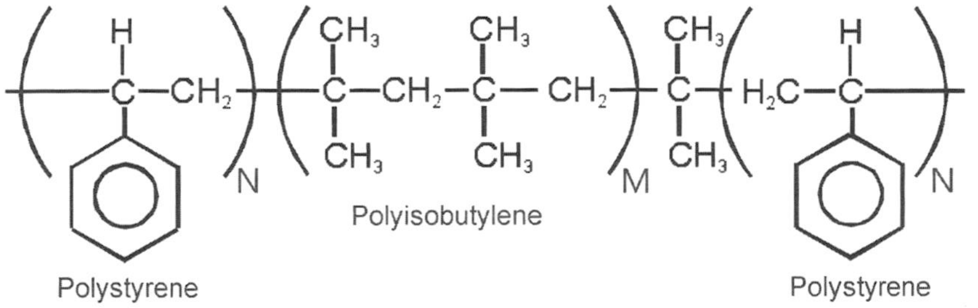

Fig. 38.1 The tri-block polymer poly(styrene-*block*-isobutylene-*block*-styrene), or "SIBS," in which the central block is polyisobutylene and the end caps are glassy segments of polystyrene that serve to hold the strands of polyisobutylene together ($M \gg N$) to form an elastomer.

Another issue was the placement of the tube. It was decided that draining to a flap under the conjunctiva and Tenon's capsule, much like the gold-standard trabeculectomy, made the most sense. The advantage of the MicroShunt would be the avoidance of cutting the sclera and suturing the scleral flap with sutures placed under the proper tension to control outflow, a process that requires significant surgical skill. In addition, the fluid dynamics of the MicroShunt could be controlled by the lumen diameter and length to minimize hypotony. And so began the development of a SIBS-based microshunt.[12,13]

The Four Iterations of the Glaucoma Device

There were three major iterations of shunt design (**Fig. 38.2**) with varied dimensions (**Table 38.1**). These three iterations were tested first in chronic rabbit eye studies at the University of Miami, Bascom Palmer Eye Institute *Ophthalmic Biophysics Center* (OBC) laboratory, and then in pilot feasibility studies over a period of 4 years to determine the best design as well as the best implant technique. All animal studies were authorized by the University of Miami Animal Care and Use Committee. All feasibility studies in humans were authorized by the appropriate government ethics committees. In France, approval was granted by AFSSAPS (Agence Française de Sécurité Sanitaire des Produits de Santé) and later by ANSM (Agence Nationale de Sécurité du Medicament et des Produits de Santé). In the Dominican Republic, approval was granted by CONABIOS (the Dominican Republic National Counsel of Bioethics and Health). Local hospital-based ethics committee approvals were also obtained where necessary.

Table 38.2 summarizes the baseline characteristics, changes in IOP, and glaucoma medication use at 1 year. The major criterion for qualified success, adopted from the Tube Versus Trabeculectomy (TVT) study,[14] is IOP ≤ 21 mmHg with a reduction from baseline of ≥ 20% with or without glaucoma medication and with no further incisional procedure.

The first-generation product was a SIBS tube (**Fig. 38.2a**) with a 1 mm × 1 mm SIBS tab jutting out of one side. It was called the MIDI-Tube (minimally invasive drainage implant). The purpose of the tab was to prevent migration of the shunt into the anterior chamber due to movement caused by globe rotation and blinking. The reason the tab was attached to one wall of the shunt, and not symmetrical about the tube, was that the device was delivered through a slotted needle inserter, in which the tab jutted out of the slot in the needle.

Professor Isabelle Riss, formerly at the Hôpital Pellegrin in Bordeaux, France, and currently at Pôle Ophtalmologique de la Clinique Mutualiste, Pessac, Cedex, France, was the first surgeon to implant the MIDI-Tube in humans in January 2006. Twenty-four advanced cases, with about half of the eyes failing previous trabeculectomy, were used in the Bordeaux I study (**Table 38.2**). Mitomycin C (MMC) was not used intraoperatively, and the qualified success rate was 42% at 1 year. In addition, there were two

occurrences of erosion (successfully patched) of the sharp corner of the tab through the conjunctiva in two patients who were extreme myopes (eye was elongated and the conjunctiva stretched thin). It was concluded that MMC would be required in this patient population to sustain the bleb and that the tab needed to be redesigned to be less erosive. It was also found that the slotted needle inserter was unreliable, as the device, being very soft and somewhat sticky, often jammed in the inserter; it was more reliable to insert the device with a forceps through a preformed needle tract than to push it through a nonlubricated tube.

A second clinical study (Bordeaux II study) of the same MIDI-Tube design was initiated in 16 patients with the application of low-dose MMC in the subconjunctival/Tenon's flap as a means of controlling healing of the conjunctiva to the sclera and loss of the bleb. MMC was applied to the scleral side of the flap only using two or three Schirmer strips, which are sponge-like strips used to absorb and measure teardrop quantity. The dose consisted of a total of approximately 0.6 mL of a 0.2 mg/mL concentration applied for 2 to 3 minutes, and the MMC was flushed from the eye with 250 mL of sterile saline. The success rate increased to 67% at 1 year in these late-stage refractory patients. These data confirmed that MMC needs to be used in conjunction with a redesigned MIDI-Tube tab in these late-stage patients. (The Bordeaux II study was in progress when the erosions were noted from the sharp tab in the Bordeaux I study.)

Nine months into the Bordeaux II study, InnFocus decided to test in parallel an alternate model called the MIDI-Ray (**Fig. 38.2b**), which was a SIBS tube (outer diameter 350 µm, lumen diameter 100 µm) with a 7-mm-diameter SIBS plate that was 350 µm thick. The device resembled a stingray; hence its name. The hypothesis was that the lack of encapsulation of the SIBS plate would facilitate fluid percolation through the sclera as well as reduce problems associated with motility and diplopia, often encountered with the large plate valves.[15] It would also obviate the need to use MMC. A 12-subject clinical study was initiated by Juan F. Batlle Pichardo in September 2007 at Centro Laser, Santo Domingo, Dominican Republic. Unfortunately, the lack of capsule formation around the MIDI-Ray SIBS plate resulted in a thin conjunctiva, which led to cystic-type blebs and a qualified success rate of only 58%. In addition, the 100-µm lumen resulted in a high incidence of acute hypotony (all cases resolved spontaneously), in which case the investigator tied off the tube with a suture until the device healed in the eye. (Tying off tubes is often practiced with the large drainage tubes such as the Baerveldt valve.)

As the data accumulated from the Bordeaux II study, showing a 67% success rate without a plate, with low-dose MMC and with no hypotony, it was decided to continue with a plateless tube, modify the tab to make it more atraumatic, and to use a broader application of MMC, which was demonstrated to be safe in the long term.[16]

This new design of the microshunt was initially called the MIDI-Arrow (**Fig. 38.2c**) as the tab was changed to an atraumatic,

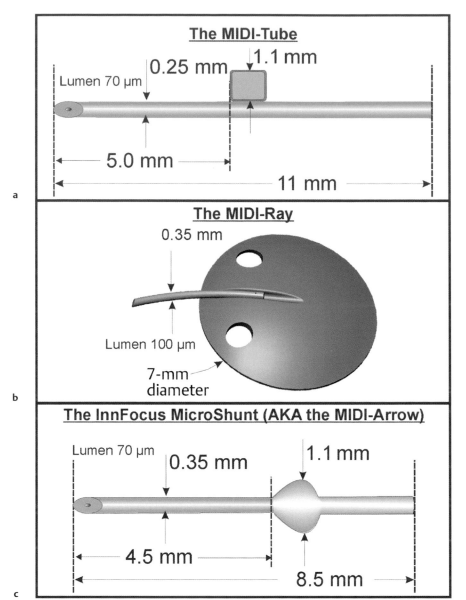

Fig. 38.2 The first three iterations of SIBS-based glaucoma shunts. **(a)** The MIDI-Tube used in the first-generation glaucoma product in the Bordeaux I and II studies. **(b)** The MIDI-Ray used in the second-generation product in the Dominican Republic I study. **(c)** The InnFocus MicroShunt® (aka MIDI-Arrow) used in the Dominican Republic II study.

planar symmetrical fin-like design that resembled the feathers on an arrow. The MIDI-Arrow name was later changed to the InnFocus MicroShunt®. The lumen of the MIDI-Arrow remained at 70 µm so as to eliminate the need to tie off the tube during the healing phase. A 23-patient feasibility trial with 0.4 mg/mL MMC applied for 3 minutes was initiated in the Dominican Republic in patients of mixed race (mixture of black, white, and aborigine) with POAG and no previous conjunctival incisions, who had failed maximum tolerated glaucoma medication. These changes to the device as well as the procedure led to a qualified success rate of 100% with a 50% drop in IOP from baseline at 1 year.

The change in IOP in the 1-year feasibility studies of the MIDI-Tube without MMC (Bordeaux I), MIDI-Tube with low-dose MMC (Bordeaux II), MIDI-Ray (Dominican Republic I), and Inn-Focus MicroShunt (Dominican Republic II) are plotted in **Fig. 38.3**. The decision was subsequently made to freeze the InnFocus MicroShunt design and extend the data set in the Dominican Republic and confirm the data with an additional set of patients in Bordeaux, France.

The following sections of the chapter discuss the refined procedure for the InnFocus MicroShunt and present a summary of 3-year follow-up results of the Dominican Republic II clinical trial introduced above and with patient characteristics described in **Table 38.2**. A more detailed report on this patient population has been submitted for publication at the time of this writing and therefore cannot be included in this chapter.

Methods

After approval of the implant protocol by CONABIOS, a prospective study was conducted by Juan F. Batlle Pichardo at Centro Laser, Santo Domingo, Dominican Republic. The major inclusion criteria included patients with POAG who had failed maximum tolerated glaucoma medication. Patients who were also undergoing cataract surgery were allowed in this study, but it was not a requirement. Patients who had failed previous conjunctiva surgeries were excluded from the study. All eligible patients in the practice of the principal investigator who would otherwise be considered for primary trabeculectomy were offered participation

Table 38.1   Comparison of the MIDI-Tube with the MIDI-Ray and the InnFocus MicroShunt® (MIDI-Arrow)

Device	MIDI-Tube	MIDI-Tube	MIDI-Ray	InnFocus MicroShunt® (aka MIDI-Arrow)
Study	Bordeaux I	Bordeaux II	DR I	DR II
Tube outer diameter (mm)	0.25	0.25	0.35	0.35
Tube lumen diameter (µm)	70	70	100	70
Total length (mm)	11	11	12	8.5
Migration restrictor type	Tab	Tab	Plate	Fin
Migration restrictor size (mm)	1 × 1	1 × 1	7 diameter	1.1 wingspan
Needle tract gauge	27	25–27	27	25–27
Introducer	Inserter	Inserter	Forceps	Forceps
Mitomycin C concentration, time (min)	None	0.2 mg/mL, 2	None	0.4 mg/mL, 3
Area of mitomycin C applied	None	Sclera	None	Entire flap
Lumen tied off?	No	No	Yes	No

Table 38.2   Summary of Baseline Characteristics and 1-Year Results

Device	MIDI-Tube	MIDI-Tube	MIDI-Ray	InnFocus MicroShunt® (aka MIDI-Arrow)
Study	Bordeaux I	Bordeaux II	DR I	DR II
Baseline characteristics				
Number of patients	24	16	12	23
Average age	65.2 ± 18.9	57.1 ± 13.5	56.8 ± 13	59.8 ± 15.3
Race	Caucasian	Caucasian	Mixed	Mixed
Status of test eye: phakic/cataract/pseudophakic	9/1/14	10/0/6	4/7/1	10/11/2
Diagnosis of primary open-angle glaucoma	19	14	12	23
Congenital	3	0	0	0
Plateau iris	1	1	0	0
Poststeroid	1	1	0	0
Previous conjunctival surgeries	12	11	0	0
Baseline intraocular pressure (with full medication regimen)	24.1 ± 7.8	21.1 ± 5.2	24.4 ± 4.4	23.8 ± 5.3
Average number of glaucoma medications	2.9 ± 1.2	1.7 ± 0.9	1.7 ± 0.8	2.4 ± 1.0
Results at 1 year				
Intraocular pressure (mm Hg)	16.2 ± 4.1	12.8 ± 3.3	14.4 ± 3.9	10.7 ± 2.8
Number of glaucoma medications	1.5 ± 1.3	0.7 ± 0.5	1.2 ± 1.1	0.3 ± 0.8
Surgical success	42%	67%	58%	100%

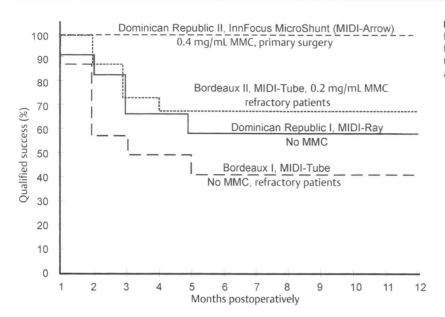

Fig. 38.3 The 1-year surgical success rate of the four InnFocus MIDI designs and iterations. The fourth-generation InnFocus MicroShunt provides the best results, with a 100% qualified success rate at 1 year.

in the study; none refused and all signed the appropriate consent forms. The patients were enrolled prospectively in the order of consent.

The MicroShunt was provided by the manufacturer, InnFocus, Inc. (Miami, FL) in a sterile packaged kit that contained (1) a ruler to measure the site of entry (3 mm from the limbus); (2) a marking pen to ink the ruler; (3) three LASIK sponges to apply MMC (0.4 mg/mL for 3 minutes; the MMC was not supplied); (4) a 1 mm × 1 mm triangular knife to incise a shallow pocket in the sclera; and (5) a 27- or 25-gauge needle to form a needle tract under the limbus to the anterior chamber. The implant procedure is shown

in **Fig. 38.4**. A light-pressure patch was used the day after surgery and nightly for 5 days thereafter.

Results: The Dominican Republic Study

Baseline demographic characteristics are listed in **Table 38.2**. Twenty-one phakic patients (11 with visually impairing cataracts) and two pseudophakic patients participated in the study. The mean baseline IOP was 23.8 ± 5.3 mm Hg (range, 19–38 mm Hg)

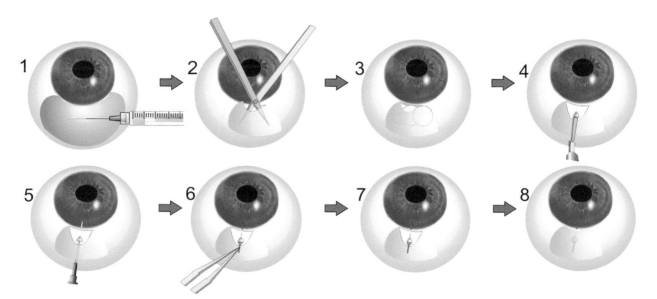

Fig. 38.4 The steps of the implant procedure: (1) Lidocaine and epinephrine are injected under the conjunctiva hydrating the Tenon's space. (2) A fornix-based flap is made under the conjunctiva and Tenon's, extending to two quadrants and posteriorly 8 mm. Bipolar diathermy is used to cauterize any bleeding blood vessels. (3) Three LASIK shields soaked in mitomycin C (MMC; 0.4 mg/mL) are placed in the flap for 3 minutes and then removed and the flap rinsed with 25 mL buffered saline. (4) A shallow pocket is in-cised in the sclera with a 1-mm-wide knife. (5) A 25-gauge needle tract is made through the pocket and under the limbus to the anterior chamber, bisecting the angle between the cornea and iris. (6) The InnFocus Micro-Shunt is fed through the pocket and needle tract. (7) The fins of the Micro-Shunt are wedged into the pocket to prevent migration and leakage around the tube. Flow is confirmed exiting the device. (8) The fornix-based flap is closed with multiple interrupted 10-0 nylon sutures on a spatula needle.

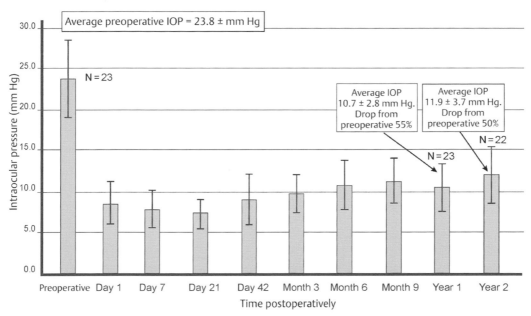

Fig. 38.5 Average intraocular pressure results of the InnFocus MicroShunt (aka MIDI-Arrow) up to 2 years (23 and 22 patients at 1 and 2 years, respectively). Data includes both the MicroShunt implanted alone (14 patients) as well as the MicroShunt implanted in combination with cataract surgery (nine patients).

In the study eye. All 23 patients had POAG with IOP that met the inclusion criteria. The mean baseline best corrected distance visual acuity was 20/60 (range, 20/20 ti light perception only). The visual field mean deviation average for both groups was −20.1 ± 12.1 dB (range, −1.7 to −33.9 dB). The mean number of glaucoma medications per patient at baseline was 2.4 ± 1.0 (range, 1–4).

Postoperative data were available for 23 patients at 1 year and 22 patients thereafter, as one patient was lost to follow-up. Fourteen patients underwent MicroShunt implantation alone, and nine underwent combined MicroShunt insertion and phacoemulsification with subsequent intraocular lens (IOL) implantation.

The mean percent reduction in IOP from baseline at 1 and 2 years was 55% and 50%, respectively. The mean IOPs were 10.7 ± 2.8 mm Hg and 11.9 ± 3.7 mm Hg, respectively. A bar chart of IOP with time is presented in **Fig. 38.5**.

The qualified success rate was 100% at 1 (23/23) and 2 years (22/22).

The mean number of preoperative glaucoma medications per patient was 2.4 ± 0.9. Glaucoma medication use per patient at 1 and 2 years was 0.3 ± 0.8 and 0.4 ± 1.0, respectively. The percent of patients whose IOP was controlled without medication at 1 and 2 years was 87% and 86%, respectively.

There were no visual acuity losses or gains greater than one Snellen line in any of the patients who had glaucoma surgery alone over the 2-year time frame tested. Three patients gained two or more lines at 1 year, and four patients at 2 years, following implantation of a MicroShunt in combination with cataract surgery.

The most common postoperative adverse events were IOP < 5 mm Hg after day 1, which occurred in three patients who had the combined surgery (3/23 [13%] of all cases) and all resolved spontaneously by day 90. Shallow anterior chambers were observed in 3/23 (13%) patients, but no patient required reformation of the anterior chamber or drainage of a choroidal effusion. Choroidal detachment was observed in two patients (8.7%) from the combined group, which resolved spontaneously. There were no sight-threatening long-term adverse events.

Figs. 38.6 and **38.7** show images of the MicroShunt at 9- and 12-month implant durations. **Fig. 38.8** shows a Visante *optical coherence tomography* (OCT) of the device at 2-year implant duration.

Discussion and Conclusions

The success of the InnFocus MicroShunt by Dr. Batlle Pichardo's group in the Dominican Republic spurred additional implantation of the MicroShunt by Dr. Riss in Bordeaux, France; however, the IOP results between Bordeaux and the Dominican Republic at first differed. The IOP values in the Bordeaux group were about 2 to 3 mm Hg higher than those in the Dominican Republic. A considerable amount of time was spent analyzing the data to determine the cause of the discrepancy. The Dominican

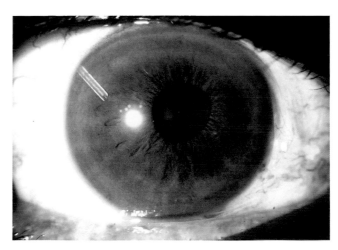

Fig. 38.6 Anterior segment photograph, right eye, 9-month follow-up. The device is in the anterior chamber; intraocular pressure (IOP) is 14 mm Hg.

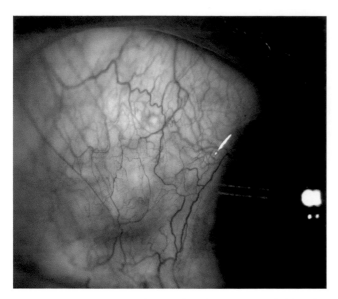

Fig. 38.7 Anterior segment photograph, right eye, 12-month follow-up. The device is in the anterior chamber; IOP is 14 mm Hg.

Republic patients were mainly of Afro-Caribbean heritage and traditionally more difficult to treat than the Bordeaux Caucasian group. However, this variation should have caused the Dominican Republic IOP data to be higher than Bordeaux, which was not the case. The second observation was that the Bordeaux group was treated predominantly with prostaglandins for several years prior to surgery, whereas the Dominican Republic group rarely used prostaglandins as they were too expensive. After careful scrutiny of the implant procedures at both sites, it was discovered that placement of MMC was a key factor; MMC placed close to the limbus, as was practiced in the Dominican Republic yielded lower IOP than MMC placed deep in the pocket, as was practiced in France. In addition, wide subconjunctival/Tenon's flaps provided lower IOP. A series of implants was initiated in Bordeaux to confirm these observations at the time of this writing, and results will be published once they are confirmed.

The development of the InnFocus MicroShunt was an educated iterative process that occurred over the course of 10 years. The process required sophisticated chemistry and engineering, including controlling the foreign-body reaction with SIBS, design-ing the shunt to be atraumatic with a lumen size that minimized hypotony, and developing a design and implant procedure that protected the conjunctiva from being eroded by the device. The fins on the shunt are held firmly in the shallow pocket formed in the sclera and act as a cork to divert aqueous humor into the lumen of the device, which, due to its hydrodynamic design, minimized hypotony. Draining to a bleb, as does the gold-standard trabeculectomy, is important, as the shunt bypasses the high resistances that can be anywhere in the drainage path for aqueous humor, such as the trabecular meshwork, Schlemm's canal, the collector channels, the aqueous veins, and the episcleral veins.

Another important factor was the placement of MMC close to the limbus. One of the proposed theories is that aqueous humor can drain through the naturally occurring microcysts in the conjunctiva[17]; that is, if the resistance through the microcysts is lower than that in the episcleral venous system, fluid will drain through the path of least resistance. MMC may prevent fibrosis or enable the occurrence of the microcysts and allow them to function in this manner. This theory would explain why relatively low IOP is achieved when MMC is placed close to the limbus as opposed to deep in the pocket, as the microcysts tend to predominate where the conjunctiva is thin. It also provides a rationale as to why a wider pocket yields a lower IOP, as it exposes aqueous humor to more microcysts.

The InnFocus MicroShunt is effective in lowering IOP by 50 to 55% and in significantly reducing the need for glaucoma medications, with no long-term adverse events. The control of IOP to a level below 14 mm Hg in over 80% of patients suggests that glaucomatous progression of vision loss will be unlikely.[18]

The advantages of the MicroShunt procedure include (1) no dissection of the sclera; (2) ease of procedure without the need for special equipment; and (3) minimal need for postoperative interventions, such as suture lysis. In addition, the soft, conforming, noninflammatory nature of the SIBS material and the use of a 3-mm-long translimbal needle track require no patch graft to prevent conjunctival erosion as needed for the large drainage valves.

The intended use of the InnFocus MicroShunt is to provide a simple alternative to primary trabeculectomy. Once its safety and effectiveness are well established, it is expected that this device will be used in the treatment of earlier stage patients as an alternative to long-term glaucoma medication where the drugs, or rather the preservatives in the drugs,[19] can wreak havoc on the cornea as well as the conjunctiva and severely limit treatment effectiveness in the future. Although the evidence is only anecdotal at this time, surgeons are successfully treating patients who failed the initial Bordeaux studies by adding a second MicroShunt in the eye. The InnFocus MicroShunt was CE Marked on January 9, 2012, in Europe and several other clinical studies are under way in Europe to increase the number of patients and to investigate the limitations of the device. In addition, a U.S. Investigational Device Exception (IDE) was granted by the Food and Drug Administration (FDA) in May 2013, and a multicenter clinical trial comparing the MicroShunt with primary trabeculectomy in patients refractory to medication is under way.

Acknowledgements

The authors wish to acknowledge Maria Consuelo Varela in the Dominican Republic and Shirley Albrespy in Bordeaux, France, as the clinical coordinators in these studies. We would also like to thank Dr. Richard K. Parrish II and Dr. Paul Palmberg for their help in designing the implant protocols. We would also like to thank John B. Martin for building the plant that produces the InnFocus MicroShunt. The authors also thank Wendy Perdomo and Odette Guzman.

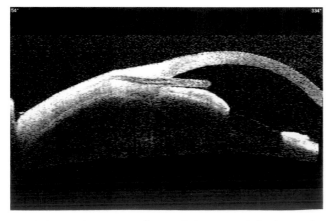

Fig. 38.8 Anterior segment photograph (Visante optical coherence tomography), right eye, 2-year follow-up. The device is in the anterior chamber; IOP is 16 mm Hg.

The Bascom Palmer Eye Institute's team is supported in part by the Florida Lions Eye Bank, an unrestricted grant from Research to Prevent Blindness, a National Institutes of Health (NIH) center grant P30-EY014801, and the Henri and Flore Lesieur Foundation. Funding for the research and development work as well as for the clinical study was provided by InnFocus, Inc., Miami FL. The authors would like to dedicate this publication to the late Dr. Francisco Fantes, co-inventor of the MicroShunt, and the inspiration behind its development. Sadly, Dr. Fantes passed away in the third year of this study.

References

1. Pinchuk L. A review of the biostability and carcinogenicity of polyurethanes in medicine and the new generation of "biostable" polyurethanes. J Biomater Sci Polym Ed 1994;6:225–267

2. Kennedy JP, Ivan B. Designed Polymers by Carbocationic Macromolecular Engineering: Theory and Practice. New York: Oxford University Press; 1991

3. Pinchuk L. Biostable elastomeric polymers having quaternary carbons. US Patent 5,741,331, April 21, 1998

4. Pinchuk L. Method of implanting biostable elastomeric polymers having quaternary carbons. US Patent 6102939, August 15, 2000

5. Pinchuk L, Wilson GJ, Barry JJ, Schoephoerster RT, Parel J-M, Kennedy JP. Medical applications of poly(styrene-block-isobutylene-block-styrene) ("SIBS"). Biomaterials 2008;29:448–460

6. Silber S, Colombo A, Banning AP, et al. Final 5-year results of the TAXUS II trial: a randomized study to assess the effectiveness of slow- and moderate-release polymer-based paclitaxel-eluting stents for de novo coronary artery lesions. Circulation 2009;120:1498–1504

7. Strickler F, Richard R, McFadden S, et al. In vivo and in vitro characterization of poly(styrene-b-isobutylene-b-styrene) copolymer stent coatings for biostability, vascular compatibility and mechanical integrity. J Biomed Mater Res A 2010;92:773–782

8. Parel JM, Stoiber J, Fernandez V, et al. Optical properties and biocompatibility of a novel polymer for intraocular implants: comparative study in the rabbit (abstract). Presented at the Ophthalmic Technologies XIV meeting, #5314-45, San Jose, CA, January 24-25, 2004

9. Acosta AC, Espana EM, Yamamoto H, et al. A newly designed glaucoma drainage implant made of poly(styrene-b-isobutylene-b-styrene): biocompatibility and function in normal rabbit eyes. Arch Ophthalmol 2006;124:1742–1749

10. Arrieta EA, Aly M, Parrish R II, et al. Clinicopathologic correlations of poly-(styrene-b-isobutylene-b-styrene) glaucoma drainage devices of different internal diameters in rabbits. Ophthalmic Surg Lasers Imaging 2011;42: 338–345

11. Fantes F, Acosta AC, Carraway J, Siddiq F, Pinchuk L, Weber BA. An independent GLP evaluation of a new glaucoma drain, the MIDI. Invest Ophthalmol Vis Sci 2006;47:3547

12. Emi K, Pederson JE, Toris CB. Hydrostatic pressure of the suprachoroidal space. Invest Ophthalmol Vis Sci 1989;30:233–238

13. Pinchuk L, Parel J-M, Fantes F, et al. Glaucoma drainage device. U.S. Patent 7,431,709, October 7, 2008

14. Gedde SJ, Heuer DK, Parrish RK II; Tube Versus Trabeculectomy Study Group. Review of results from the tube versus trabeculectomy study. Curr Opin Ophthalmol 2010;21:123–128

15. Gedde SJ, Schiffman JC, Feuer WJ, Herndon LW, Brandt JD, Budenz DL; Tube Versus Trabeculectomy Study Group. Three-year follow-up of the tube versus trabeculectomy study. Am J Ophthalmol 2009;148:670–684

16. Wells AP, Cordeiro MF, Bunce C, Khaw PT. Cystic bleb formation and related complications in limbus- versus fornix-based conjunctival flaps in pediatric and young adult trabeculectomy with mitomycin C. Ophthalmology 2003;110:2192–2197

17. Morita K, Gao Y, Saito Y, et al. In vivo confocal microscopy and ultrasound biomicroscopy study of filtering blebs after trabeculectomy: limbus-based versus fornix-based conjunctival flaps. J Glaucoma 2012;21:383–391

18. The AGIS Investigators. The Advanced Glaucoma Intervention Study (AGIS): 7. The relationship between control of intraocular pressure and visual field deterioration. Am J Ophthalmol 2000;130:429–440

19. Huang C, Wang H, Pan J, et al. Benzalkonium chloride induces subconjunctival fibrosis through the COX-2-modulated activation of a TGF-β1/Smad3 signaling pathway. Invest Ophthalmol Vis Sci 2014;55:8111–8122

39 Combining Minimally Invasive Glaucoma Surgery Procedures

Mohammad Hamid and Paul Harasymowycz

Case Presentation

A 65–year-old man with a history of pseudoexfoliation syndrome presented with gradual vision loss in his right eye. Initial examination demonstrated classic pseudoexfoliative (PXE) material on the anterior capsule and pupillary margin (**Fig. 39.1**). His right eye had moderate cataract with phacodonesis, pigment peppering on the iris stoma, and iris transillumination defects more prominent inferiorly. Gonioscopy showed appositional angle closure in his right eye and a double hump configuration of the iris noted bilaterally, with 2–3+ trabecular meshwork pigmentation. Fundus examination showed excavation of both optic nerves with an inferior notch in the right eye. Although the patient was initially treated with glaucoma medication, his intraocular pressure (IOP) remained above target and his visual fields were progressing.

The diagnosis was pseudoexfoliation glaucoma with phacodonesis from zonular dehiscence, as well as appositional angle closure from a combination of plateau iris and an anteriorly shifted lens. A combined ICE (iStent, cataract extraction, and endocyclophotocoagulation) and MIGS (minimally invasive glaucoma surgery) procedure was planned (**Fig. 39.2**). A femtosecond laser–assisted cataract extraction with a capsular tension ring was performed, with a central deepening of the anterior chamber noted after lens extraction. With the intraocular lens (IOL) in place, two trabecular bypass stents were inserted in the nasal quadrant next to pigmented areas of trabecular meshwork and adjacent collector channels. Finally, endocycloplasty was performed to further open up the angles and reduce aqueous humor production.

This case demonstrates the utility of combining MIGS procedures to properly target the multiple mechanisms causing glaucoma and minimizing the risks of penetrating surgery (**Table 39.1**).

The Procedures

Traditionally, glaucoma surgeons have relied on a handful of procedures, the most notable being trabeculectomy, a filtering procedure that reroutes aqueous humor from the anterior chamber to the sub-Tenon's and subconjunctival space. Another widely used procedure is the implantation of valved or nonvalved glaucoma drainage devices such as the Ahmed or Baerveldt implants. Although these surgeries may be effective in lowering the IOP, significant postoperative risks exist and aggressive healing may impede surgical success.[1]

Recently, a new paradigm in glaucoma management was introduced and coined as MIGS.[2] These newer techniques are changing glaucoma surgery in a similar fashion to the way that small incision phacoemulsification changed cataract surgery, in that MIGS procedures by nature are less invasive and use micro-incisions. The newer materials, smaller devices, and microinstrumentation have changed the traditional ab externo approach to an ab interno one, thus sparing the conjunctival tissue for future surgeries.

Commonly used MIGS procedures target the trabecular outflow pathway, the most common of which is the iStent Trabecular Micro-Bypass (Glaukos Corp., Laguna Hills, CA). However, newer procedures are being developed and utilize other glaucoma outflow pathways. **Table 39.1** categorizes the current MIGS procedures.

Categorizing MIGS procedures by their main mechanism of IOP reduction enables surgeons to more effectively combine them and target the different underlying mechanisms of the patient's disease.

Aqueous Humor Reduction

Historically, medications and transscleral cyclophotocoagulation were used to decrease aqueous humor production to treat glaucoma. However, with the development of endocyclophotocoagulation (ECP), surgeons can now utilize this minimally invasive technique to create focalized treatment of the ciliary body. In contrast to other MIGS procedures, ECP decreases aqueous humor production. This approach can easily be employed in combination with other MIGS procedures that act on different glaucoma pathways and ultimately reduce the IOP to the desired level.

Usually, ECP can be used in all cases of open- or closed-angle glaucoma. However, one may wish to avoid it in uveitic patients or patients prone to ciliary body shutdown.

Narrow Angle

Plateau iris syndrome is characterized by anteriorly rotated or large ciliary processes that displace the iris and close the angle. Clinically, this syndrome does not resolve with peripheral laser iridotomy. Ophthalmologists have developed the endocycloplasty procedure to shrink the ciliary processes. Combined with cataract extraction, this procedure helps to open the angle.

Cataract extraction can be regarded as one of the first MIGS procedures. It has been hypothesized that phacoemulsification reduces IOP by increasing aqueous outflow facility.[3,4] However its effect is more important on angle-closure glaucoma.[5] Thus, one may advocate utilizing lens extraction as a MIGS procedure in acute and chronic angle closure, phacomorphic glaucoma, plateau iris syndrome, pseudoexfoliative glaucoma, or any cause of phacodonesis resulting in an anteriorly displaced lens.

Lastly, goniosynechialysis can also be considered as a MIGS procedure, especially for patients who previously had an acute

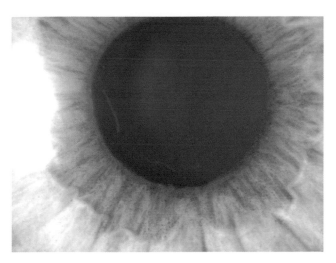

Fig. 39.1   Pseudoexfoliation syndrome. Classic pseudoexfoliative (PXE) material is visualized on the anterior capsule and pupillary margin. One can notice pigment peppering on the pupillary border, most notably on the inferior portion of the iris.

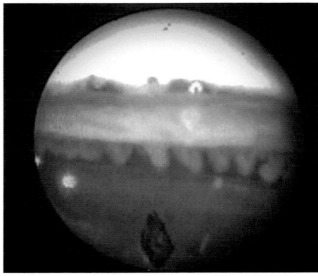

Fig. 39.2   Combined ICE (iStent, cataract extraction, and endocyclophotocoagulation) and MIGS (minimally invasive glaucoma surgery) procedure. Preoperative visualization of the ciliary body and nasal angle with two properly place iStents after cataract extraction and intraocular lens implantation using the endocyclophotocoagulation probe.

episode of angle-closure glaucoma and have recent peripheral anterior synechiae (PAS).[6]

Trabecular Outflow

In contrast to other procedures, MIGS procedures targeting the trabecular meshwork have the advantage of utilizing the natural conventional outflow pathway. Existing procedures in this category are trabecular bypass stenting with the iStent and trabeculotomy ab interno with the Trabectome (NeoMedix, Tustin, CA). Other procedures and devices that utilize this mechanism of action are currently in development.[7] These trabecular bypass devices can be used for all primary or secondary open-angle glaucomas. One may also advocate their use in patients with mixed-mechanism glaucoma whose angles have opened after lens extraction. However, their use in patients suspected of having elevated episcleral venous pressures or diseased distal outflow pathways pathologies (nonfunctional collector drainage system) should be avoided.

Suprachoroidal Shunts

Prostaglandin analogue drops have extensively been used to exploit the uveoscleral outflow pathway. Although it is not the main mechanism by which aqueous humor drains, it constitutes a second natural pathway for IOP reduction. Thus, newer MIGS devices such as the CyPass Micro-Stent (Transcend Medical Inc., Menlo Park, CA) and the iStent Supra are being developed to utilize the suprachoroidal space. This potential space has a negative pressure compared with the anterior chamber, thus creating a gradient for aqueous humor to egress.[8]

This alternative surgical option can be useful in patients with poorly functioning trabecular outflow pathways, scarred subconjunctival tissue, or poor integrity of conjunctiva tissue,

Table 39.1   Categorization of Current Minimally Invasive Glaucoma Surgery Procedures

Aqueous Humor Reduction	Narrow Angle	Trabecular Outflow	Suprachoroidal Shunt	Transconjunctival Filtration
ECP	Lens extraction	Trabectome	Glaukos G3	AqueSys XEN
	Geniosynechialysis	iStent G2	Cypass	InnFocus MicroShunt
	Endocydoplasty	Hydrus		
		Lens extraction		
		GATT		
		TRAB360		
		ELT		

Abbreviations: ECP, endocyclophotocoagulation; ELT, excimer laser trabeculostomy; GATT, gonioscopy-assisted transluminal trabeculotomy.

and in patients at high risk for scarring. Similarly to trabecular bypass devices, patients with suspected elevated episcleral venous pressures are also poor candidates for this category of MIGS procedures.

Transconjunctival Filtration

Ultimately when the natural pathways of the eye are not functioning properly, an alternative pathway needs to be created. For years now, ophthalmologists have rightfully depended on trabeculectomies and aqueous drainage devices to reduce IOP. Currently, new promising MIGS procedures such as the AqueSys XEN (AqueSys, Aliso Viejo, CA) and the InnFocus MicroShunt (InnFocus, Miami, FL) are being developed to effectively drain aqueous humor to the subconjunctival space. In contrast to the traditional ab externo surgeries, these procedures have the advantages of being ab interno, less invasive, and sparing of the conjunctival tissue while offering the potential for significant IOP reduction. These devices could be used for uncontrolled open-angle glaucoma patients. Targeting this mechanism of IOP reduction can be especially beneficial in patients with elevated episcleral venous pressures. Similar to trabeculectomy, patients with subconjunctival tissue scarring or with poor tissue integrity are not good candidates. In addition, transconjunctival filtration devices should be used with caution in patients wearing contact lenses and who have moderate to severe ocular surface disease.

Rationale Behind the Procedures

Whenever a surgical procedure is being discussed with a patient, the risks and benefits should always be described and evaluated. This should be no different when a combination of MIGS procedures is being considered. The overall benefits of combining MIGS procedure are as follows:

- Greater IOP reduction
- Reduction in the number of glaucoma medications
- Increased compliance
- Fewer follow-up appointments
- Fewer postoperative complications
- Lower cost
- Targeting of multiple glaucoma mechanisms

Intraocular Pressure Reduction

The main reason to combine MIGS procedures is to have a significantly greater IOP reduction. In patients with advanced glaucoma requiring an IOP in the low teens, one MIGS procedure may not be sufficient to attain the required IOP. Combining MIGS procedures could provide adequate IOP reduction while carrying lower complication rates than traditional penetrating surgeries. Therefore, by combining complementary MIGS surgeries one may achieve ideal IOP while minimizing patient's risks.

Reduction in the Number of Glaucoma Medications

Ocular drops are not harmless. Allergies, intolerance, secondary effects, dry eyes, and benzalkonium chloride (BAK)-related toxicities are several problems associated with the use of glaucoma medications. Performing one MIGS procedure supplemented with a topical glaucoma medication might provide adequate IOP control of a patient's glaucoma. However, combining MIGS proce-

dures could potentially reduce the IOP to a level where no or less glaucoma drops are required.[9]

Increased Compliance

Compliance with medical therapy in glaucoma is a serious problem. A recent study using a computerized device demonstrated that ~ 50% of patients were not compliant with their glaucoma treatment.[10] A noncompliant patient with progressing disease could be an excellent candidate for multiple MIGS procedures in contrast to traditional penetrating surgeries. MIGS would help control IOP, limit postoperative risks, and reduce the burden of using drops.

Fewer Follow-Up Appointments

Ab externo filtering procedures usually necessitate frequent follow-up appointments. Adjunctive laser suture lysis, ocular massage, and subconjunctival injections of anti-fibrotics or anti–vascular endothelial growth factor (VEGF) agents are often required to modulate the success of bleb-filtering procedures. This requires multiple visits to the doctor's office. In contrast, MIGS procedures are less arduous on patients, require fewer postoperative interventions, and provide faster recovery time. Such advantages are important to consider in patients with mobility restrictions and those having limited access to health care facilities.

Fewer Postoperative Complications

One of the main reasons to consider MIGS over traditional glaucoma surgeries is their safety profile. Serious and visually impairing complications such as endophthalmitis, suprachoroidal hemorrhage, choroidal effusions, hypotony, diplopia, and corneal decompensation are significantly reduced in comparison with penetrating ab externo procedures.[2,11] Thus one might prefer MIGS procedures in higher risk patients, including older patients, those on anticoagulants medications, and those with uncontrolled systemic hypertension.

Lower Cost

In every treatment prescribed, the issue of cost is relevant. The same consideration applies to MIGS procedures. Economic studies are multifactorial, and long-term results are difficult to obtain. However, one Canadian study examined the cost of implanting two iStents or a Trabectome or performing ECP versus medical therapy. At 6 years, all three procedures showed modest cost savings when compared with the cost of glaucoma medications.[12] Although no study has addressed the cost of MIGS procedures versus traditional surgeries, certain factors need to be considered. Combining MIGS procedures can entail a significant initial cost, but it may reduce the need for additional medical therapy, additional MIGS procedures, and additional ab externo glaucoma surgeries. Further studies pertaining to direct and indirect costs for patients and society are required to better clarify this issue.

Targeting of Multiple Glaucoma Mechanisms

Traditionally filtration surgeries have relied on transconjunctival filtration as a "one method fits all" approach to reduce the IOP. However, with the advent of MIGS procedures, one may target the specific pathophysiology in question. Thus, one may utilize and combine categories of MIGS as a customable arsenal for glaucoma therapy.

Combination with Cataract Extraction

Modern microincisional phacoemulsification may be considered the first MIGS procedure as a means to lower the IOP. A recent large investigation conducted in the Ocular Hypertension Treatment Study (OHTS) addressed IOP change in ocular hypertensive patients undergoing cataract extraction. It showed a statistically significant IOP reduction of 16.5% with a follow-up of 3 years.[13] Although the precise mechanism of IOP reduction remains uncertain, there are some interesting factors to consider. Eyes with a higher preoperative IOP had a higher IOP reduction.[13] Eyes with a narrow-angle anterior chamber had a larger IOP reduction after phacoemulsification, thus prompting the idea of a simple mechanical theory where a narrow angle becomes more open.[3] However, in the Mansberger et al[13] study, all patients had open angles. The report evokes the hypothesis that phacoemulsification and lens implantation increases outflow facility by increasing the mechanical tension on lens zonules, widening the intertrabecular space and thus improving outflow facility.

For the reasons mentioned above, lens extraction should also be considered a MIGS procedure, and can easily be combined with one or two additional MIGS surgeries to achieve a lower target IOP. It is highly probable that with the current advances in MIGS technologies, traditional ab externo surgery will be performed less frequently.

Complications Specific to the Procedures

The MIGS procedures usually have complications rates similar to those of standard phacoemulsification,[7] but specific complications may arise. These include rare but significant IOP spikes in surgeries involving the trabecular meshwork, including the use of iStents and the Trabectome. There seems to be a significant steroid response that may occur due to the easier access of steroid molecules to Schlemm's canal and the outflow system. PAS and membranes growing over the cleft after Trabectome surgery have also been observed, and may require yttrium-aluminum-garnet (YAG) membranectomy.[14] Uveitis, pigment dispersion, and hypotony have also been described after ECP.[15]

Combining MIGS procedure can incur specific complications. For example, in the ICE procedure, to avoid uveitis from ciliary body ablation, higher doses and longer duration of steroids may incur more episodes of IOP spikes if combined with Trabectome or iStent surgery. In addition, pigment shedding from an ECP procedure may block smaller trabecular bypass devices, and increased postoperative inflammation may encourage more aggressive ab interno healing with increased PAS and inflammatory membrane formation. Thus one may advocate the use of a weaker corticosteroid and a faster taper. Increased nonsteroidal anti-inflammatory drug (NSAID) use and IOP-lowering therapy in the early postoperative period may be necessary when combining MIGS procedures, and careful topical steroid tapering and IOP monitoring may be required.

When combining a Trabectome or trabecular bypass procedure with a transconjunctival filtering device, other specific complications may also occur. Blood reflux from collector channels, hyphema from small vessels, pigment granules, and inflammatory mediators either obstruct the transconjunctival filtering device and may also egress into the subconjunctival space and create additional inflammation and scarring. Inflammatory media-

ators and pigment from ECP or trabecular surgery may also enter the suprachoroidal space, and may also increase rates of scarring and membrane formation.

Although rare with a single MIGS procedure, hypotony could also become a potential complication when combining MIGS procedures especially if a cyclodialysis cleft results from trabecular or suprachoroidal procedures and are then coupled with a transconjunctival device (AquaSys XEN) or ECP.

Recognizing Complications

Complications are an inherent part of surgery. Some are bound to occur even with an uneventful procedure, so surgeons should expect them and prepare a management plan. As for combining MIGS procedures, it would advisable to take a thorough history of the patient's systemic and ocular findings to identify any risk factors for serious complications. The following pertinent preoperative factors and their surgical implications should be assessed preoperatively:

1. Uncontrolled arterial pressure → increased risk of suprachoroidal hemorrhage
2. Anticoagulation medication → increased risk of blood reflux, suprachoroidal hemorrhage
3. Increased skin pigmentation → increased risk of conjunctival bleb scarring
4. Rosacea, severe blepharitis → increased risk of conjunctival scarring
5. Chronic use of miotics → increased risk of conjunctival scarring
6. History of uveitis → increased risk of hypotony, inflammation, pressure spikes
7. High myopia → increased risk of hypotony, suprachoroidal hemorrhage
8. High hyperopia, angle-closure glaucoma → increased risk of shallow anterior chamber, malignant glaucoma
9. Elevated episcleral pressure → increased risk of blood reflux
10. Vitrectomized eye → increased risk of hypotony
11. History of steroid responder → increased risk of pressure spikes

Once noted, these factors need to be addressed if possible. One may consult with the patient's general practitioner about controlling the vital signs. For MIGS, anticoagulation medications are usually not stopped, but they should be considered when discussing the procedures with the patients. Treating blepharitis is indicated preoperatively, such as minocycline 100 mg twice a day for a month, tapering to once a day for a second month. The addition of topical corticosteroids 1 week preoperatively can also help diminish the blepharitis. Chronic use of miotics and BAK-containing glaucoma medications have been implicated in bleb failures.[16] Thus, one may stop miotics preoperatively and switch to preservative-free glaucoma mediation when possible. The reversal of conjunctival inflammation has been demonstrated when stopping sympathomimetic drops and adding a 1-month treatment of topical corticosteroids.[8] Patients with a history of uveitis should be controlled at least 3 months preoperatively. Nevertheless, the surgeon's awareness of risks and preparation for them are essential in reducing the risk of serious complications.

Postoperative Management

Postoperative care is usually tailored to each patient by considering the underlying glaucoma mechanism, ocular history, target

IOP, and type of surgery. However, there are some general considerations to address for all patients.

When performing procedures with trabecular bypass devices, such as iStents, a Hydrus (Ivantis, Irvine, CA), or a Trabectome, one may use weaker topical corticosteroids, loteprednol 0.5% (Lotemax, Bausch and Lomb, Bridgewater, NJ), with a faster taper: four times daily for 4 days and then taper every 4 days based on observed inflammation, or consider no steroid drops at all. In the event of severe inflammation, one may use short-term oral corticosteroids and reduce the significant steroid response. Anecdotally, 250 mg of oral acetazolamide postoperatively and at bedtime on the day of the surgery can be prescribed when trabecular bypass devices are implanted. The use of nepafenac NSAID drops (Nevanac, Alcon, TX) for a month postoperatively is also advocated as a means to control inflammation while minimizing steroid response.

Gonioscopic examination is an important element in the postoperative management of MIGS procedures. Verifying the status of the angle and the correct placement of any devices, controlling any formation of membranes that may impede the efficacy of the implant, and determining the presence of PAS should be done routinely in the postoperative period.

Before surgery, a target IOP should be determined to guide the change of postoperative glaucoma medications. Although no universal rule applies to all patients, one may initially stop any prostaglandin analogue medication, and further medications can be stopped if the IOP is below target on two consecutive visits.

Conclusion

The advent of MIGS procedures is changing the way in which we approach many of our glaucoma patients. By combining a single MIGS procedure with phacoemulsification cataract extraction, or with another MIGS procedure that lowers the IOP via a different mechanism, we can target lower IOPs after surgery and a reduced dependence on glaucoma medications.

References

1. Gedde SJ, Schiffman JC, Feuer WJ, Herndon LW, Brandt JD, Budenz DL; Tube versus Trabeculectomy Study Group. Treatment outcomes in the Tube Versus Trabeculectomy (TVT) study after five years of follow-up. Am J Ophthalmol 2012;153:789–803.e2

2. Saheb H, Ahmed II. Micro-invasive glaucoma surgery: current perspectives and future directions. Curr Opin Ophthalmol 2012;23:96–104

3. Shrivastava A, Singh K. The effect of cataract extraction on intraocular pressure. Curr Opin Ophthalmol 2010;21:118–122

4. Wang N, Chintala SK, Fini ME, Schuman JS. Ultrasound activates the TM ELAM-1/IL-1/NF-kappaB response: a potential mechanism for intraocular pressure reduction after phacoemulsification. Invest Ophthalmol Vis Sci 2003;44:1977–1981

5. Hayashi K, Hayashi H, Nakao F, Hayashi F. Effect of cataract surgery on intraocular pressure control in glaucoma patients. J Cataract Refract Surg 2001;27:1779–1786

6. White AJ, Orros JM, Healey PR. Outcomes of combined lens extraction and goniosynechialysis in angle closure. Clin Experiment Ophthalmol 2013; 41:746–752

7. Craven ER, Katz LJ, Wells JM, Giamporcaro JE; iStent Study Group. Cataract surgery with trabecular micro-bypass stent implantation in patients with mild-to-moderate open-angle glaucoma and cataract: two-year follow-up. J Cataract Refract Surg 2012;38:1339–1345

8. Broadway DC, Grierson I, Stürmer J, Hitchings RA. Reversal of topical antiglaucoma medication effects on the conjunctiva. Arch Ophthalmol 1996;114:262–267

9. Fea AM, Belda JI, Rękas M, et al. Prospective unmasked randomized evaluation of the iStent inject (®) versus two ocular hypotensive agents in patients with primary open-angle glaucoma. Clin Ophthalmol 2014;8: 875–882

10. Nordmann JP, Baudouin C, Renard JP, et al. Measurement of treatment compliance using a medical device for glaucoma patients associated with intraocular pressure control: a survey. Clin Ophthalmol 2010;4:731–739

11. Gedde SJ, Herndon LW, Brandt JD, Budenz DL, Feuer WJ, Schiffman JC; Tube Versus Trabeculectomy Study Group. Postoperative complications in the Tube Versus Trabeculectomy (TVT) study during five years of follow-up. Am J Ophthalmol 2012;153:804–814.e1

12. Iordanous Y, Kent JS, Hutnik CM, Malvankar-Mehta MS. Projected cost comparison of Trabectome, iStent, and endoscopic cyclophotocoagulation versus glaucoma medication in the Ontario Health Insurance Plan. J Glaucoma 2014;23:e112–e118

13. Mansberger SL, Gordon MO, Jampel H, et al; Ocular Hypertension Treatment Study Group. Reduction in intraocular pressure after cataract extraction: the Ocular Hypertension Treatment Study. Ophthalmology 2012;119:1826–1831

14. Wang Q, Harasymowycz P. Goniopuncture in the treatment of short-term post-Trabectome intraocular pressure elevation: a retrospective case series study. J Glaucoma 2013;22:e17–e20

15. Kaplowitz K, Kuei A, Klenofsky B, Abazari A, Honkanen R. The use of endoscopic cyclophotocoagulation for moderate to advanced glaucoma. Acta Ophthalmol (Copenh) 2014

16. Lavin MJ, Wormald RP, Migdal CS, Hitchings RA. The influence of prior therapy on the success of trabeculectomy. Arch Ophthalmol 1990;108: 1543–1548

40 Incorporating Minimally Invasive Glaucoma Surgery Procedures Into One's Practice

Iqbal Ike K. Ahmed and Manjool Shah

Minimally invasive glaucoma surgery (MIGS) offers a new avenue for interventional treatment for glaucoma patients. Instead of waiting until patients have severe disease with advanced surgical requirements, MIGS procedures can be performed on their own or combined with cataract surgery to provide additional intraocular pressure (IOP) lowering or reduction in the number of topical hypotensive agents. Prior to beginning down the pathway of incorporating MIGS into your surgical repertoire, it is important to adequately prepare yourself and your practice.

Deciding on a Minimally Invasive Glaucoma Surgery Procedure

The decision of which MIGS device to proceed with is largely based on patient selection, disease type, and planned surgical procedures that will accompany the MIGS procedure. Furthermore, capital costs for relevant equipment may play a role in some device or procedure selection. Consideration of the type of glaucoma and the desired IOP target should also help to determine which device or modality to choose for a given patient. Although this book described numerous devices and procedures that fall under the rubric of "MIGS," the discussion below focuses on the choice between the Trabectome and iStents.

Trabectome

Trabectome™ (NeoMedix, Tustin, CA) is a single-use bipolar cautery device with irrigation and aspiration that enables the surgeon to perform ab interno trabeculotomy (**Figs. 40.1** and **40.2**). It is used for the management of open-angle glaucoma, but has also been used in the setting of angle-closure glaucoma after goniosynechiolysis and lens extraction. Given a moderate IOP reduction found with the Trabectome, the technique is used for mild-to-moderate glaucoma disease burden.[1] The technique can be performed on its own or typically in combination with clear corneal phacoemulsification; studies indicate that the combination surgery results in improved IOP reduction as compared with phacoemulsification alone.

The learning curve associated with the Trabectome primarily entails gaining familiarity with angle surgery itself. There is indeed a learning curve associated with correctly performing intraoperative gonioscopy. Appropriate patient selection for the first several cases will optimize surgeons' ability to quickly familiarize themselves with the nuances of intraoperative angle visualization and manipulation.

There are capital costs associated with setting up your practice to use the Trabectome. One must acquire the Trabectome system itself, along with an appropriate goniolens and individual procedure packs.

iStent

The iStent® Trabecular Micro-Bypass (Glaukos, Laguna Hills, CA) is the world's smallest implant approved for human use. It is a 1-mm titanium microstent that is implanted directly into Schlemm's canal, thereby enabling aqueous humor to bypass the high-resistance juxtacanalicular trabecular meshwork (**Figs. 40.3** and **40.4**). The iStent is indicated for the treatment of primary open-angle glaucomas in combination with cataract extraction, and, as with other MIGS procedures, it is recommended for mild-to-moderate disease.[2,3] iStent implantation has been used to augment cataract surgery in patients with angle-closure glaucoma, and some surgeons have performed iStent implantation as a solo procedure.

Surgeons note a steep but relatively short learning curve with the iStent. In addition to familiarity with intraoperative gonioscopy, successful surgery involves fine movements and angulations of the fingers and wrists to achieve implantation and maintain adequate visualization (**Figs. 40.5** and **40.6**). Patient head positioning and microscope positioning are essential to obtain the proper viewing angle for iStent placement, and comfort with these skills is part of the steep learning curve associated with this device.

Capital costs associated with the iStent are minimal. In addition to a microscope that is capable of tilting, the main capital investment required in iStent implantation is in a high-quality intraoperative gonioscopy lens. Direct gonioprisms such as a Swan-Jacobs lens are ideal, as high magnification is of benefit. Anterior-segment microinstrumentation is often also helpful to have available in the event of a malpositioned iStent.

Patient Selection

Early in the incorporation of MIGS into your practice, stringent patient selection will maximize the potential for successful integration of MIGS modalities and will enable a more optimized learning curve. There are several key points to consider in terms of selecting the ideal patient to begin using any of the above-described MIGS devices or modalities upon.

Patient selection should begin with the demeanor of the patient. As all of these modalities and surgical approaches will be new to you, having an appropriate patient will be essential. The patient should be cooperative and able to follow the surgeon's directions, as adequate visualization of the relevant anatomy may require certain head or eye movements on the patient's part. Furthermore, your early cases may require more surgical time than patients are often used to, and as a result a patient who is aware of the need for attentiveness and cooperation is key.

For these MIGS procedures, adequate visualization requires the turning of the patient's head and eye away from the surgeon

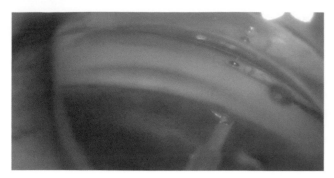

Fig. 40.1 The Trabectome device under direct gonioscopic visualization approaching the nasal angle.

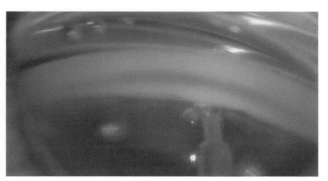

Fig. 40.2 Typical view of the Trabectome unit performing ab interno cautery and ablation of the nasal trabecular meshwork.

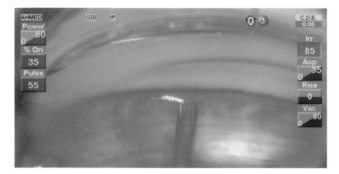

Fig. 40.3 A left-facing iStent under direct gonioscopic visualization. For the right-handed surgeon, the left-facing stent is implanted with a "forehand" technique that is often easier.

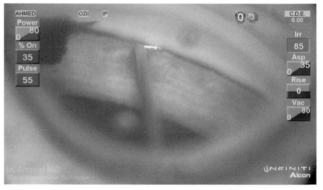

Fig. 40.4 A right-facing iStent under direct gonioscopic visualization. For the right-handed surgeon, implantation of the right-facing stent requires a "backhand" technique that may be slightly more technically challenging.

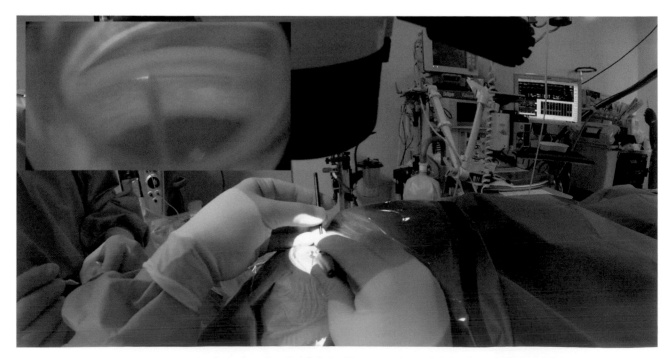

Fig. 40.5 Hand position and gonioscopic view for implantation of a left-facing iStent. Note the gentle hold of the gonioprism with the left hand, and a light "cigar"-type grip of the iStent injector with the right hand. This grip facilitates adequate hand and wrist turning required to insert the stent.

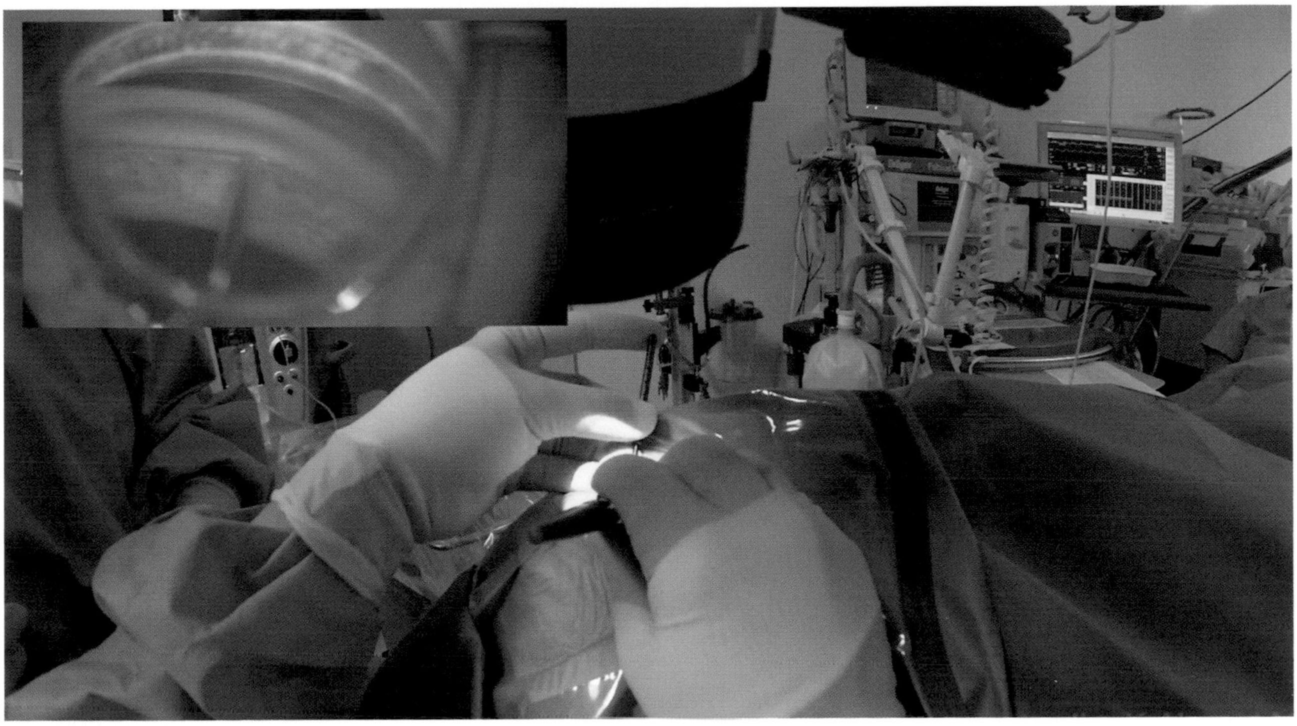

Fig. 40.6   Hand position and gonioscopic view for implantation of a right-facing iStent. Again, the gonioprism is held in the nondominant left hand, taking care to avoid undue pressure on the cornea. The hand position and grip result in the injector being more tilted, facilitating the wrist flexion and finger rotation that will be required for successful insertion.

(Fig. 40.7). As a result, it is important in early cases to avoid patients with limited cervical mobility or patients with back pain.

Importantly, familiarity with the anatomy of the anterior chamber angle, iris, and ciliary processes is absolutely essential. Selection of patients with good anatomic landmarks is key to maximizing early experiences with MIGS procedures. Early cases of Trabectome or iStent procedures should be limited to open-angle glaucomas with well-pigmented trabecular meshworks, so as to facilitate intraoperative identification of target tissues during intraoperative gonioscopy. Patients with preexisting peripheral anterior synechiae should be avoided. Patients with corneal scars or other anterior media opacities would also be less than ideal as early cases in your practice.

As your early IOP-lowering results may vary as your technique improves, it is advisable to begin your integration of MIGS procedures with patients with mild or moderate glaucoma disease burden. Ideal candidates are those with minimal visual field compromise who are hoping to reduce some topical medication burden through surgery. It would also be advisable early on to combine your MIGS procedure with planned cataract extraction. There appears to be synergistic lowering of IOP with cataract extraction,[2] and your patients will be more likely to experience a tangible benefit from surgery. With added familiarity with the procedures, surgeons may wish to extend their criteria somewhat to patients with more advanced disease or patients on more preoperative medications.

Informed Consent

The process of obtaining informed consent from the patient should begin with a clear discussion of the role of surgery. It is important to specify that the goal of performing a MIGS procedure is to reduce, but not necessarily eliminate, the patient's chronic topical medication requirement for glaucoma control.

There is evidence to support the claim that these MIGS procedures lower IOP more than cataract surgery alone, but they do not necessarily reduce IOP to levels similar to traditional, more invasive glaucoma surgeries. As a result, if the patient's glaucoma continues to progress, or if these devices inadequately control IOP at a disease-appropriate target level, it is important to discuss the possibility that additional glaucoma surgery may be needed in the future. Fortunately, one of the hallmarks of MIGS procedures is that they do not preclude the possibility of traditional glaucoma surgeries in the future should they be required.

Patients are often enthralled by the idea of having the "latest and greatest" surgical modality, and as a physician it is important to temper this excitement to some degree. New does not necessarily mean better, and in the spectrum of glaucoma surgeries, MIGS devices do not offer better IOP reduction. Patients should not be led to assume that the "next great thing" in glaucoma surgery will cure their disease, restore damage from prior visual field loss, or fulfill other fantastical claims.

An appropriate patient to select is one who understands what the recent availability of these procedures means, namely that you are in the process of incorporating these new technologies into your practice. You and your patients can feel confident that you have prepared thoroughly for this new modality, through readings, discussions, wet laboratories, and relevant courses. Withholding this information from your patients can result in a grave loss of confidence and degradation of the therapeutic relationship if it were ever to be unearthed, so it is best to address the issue head on.

Preparing for Surgery

Preparing for your first attempts with MIGS procedures can seem like a daunting task. These procedures often involve visualization and manipulation of parts of the eye that are often overlooked.

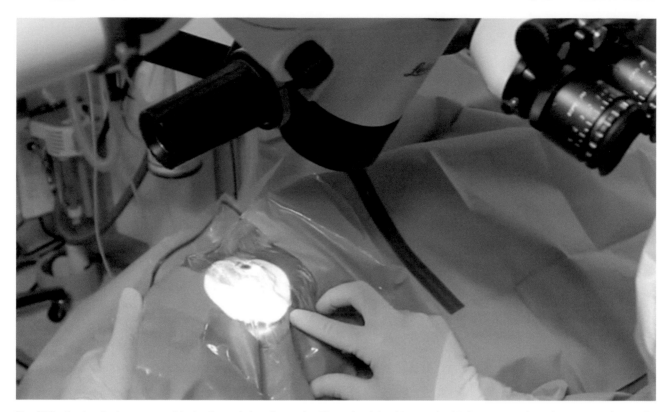

Fig. 40.7 Head and microscope positioning for angle-based surgeries. The patient's head is turned ~ 30 degrees away from the surgeon, whereas the microscope is tilted ~ 30 to 40 degrees to create an en face view of the angle with direct gonioscopy.

Familiarization of some key pearls will help ease the way toward surgical success.

First, it cannot be stated too often: knowledge of anatomic landmarks is key. Be sure to take the time to be familiar with the angle for your first angle-based MIGS cases. In the office, you can practice your gonioscopy skills and get comfortable handling a gonioprism with a light touch so as to minimize corneal striae. This skill will be invaluable during Trabectome or iStent cases. A good way to begin to familiarize oneself with intraoperative gonioscopy and accessing the angle is to end a routine clear corneal phacoemulsification case with the head and scope position changes required for MIGS procedures. A gonioprism can be applied and a cannula or a Sinskey hook can be inserted through the temporal clear corneal incision under direct gonioscopic visualization to get a sense for the approach required to access the trabecular meshwork. This controlled setting offers the surgeon an introduction to the subtleties of hand, head, and microscope positioning that is another key to MIGS success.

Plan your surgical day around the new MIGS procedure you are implementing. In an effort to optimize and accelerate your learning curve, it would be ideal to group a series of patients undergoing the same procedure on the same surgical day. There is no better way to integrate knowledge and develop the proprioceptive and fine motor skills of MIGS surgery than with repetition and review. Learning and implementing a new set of techniques or skills can be tiring, however, so make sure not to overburden your schedule; accommodate the significantly longer surgical times needed for MIGS procedures than for standard cataract extraction, at least early on.

Consider the order with which you will proceed with the MIGS portion of your procedure versus cataract extraction. For the Trabectome and iStents, experienced surgeons are of mixed opinion as to whether the MIGS procedure should come before or after phacoemulsification. Arguments in favor of performing the MIGS procedure first are that with a firmer eye and a clearer cornea, as well as a fresher patient and surgeon, the setting is best for optimum visualization and performance. Arguments in favor of performing cataract extraction first are to enable surgeons to "warm up" with a technique they are familiar with, and in some eyes the angle may become significantly more open after phacoemulsification. But ideally such an eye would not be part of one's initial cohort of MIGS patients.

Prior to arrival in the operating room, it is helpful to remind the patients of the fact that their cooperation will be necessary for the successful completion of the case. Ensuring that patients are comfortable, positioned well, and aware of the movements and positions that will be required of them is essential. Some surgeons review the head and eye turns required for angle-based surgeries prior to arrival in the operating room. Be sure to have a discussion with the anesthesia care provider to ensure that the patient is not oversedated and able to comprehend the surgeon's orders.

Lastly, in addition to familiarization with the surgical techniques themselves, be aware of the potential pitfalls and roadblocks that might arise, and have the relevant surgical tools at your disposal to handle them. Incision placement that avoids the corneal limbal vasculature will decrease the chance of blood obscuring your gonioscopic view. Having access to extra viscoelastic agents (typically cohesive agents) is beneficial for visualization during angle surgeries. There is typically some blood reflux expected during angle-based surgeries, and the presence of blood is often considered a good sign that potency to the distal outflow system has been established (**Fig. 40.8**). Judicious use of additional cohesive viscoelastic agents can ensure that visualization is maintained in spite of blood reflux. Microsurgical devices such as microforceps can be useful to retrieve an errantly placed iStent.

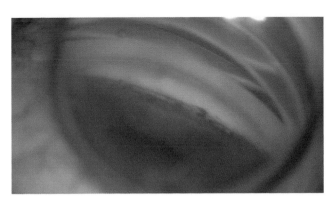

Fig. 40.8 Blood reflux after successful Trabectome-assisted ablation has been performed, demonstrating unimpaired access of aqueous humor to the distal outflow system. Similar blood reflux is often noted with successful iStent insertion. Cohesive viscoelastic agents can be used to tamponade this blood to ensure adequate visualization during surgery.

Reimbursement

When preparing your practice for the incorporation of MIGS procedures, having an understanding of reimbursement structures is crucial. Often, newer devices and procedures are released prior to established reimbursement by national and private insurances. Therefore, a billing code may not be available, or a company or government may decide not to pay for a Food and Drug Administration (FDA)-approved or CE Marked procedure for no apparent reason besides cost containment. Surgeons need to be prepared to have patients sign an Advanced Beneficiary Notice (ABN), which acknowledges that a patient will need to pay out-of-pocket for whatever costs are not reimbursed by the government or their insurance. In the future, the use of multiple MIGS devices, such as the use of more than one iStent,[4] or using one or two canal-based stents combined with a suprachoroidal stent, will further complicate reimbursement matters, but will allow surgeons to better personalize the care given to each patient.

Trabectome

Reimbursement for the Trabectome is not very straightforward, unfortunately. As it stands, in the United States there is no Current Procedure Terminology (CPT) code for the Trabectome or trabeculotomy ab interno, so instead, billers have resorted to using CPT codes for goniotomy. Time will tell if a specific CPT code and reimbursement structure for the Trabectome procedure will be developed.

iStent

Single iStent implantation utilizes CPT code 0191T, with professional reimbursement rates set by local Medicare contractors. Reimbursements are all-inclusive, meaning payment includes the cost of the implant as well. In the United States, as of January 1, 2015, a new CPT code of 0376T is used for the implantation of multiple stents. However, the facility fees set by Medicare for this code is $0.[5] Currently, patients seeking additional iStents routinely pay out-of-pocket for this added service at rates determined by their surgeons. Local Medicare contractors may yet set a professional fee for additional iStent implantation. Until that time, however, it may be prudent to establish an ABN with Medicare patients. Furthermore, as multiple stents remain "off label" at the present, it may be prudent to amend the standard informed consent documentation and discussion with provisions to that effect. It is important to note that iStent insertion is indicated only when combined with cataract extraction, and only indicated in mild-to-moderate open-angle glaucoma. As of yet, solo iStent implantation or implantation in the setting of other types of glaucoma may be considered experimental or investigational, and as a result may not be reimbursed.

References

1. Minckler D, Mosaed S, Dustin L, Ms BF; Trabectome Study Group. Trabectome (trabeculectomy-internal approach): additional experience and extended follow-up. Trans Am Ophthalmol Soc 2008;106:149–159, discussion 159–160

2. Samuelson TW, Katz LJ, Wells JM, Duh YJ, Giamporcaro JE; US iStent Study Group. Randomized evaluation of the trabecular micro-bypass stent with phacoemulsification in patients with glaucoma and cataract. Ophthalmology 2011;118:459–467

3. Craven ER, Katz LJ, Wells JM, Giamporcaro JE; iStent Study Group. Cataract surgery with trabecular micro-bypass stent implantation in patients with mild-to-moderate open-angle glaucoma and cataract: two-year follow-up. J Cataract Refract Surg 2012;38:1339–1345

4. Belovay GW, Naqi A, Chan BJ, Rateb M, Ahmed II. Using multiple trabecular micro-bypass stents in cataract patients to treat open-angle glaucoma. J Cataract Refract Surg 2012;38):1911–1917

5. iStent Trabecular Micro-Bypass Stent Reimbursement Guide. Laguna Hills, CA: Glaukos; revised April 29, 2014

Index

Note: Page references followed by *f* or *t* indicate figures or tables, respectively

195